H. Pokieser, G. Lechner (Eds.)

Advances in CT III

3rd European Scientific User Conference SOMATOM PLUS
Vienna, April 1994

With 173 Figures and 48 Tables

Springer-Verlag
Berlin Heidelberg New York
London Paris Tokyo
Hong Kong Barcelona Budapest

Professor Dr. H. Pokieser
Professor Dr. G. Lechner

AKH Vienna
Department of Radiology,
University Hospital Vienna,
Währinger Gürtel 18–20, A-1090 Vienna
Austria

ISBN-13: 978-3-642-79118-5 e-ISBN-13: 978-3-642-79116-1
DOI: 10.1007/ 978-3-642-79116-1

Library of Congress Cataloging-in-Publication Data
European Scientific User Conference Somatom Plus (3rd : 1994 : Vienna, Austria)
Advances in CT III : 3rd European Scientific User Conference SOMATOM PLUS, Wien, April, 1994 / H. Pokieser, G. Lechner (eds.).
Includes Index.
ISBN-13: 978-3-642-79118-5
1. Tomo-graphy-Gongresses. I. Pokieser, Herbert. II. Lechner, G. (Gisbert). III. Title.
RC78.8.T6E92 1994 616.07'572 – dc20

Softcover reprint of the hardcover 1st edition 1994

Typesetting: Fotosatz-Service Köhler OHG, Würzburg
SPIN: 10426931 21/3020 - 5 4 3 2 1 0 Printed on acid-free paper

Preface

In nearly all areas of technology our generation is experiencing the phenomena of fast paced innovation and great bursts in development. Besides the completely new techniques, the "experienced user" is astonished when obviously good and apparently matured technology such as the next to last generation of CT equipment undergoes further development, such as is the case with the spiral CT technique.

The enormous potential of spiral CT suddenly became apparent, stimulating and giving rise to a wide range of research on its clinical application. Yet again we can see in the field of imaging how great advances in one method competitively affect the range of application in another. Hence it is extremely valuable and necessary to appraise the current situation now. Both physicians – who use the equipment – and the health system and with this the patient – which finances it – have the obligation and the right to permanent optimization of the application strategies of diagnostic procedures.

Not least, this symposium also meant to fit the new voice of spiral CT harmoniously into the symphonic score of diagnostic procedures. The large radiodiagnostic department of the university clinics which has been established at the Neues Allgemeines Krankenhaus in Vienna, Austria, is proud to have jointly arranged this user symposium with Siemens.

Vienna, June 1994 *H. Pokieser, G. Lechner*

Contents

CT Angiography I
Chairmen: A. L. Baert, M. Langer

CT Angiography II
Chairmen: M. Heller, J. Lammer

Lung

Chairmen: R. Rienmüller, D. Hahn

Chairmen

Prof. Dr. A. L. BAERT
Universitaire Ziekenhuis Gasthuisberg
Herestraat 49
B-3000 Leuven

Prof. Dr. C. D. CLAUSSEN
Eberhard-Karls-Universität Tübingen
Radiologische Universitätsklinik
Hoppe-Seyler-Strasse 3
D-72016 Tübingen

Dr. A. K. DIXON
University Department of Radiology
University of Cambridge
and Addenbrooke's Hospital
GB-Cambridge CB2 2QQ

Doz. Dr. W. DOCK
Allgemeines Krankenhaus der Stadt Wien
Universitätsklinik für Radiodiagnostik
Währinger Gürtel 18–20
A-1090 Wien

Prof. Dr. D. HAHN
Universitätsklinik im Luitpoldkrankenhaus
Institut für Röntgendiagnostik
Josef-Schneider-Strasse 2
D-97080 Würzburg

Prof. Dr. M. HELLER
Klinikum der Christian-Albrechts-Universität zu Kiel
Klinik für Radiologische Diagnostik
Arnold-Heller-Straße 9
D-24105 Kiel

Univ.-Doz. Dr. W. HRUBY
Institut für Röntgendiagnostik
im Donauspital
Langobardenstrasse 122
A-1220 Wien

Prof. Dr. W. KALENDER
Siemens AG
Bereich Medizinische Technik
Henkestrasse 127
D-91050 Erlangen

Prof. Dr. J. LAMMER
Allgemeines Krankenhaus der Stadt Wien
Universitätsklinik für Radiodiagnostik
Währinger Gürtel 18–20
A-1090 Wien

Prof. Dr. M. LANGER
Klinikum der Albert-Ludwigs-Universität
Radiologische Universitätsklinik
Hugstetter Strasse 55
D-79106 Freiburg

Univ. Doz. Dr. V. METZ
Allgemeines Krankenhaus der Stadt Wien
Universitätsklinik für Radiodiagnostik
Abteilung für Chirurgische Fächer
Währinger Gürtel 18–20
A-1090 Wien

Prof. Dr. R. RIENMÜLLER
Universitätsklinik für Radiologie
und Zentralröntgeninstitut
Auenbruggerplatz 9
A-8036 Graz

Speakers

Dr. W. Anzboeck
Institut für Röntgendiagnostik
im Donauspital
Langobardenstrasse 122
A-1220 Wien

Dr. A. Blum
Centre Hospitalier Universitaire
Hôpitaux des Brabois
Départment de Radiologie
rue du Morvan
F-54511 Vandœuvre CEDEX

Dr. R. Braunschweig
Eberhard-Karls-Universität Tübingen
Radiologische Universitätsklinik
Abteilung für Radiologische Diagnostik
Hoppe-Seyler-Strasse 3
D-72026 Tübingen

Dr. C. H. Buitrago-Téllez
Albert-Ludwigs-Universität
Abteilung Röntgendiagnostik
Radiologische Universitätsklinik
Hugstetter Strasse 55
D-79106 Freiburg

Dr. K. Cederlund
Department of Thoracic Radiology
Karolinska Hospital
Box 110
S-171 76 Stockholm

Dr. A. Dickschas
Bezirkskrankenhaus Erlangen
Chefarzt der Neurologie
Am Europakanal 71
D-91056 Erlangen

Dr. A. K. Dixon
Department of Radiology
University of Cambridge
and Addenbrooke's Hospital
GB-Cambridge CB2 2QQ

Doz. Dr. W. Dock
Allgemeines Krankenhaus der Stadt Wien
Universitätsklinik für Radiodiagnostik
Währinger Gürtel 18–20
A-1090 Wien

Dr. R. Dore
Via Lombroso n. 3
I-27100 Pavia

Dr. M. Dragani
Istituto di Scienze Radiologiche
Osp. "SS. Annunziata"
Via P. A. Valignani
I-66100 Chieti

Dr. C. Ehritt-Braun
Albert-Ludwigs-Universität
Radiologische Universitätsklinik
Abteilung Röntgendiagnostik
Hugstetter Strasse 55
D-79106 Freiburg

Dr. L. P. Emde
Christian-Albrechts-Universität zu Kiel
Klinik für Radiologische Diagnostik
Arnold-Heller-Strasse 9
D-24105 Kiel

Dr. F. J. Ferstl
Albert-Ludwigs-Universität
Radiologische Universitätsklinik
Abteilung Röntgendiagnostik
Hugstetter Strasse 55
D-79106 Freiburg

Dr. T. Fleiter
Eberhard-Karls-Universität Tübingen
Radiologische Universitätsklinik
Abteilung für Radiologische Diagnostik
Hoppe-Seyler-Strasse 3
D-72026 Tübingen

Dr. M. Freund
Klinikum der Christian-Albrechts-Universität zu Kiel
Klinik für Radiologische Diagnostik
Arnold-Heller-Strasse 9
D-24105 Kiel

Prof. Dr. M. Galanski
Medizinische Hochschule Hannover
Abteilung Diagnostische Radiologie
Konstanty-Gutschow-Strasse 8
D-30623 Hannover

Dr. U. Golin
Institut für Radiologie und Nuklearmedizin
Knappschaftskrankenhaus
Bochum-Langendreer
– Universitätsklinik –
in der Schornau 23/25
D-44892 Bochum

Dr. O. Graf
Allgemeines Krankenhaus der Stadt Wien
Universitätsklinik für Radiodiagnostik
Abteilung für Chirurgische Fächer
Währinger Gürtel 18–20
A-1090 Wien

Dr. D. Hentschel
Siemens Medical Systems, Inc.
186 Wood Avenue South
Iselin, New Jersey 08830 USA

Prof. Dr. H. Hirschfelder
Orthopädische Universitätsklinik
Rathsberger Strasse 57
D-91054 Erlangen

Prof. Dr. U. Hirschfelder
Universität Erlangen
Abteilung für Orthodentik
D-91054 Erlangen

Dr. P. E. Huppert
Eberhard-Karls-Universität Tübingen
Radiologische Universitätsklinik
Abteilung für Radiologische Diagnostik
Hoppe-Seyler-Strasse 3
D-72026 Tübingen

Prof. Dr. W. Kalender
Siemens AG
Bereich Medizinische Technik
Henkestrasse 127
D-91050 Erlangen

Dr. R. Kloeppel
Universitätsklinikum Leipzig
Klinik für Diagnostische Radiologie
Liebigstrasse 20a
D-04103 Leipzig

Dr. A. Koehler
Medizinische Hochschule Hannover
Abteilung Diagnostische Radiologie
Konstanty-Gutschow-Strasse 8
D-30623 Hannover

Dr. R. Kursawe
Medizinische Fakultät
der Humboldt-Universität zu Berlin
Abteilung für Diagnostische Radiologie
Schumannstrasse 20/21
D-10117 Berlin

Prof. Dr. J. Lammer
Allgemeines Krankenhaus der Stadt Wien
Universitätsklinik für Radiodiagnostik
Abteilung für Radiologie und
Interventionelle Radiologie
Währinger Gürtel 18–20
A-1090 Wien

Dr. A. Nilles
Albert-Ludwigs-Universität
Radiologische Universitätsklinik
Abteilung Röntgendiagnostik
Hugstetter Strasse 55
D-79106 Freiburg

Dr. M. Oldendorf
Klinikum Nord
Abteilung für Diagnostische
und Interventionelle Radiologie
Flurstrasse 17
D-90340 Nürnberg

Dr. M. Oudkerk
Dr. Daniel den Hoed Cancer Center
and Rotterdam Radio-Therapeutic Institute
Postbus 5201
NL-3008 AE Rotterdam

Dr. M. Prokop
Medizinische Hochschule Hannover
Abteilung Diagnostische Radiologie
Konstanty-Gutschow-Strasse 8
D-30623 Hannover

Dr. J. Regn
Siemens AG
Bereich Medizinische Technik
Hartmannstrasse 16
D-91052 Erlangen

Dr. M. Reuter
Klinikum der Christian-Albrechts-Universität zu Kiel
Klinik für Radiologische Diagnostik
Arnold-Heller-Strasse 9
D-24105 Kiel

Dr. C. S. Richter
Strahlenklinik und Poliklinik
Klinikum Rudolf Virchow
Freie Universität Berlin
Standort Charlottenburg
Spandauer Damm 130
D-14050 Berlin

Prof. Dr. R. Rienmüller
Universitätsklinik für Radiologie
und Zentralröntgeninstitut
Auenbruggerplatz 9
A-8036 Graz

Dr. H. Rytkönen
Department of Clinical Radiology
University Hospital
P. O. Box 1777
SF-70211 Kuopio

Dr. C. Schaefer-Prokop
Medizinische Hochschule Hannover
Abteilung Diagnostische Radiologie
Konstanty-Gutschow-Strasse 8
D-30623 Hannover

Dr. R. Sokiranski
Eberhard-Karls-Universität Tübingen
Radiologische Universitätsklinik
Abteilung für Radiologische Diagnostik
Hoppe-Seyler-Strasse 3
D-72026 Tübingen

Dr. M. Storto
Istituto di Scienze Radiologiche
Osp. "SS. Annunziata"
Via P. A. Valignani
I-66100 Chieti

Priv.-Doz. Dr. S. Tuengerthal
Thoraxklinik Heidelberg
Amalienstrasse 5
D-69126 Heidelberg

Dr. L. van Hoe
University Hospital K. U. L.
Department of Radiology
Herestraat 49
B-3000 Leuven

Dr. A. B. van Rossum
Department of Radiology
Leyenburg Hospital
Leyweg 275
NL-2545 CH The Hague

Dr. G. Wittenberg
Institut für Röntgendiagnostik
der Universität Würzburg
Josef-Schneider-Strasse 2
D-97080 Würzburg

Dipl.-Ing. W. Wittmoser
Institut für Radiologie
der Universität Erlangen
Krankenhausstrasse 12
D-91054 Erlangen

CT Angiography I

Chairmen: A. L. Baert, M. Langer

Basics of CT Angiography

J. Regn, J. Ezrielev, R. Hupke, W. A. Kalender, K. Maatsch

Computed tomographic angiography (CTA) is a new tool for the volumetric display of contrast-filled vessels from Spiral CT data. It is a software package developed by SIEMENS Medical Systems for the SOMATOM Plus family.

Spiral scanning is a prerequisite for CTA, because it allows the fast scanning of large anatomic volumes to follow the injected bolus of contrast material through the volume of interest. With spiral CT the data acquisition can be achieved during one breath hold, which gives the certainty that small lesions won't be missed due to breathing motion. Since spiral scanning is much faster than scanning single slices an optimal utilization of contrast is achieved. The utilisation is further optimized with the use of the double spiral.

As data of the complete volume is acquired using spiral scanning, retrospective reconstructions are possible with arbitrary slice increments. To achieve excellent image quality in 3D evaluations, the reconstruction of overlapping slices is possible without the need for overlapping scans.

CTA is building upon the basis of spiral scanning, adding the appropriate volume rendering techniques. With the acquisition of a spiral CT data set, different 3D evaluations are possible:

1. Shaded surface display (SSD) (Fig. 1): In the viewing direction, the first voxel along each ray with a CT value above a definded density threshold or within a density range is considered. Then a surface is calculated as if the structure would be illuminated by a light source to achieve the 3D impression via shading. But here density information is lost.
2. Maximum intensity projection (MIP) (Fig. 2): Parallel rays are traced through the volume and the voxel with the maximum density value is projected to an output image. These maximum intensity voxel values form the image matrix. With this technique the depth information is lost, but the density information is kept.

CTA is an economical method in respect to patient management (Table 1). The major differences are that for CTA there are no lab tests, local anesthesia or catheter placement. While mostly intra-aterial contrast is necessary for conventional angiography, CTA requires merely intra-venous contrast application, making it only minimally invasive. With CTA the patient is scanned once for all the projections. For conventional angiography they take one ore more image sets. With CTA there is no resting period necessary for the patient.

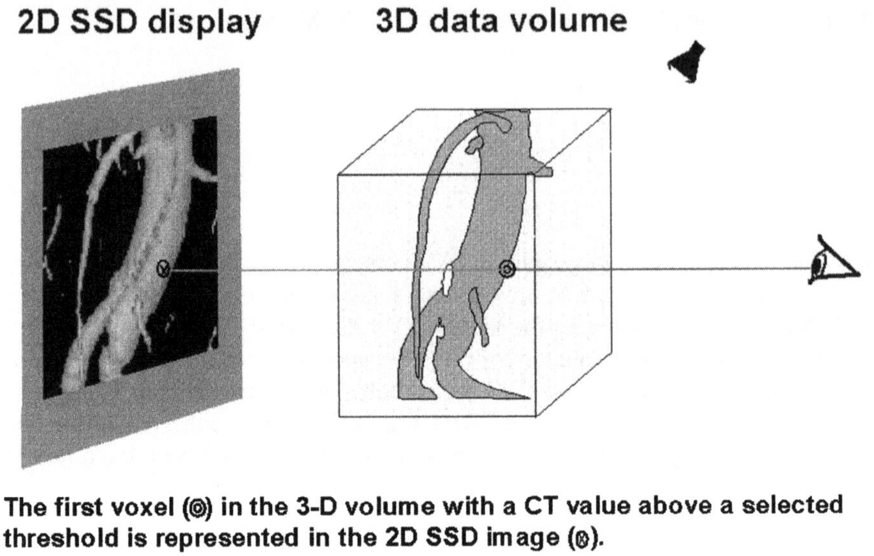

Fig. 1. Principle of SSD (Kalender et al. 1994)

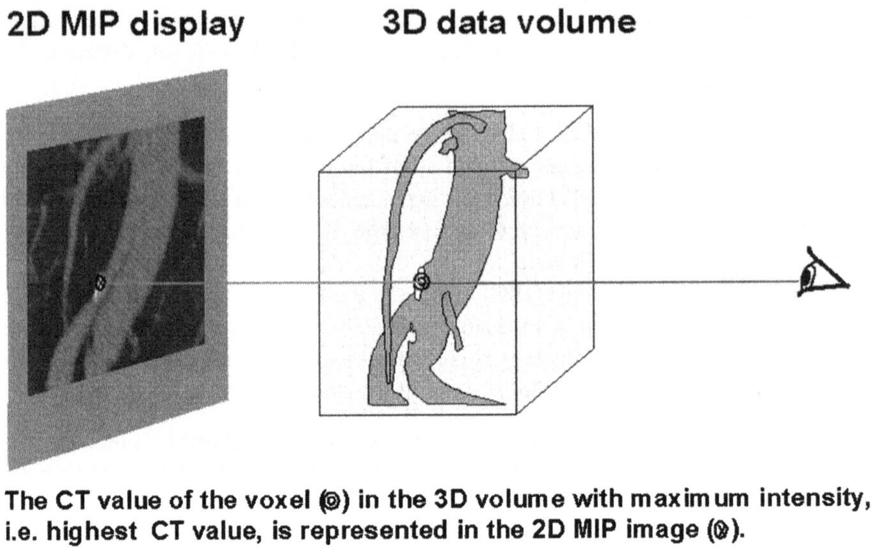

Fig. 2. Principle of MIP (Kalender et al. 1994)

Table 1. Comparison between CTA and conventional film-screen angiography (Oates 1993)

Patient flow chart (outpatient)	
Spiral CTA	Conventional angiography
Check in	Check in (daycare)
	Lab tests
	Premedication and local anesthesia, catheter is placed
IV contrast	IA contrast
Patient is scanned	One/two image sets are taken Catheter is withdrawn Patient rests (6 h)

CTA, computed tomographic angiography

If dense bone and contrast filled vessels lie along one ray the bone's value will be displayed in the projection and not the contrast filled vessel, since the bone is at a higher density than contrast. It therefore becomes necessary to remove the bones from the images using an editor.

With the slice editor each slice of the stack has to be edited separately one after the other. This can be quite time consuming, but extremely valuable when anatomy changes rapidly in the scanning direction.

The slice editor includes functionalities like:

- ROI: A region of interest can be drawn in the image; its contents is either retained or removed.
- Pathfinder: A path is automatically drawn between two dense structures; it can then be used as an ROI. This is useful, for example, to make the separation of the spine and the aorta easier.
- Paint: The paint feature is used for replacing certain pixels in the image by pixels of defined values.
- Threshold: Thresholding retains all the pixels in a predefined CT-density range and replaces the rest by a predefined CT value.
- Region growing: Region growing is a regional thresholding and is used to remove certain structures in a density range (Fig. 3).

The slab editor (Fig. 4) the possibility to quickly remove bones out of a stack of images. The transaxial images defining the volume are used to calculate a lateral MIP as a reference. This lateral MIP shows the gross anatomy in the z-direction, and can be used to divide the volume into subvolumes (slabs) (Fig. 4a). One slab consists of several transaxial slices of similar anatomy in the z-direction. Once the slabs are defined, an axial MIP for every slab is calculated (Fig. 4b). In each projection a region of interest can be determined around the structures to be viewed (Fig. 4c). The ROI of the previous slab is retained for the current slab and can be changed

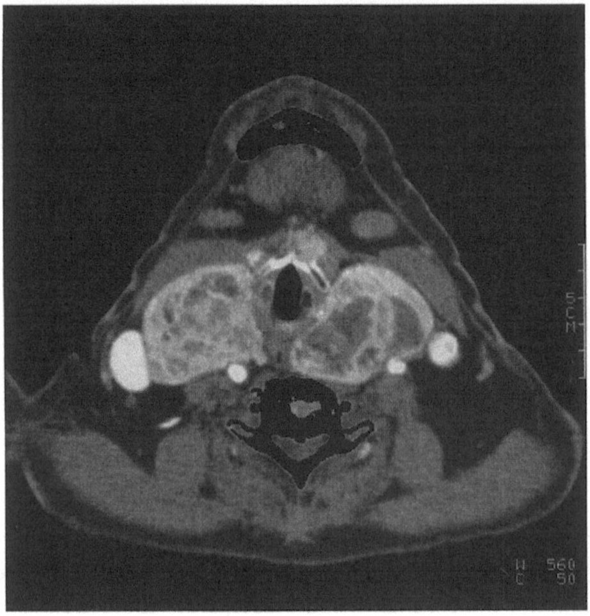

Fig. 3. Regional thresholding is used to remove the teeth and the spine in the slice

using the mouse. Only the content of the image within the ROIs is used to calculate the 3Ds (Fig. 4d). The edited images can be automatically stored to disk.

Now that the edited images have been created, 3D displays can be calculated:

While SSD gives a real volumetric impression of the morphology of the vessels, a precise definition of the thresholds is necessary (Fig. 5).

Using a low threshold (Fig. 5a), small blood vessels can be seen, but unwanted structures might appear and merge with the vessels. Conversely, using a high threshold (Fig. 5c), there might appear a threshold-dependent occlusion. As there is no density information in the surface image it is impossible to distinguish calcifications and vessels. The MIP algorithm preserves the attenuation values, therefore a difference between the intraluminal contrast and the calcifications is visualized in the output image.

Advantages of CTA (Semba and Dake 1993):

- Provides rapid, relatively non-invasive method for assesing the abdominal aorta and major branch vessels.
- Has superior resolution than magnetic resonance angiography and metallic clips do not represent a problem.
- It is faster to perform than ultrasound or magnetic resonance angiography.
- It is not operator dependent as opposed to ultrasound or conventional angiography.
- It can provide views of the abdominal vasculature which are simply not possible with any other modality.

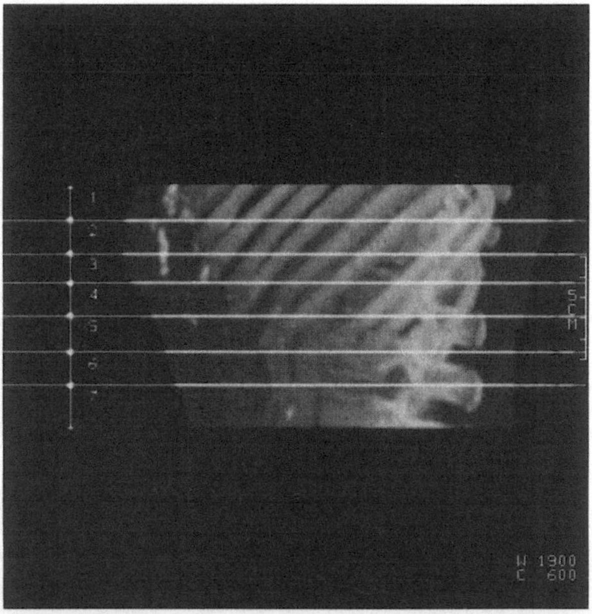

a

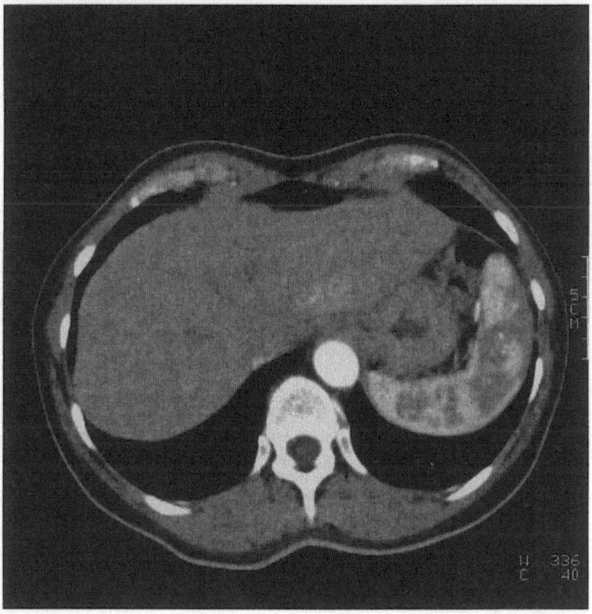

b

Fig. 4 a – d. Slab editor: lateral MIP with slabs marked (**a**), MIP of a slab (**b**), ROI in one slab (**c**), edited image (**d**)

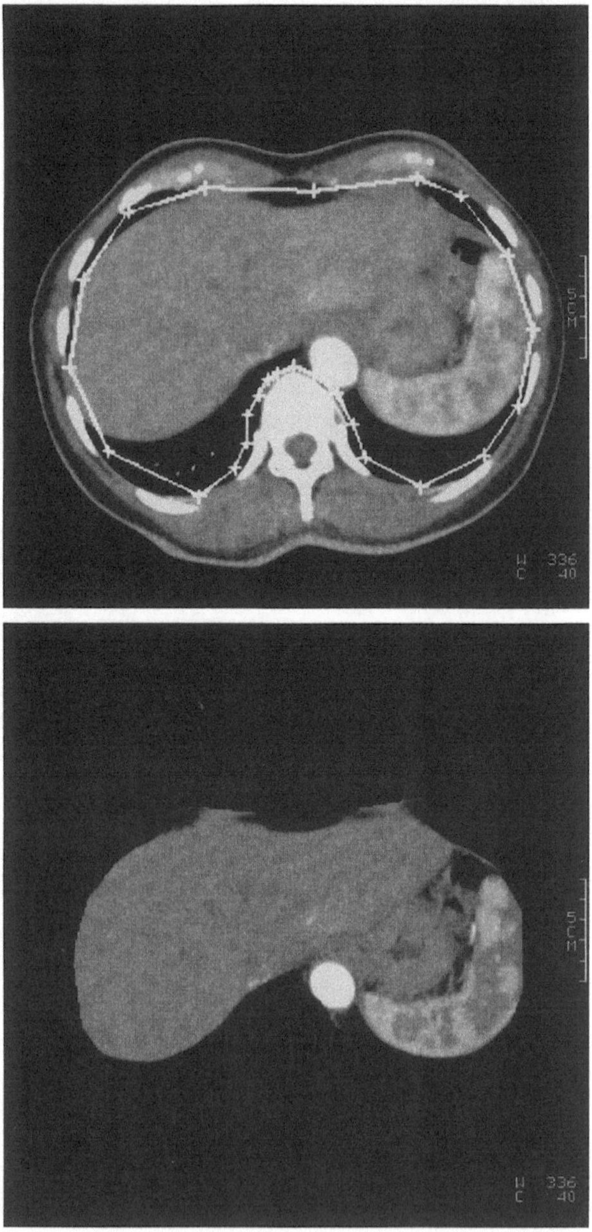

c

d

Fig. 4c, d

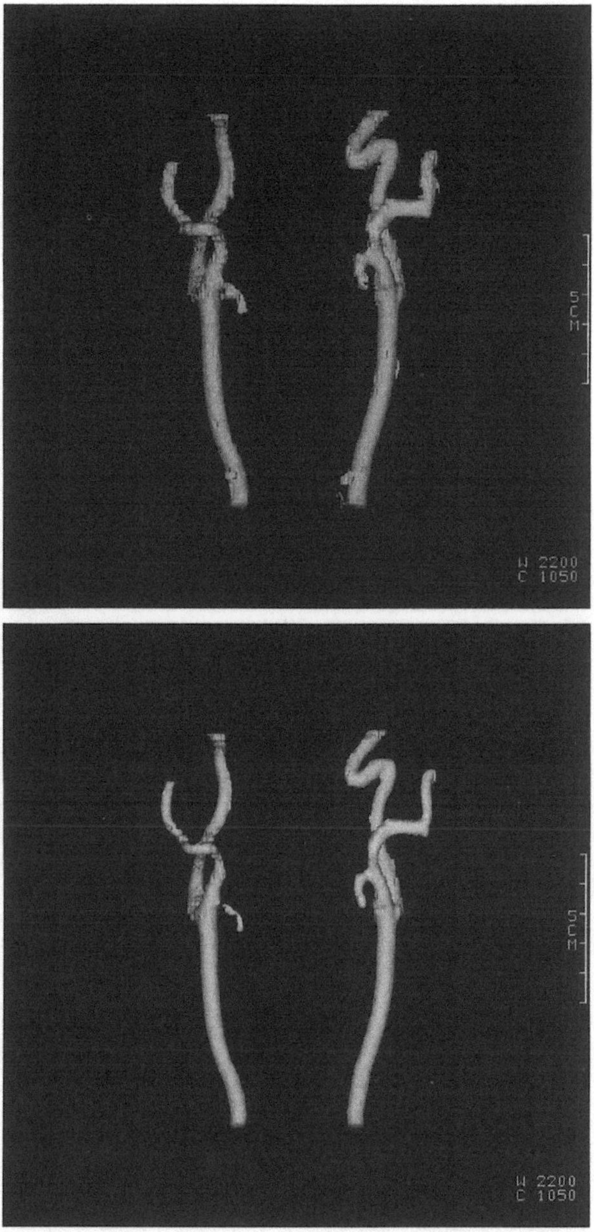

a

b

Fig. 5 a – d. Threshold dependence of the SSD algorithm (low → high: **a** – **c**). For comparison an MIP image is shown (**d**)

c

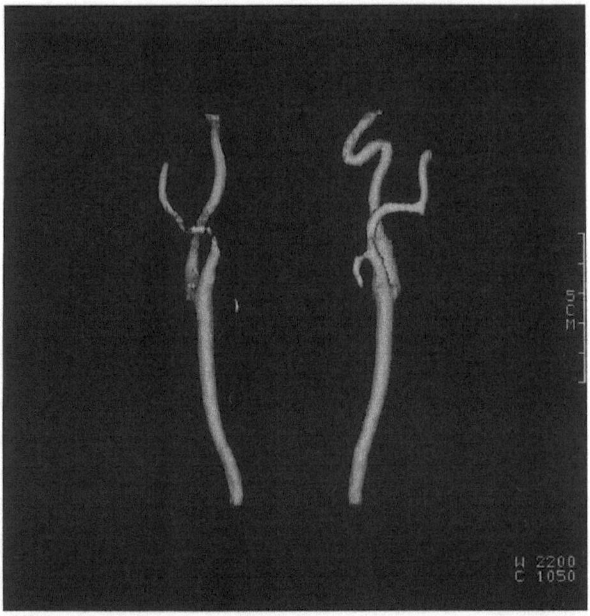

d

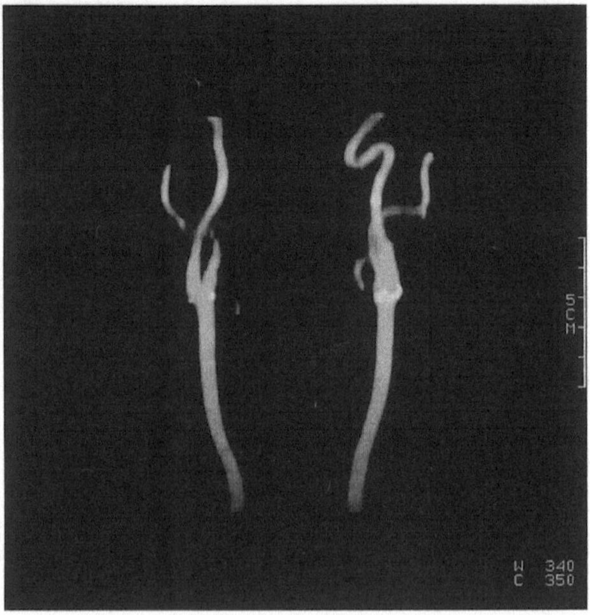

Fig. 5c, d

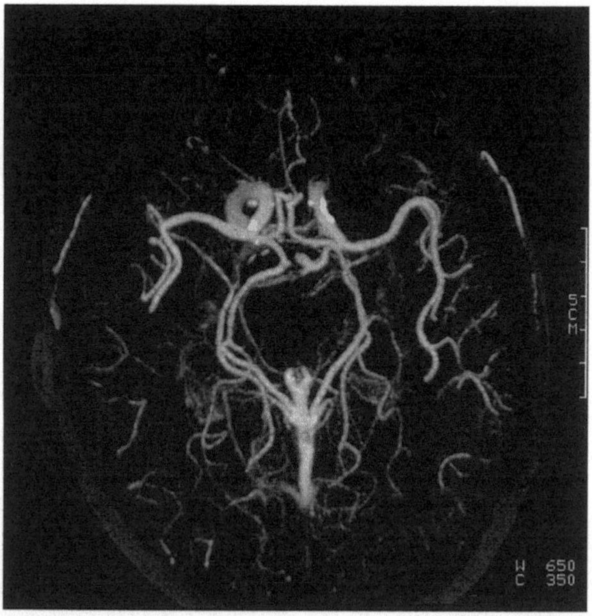

Fig. 6. CTA of a circle of Willis

- It provides three different imaging formats from a single scan acquisition – standard CT cross-sectional views, shaded surface display (SSD), and MIP.
- The scanner can be used non-angiographically for fast routine CT examinations of the head, chest, or abdomen, thus improving exam efficiency and patient throughput within the radiology department.

CTA is suitable for several clinical applications:

- Screening for vascular disease
- Screening for surgical planning
- Follow-ups of stent placements
- Vascular graft patency
- Renal artery stenoses
- Abdominal aortic aneurysms
- Hepatic vascularity
- Circle of Willis or
- Carotids

In Fig. 6, the maximum intensity projection of a circle of Willis with coiling is shown. Small brain vessels can be seen in the image as well. This view is an x-projection and the bone has been removed from the transaxial images by using the slice editor with the grow functionality.

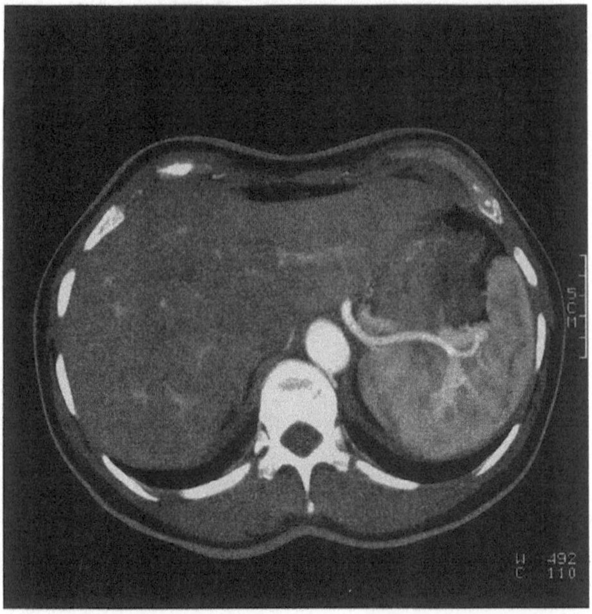

a

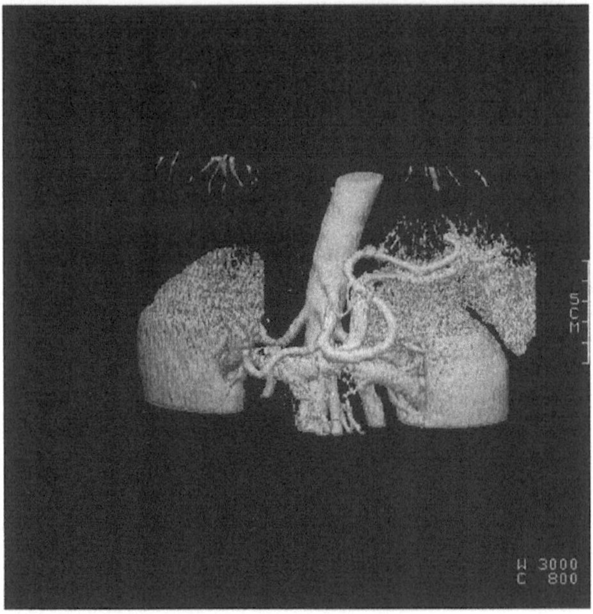

b

Fig. 7a–d. Thin slab MIP (**a**) to represent the data set, SSD (**b**), MIP (**c**), and MPR (**d**) of the same data set

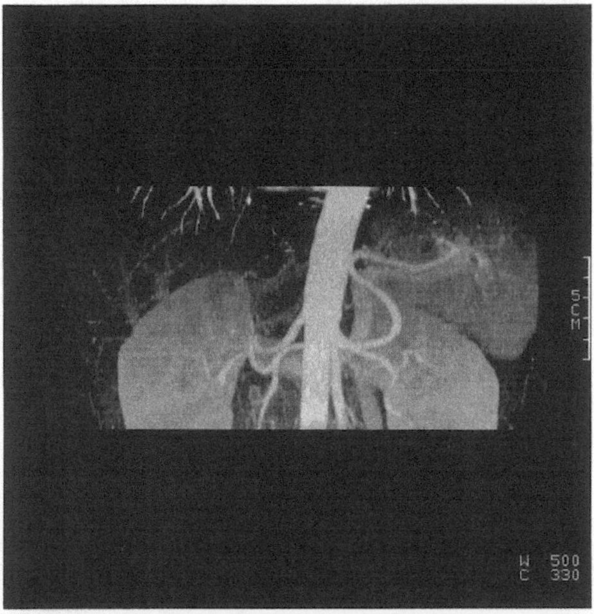

c

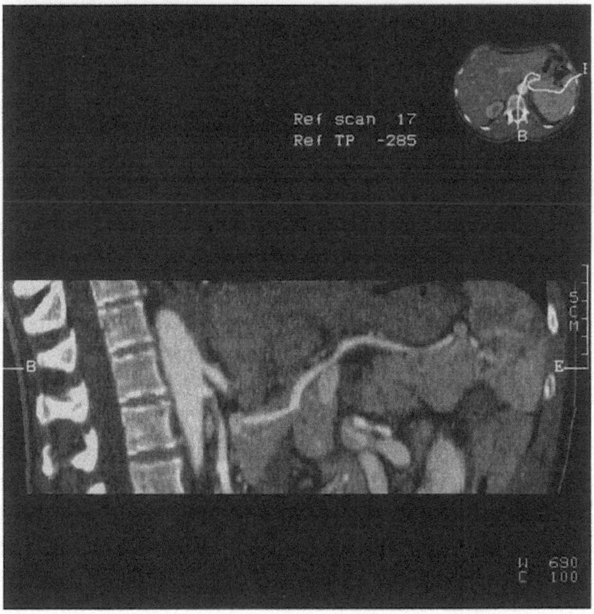

Fig. 7c, d

d

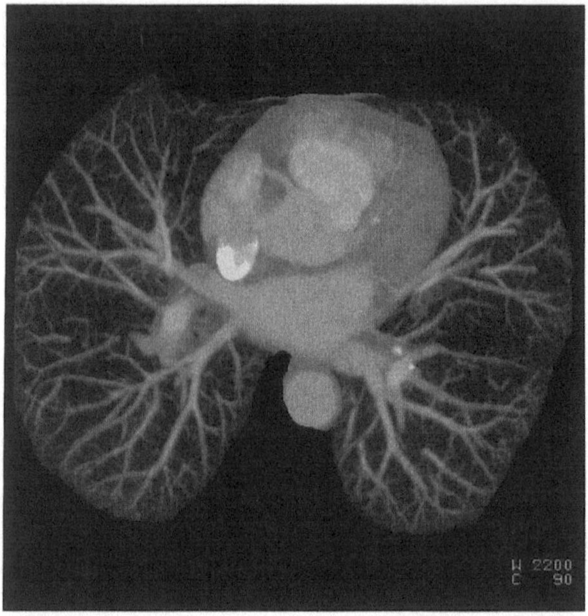

Fig. 8. CTA of a heart scanned with electron beam tomography

Conclusion

Once having aquired a volume data set with contrast material using the Spiral CT technique – all the possibilities are available for 3D evaluations:

With one data set (Fig. 7a), a surface shaded image (Fig. 7b) can be calculated to clearly see the 3D morphology of the vessels. To display calcifications and contrast in the vessels and to avoid threshold effects, maximum intensity projections (Fig. 7c) can be evaluated and then, having detected some pathology, multi-planar reformats (Fig. 7d) can be extracted from the same data set. This helps to save time for the patient and enables the radiologist to receive all the information of the volume and present it in an appropriate manner to others (i.e. the surgeon).

Figure 8 shows that CTA and MIP are also useful for moving organs like the heart: This heart was scanned with Electron Beam Tomography and evaluated with the MIP algorithm.

References

Kalender WA et al. (1994) Grundlagen der Gefäßdarstellung mit Spiral-CT. Aktuelle Radiologie, submitted for publication

Oates M (1993) Spiral Computed Tomography Angiography vs. Conventional Angiography. Administrative Radiology 7 : 41 – 43

Semba CP, Dake MD (1993) Point-Couterpoint. Administrative Radiology 11 : 15

Spiral CT Angiography of Extracranial Cerebral Vessels

A. Dickschas, M. Mönius, H. Zeiner, P. Weber

Introduction

In this study the diagnostic potential of spiral computed tomographic angiography (SCTA) for the display of extracranial cerebral vessels is presented in light of the present state of development, based on several sets of images.

We gave a preliminary report on our first experiences with this new diagnostic chance for the Neuroradiology at the 8th European congress of Radiology in September 1993 in Vienna (Dickschas 1993).

Material and Methods

This actual study is based on meanwhile 51 CT examinations we performed for two years and six months, since October 1991. Although a digital subtraction angiogram was additionally performed in 15 cases.

The scanning technique selected, made use of the Spiral CT mode offered by the Somatom Plus.

Cervical vessels were displayed three-dimensionally (Fig. 1) using the shaded surface display (SSD) coupled with maximum intensity projection (MIP) (Napel et al. 1992; Magnusson et al. 1991).

We employed a 3 mm slice thicknes with a 6 mm table feed. The reconstruction of the conventional transversal slices was performed with 1 to 2 mm overlapping.

The planimetric determination of vascular lumina, and particularly of stenoses, was performed in the transaxial slices using conventional distance- and planimetric measurement techniques.

In the correlating transaxial slices of an angiostenosis localized in the 3D or MIP angiogram, the absolute reduction in the area of the constricted lumen is measured with planimetric precision and the percentile reduction in area is calculated in relation to the area of the original lumen.

The degree of stenosis was calculated by the formula $(1 - As/An) \times 100\%$ (Fürst et al. 1993)

The contrast medium was administered periphero-venously. We used a volume-controlled CT injector to inject a highly concentrated, non-ionic contrast medium in a total volume of 100 ml at a constant flow rate of 4 ml/sec. The Spiral-CT was used for patients with average blood pressure values, following a delay of 12 sec. after the beginning of injection.

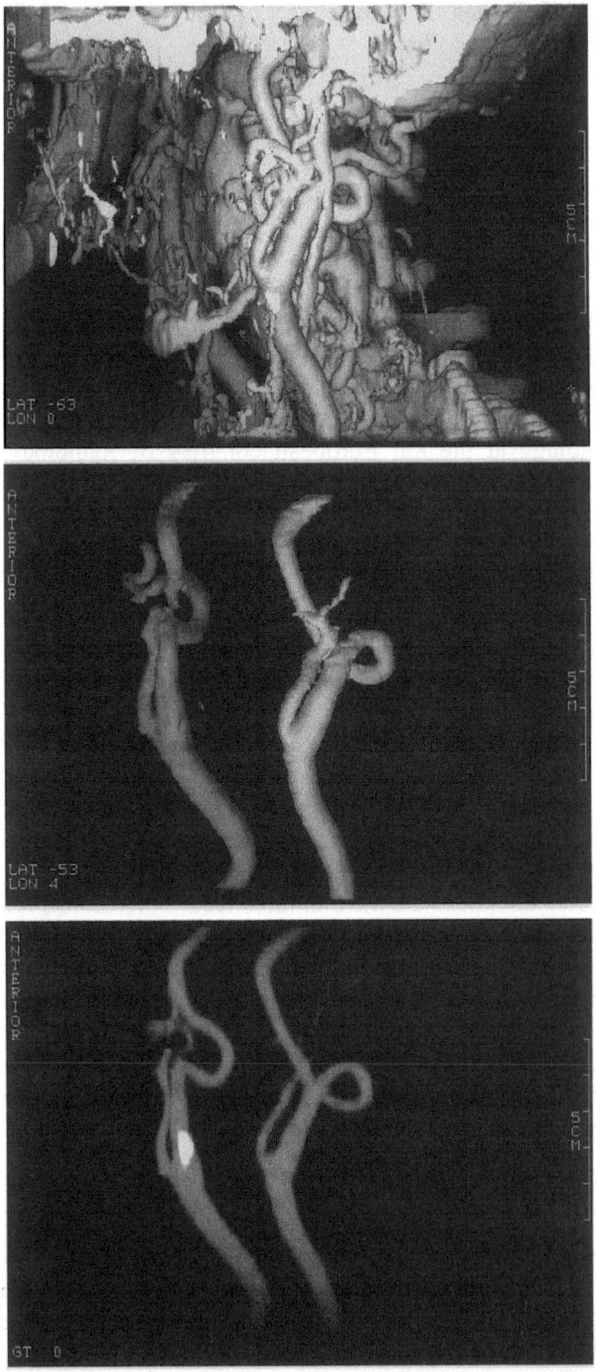

Fig. 1 a–c. Tortuosity of both internal carotid arteries in a 60-year-old patient suffering from syncopes. Three-dimensional display using the shaded surface display (**a, b**) and maximum intensity projection (**c**). Through image **c** a focal calcification in the wall of right internal carotid artery is shown

In cases involving a hypertensive initial condition, it is advisable to use a test bolus of 10 ml to determine the delay time.

Thus, the total examination time amounts to 42 sec., including 30 s scan time.

The bone structures must be removed from the transaxial slices prior to 3D- or MIP- image reconstruction with the aid of an editing program.

Results and Discussion

For these minimally invasive studies we obtained images of the vascular ROIs with good diagnostic quality. A three-dimensional display of vessels complied well with our physiological 3D vision and registration of anatomic structures. The vascular ROIs could also be displayed together with the adjucant skeletal structure.

This possibility improves the anatomic survey and the topic localisation of vascular findings (Fig. 2). Moreover, the underlying transaxial slices permit a planimetric evaluation of the interesting vascular lumina and therefore provide exact quantitative information concerning the extent of stenosis, not possible with any other method (Fig. 3).

Either concentric or irregular, i.e. eccentric stenoses can be detected equally well and with metric certainty.

Via conventional angiographic methods only a concentrically configured stenosis permits a reliable, gradual assessment in each beam path. The extent of excentrically and irregularily configured stenoses sometimes is only approximately estimated. Eccentric constrictions tend to result in underestimation of the extent (Büdingen et al. 1982).

With the aid of the MIP program, SCTA of extracranial cerebral vessels can be used as a further specific diagnostic enhancement to the display of intravascular calcifications (Moran et al 1991). Using this software program, it is possible to indicate and precisely locate intravascular calcifications, thus supplying important additional information on the type of stenosis (Figs. 4+6).

This knowledge is important for the therapeutic concept especially in cases involving ventilation of the indication for an operation or for vasodilatation.

The three-dimensional display also is particulary suitable for spatial display of the irregularities of the vascular walls (Figs. 4+6) since the vessels are reconstructed through the contrast medium volume contained in the lumina.

SCTA also permits the examiner to view the vascular network in all of the positions previously not displayable with conventional angiography (Fig. 5).

Thus for example, disturbing vascular convolutions like the ones occasionally encountered in angiograms can be freely broken down through rotation of the reconstructed vascular network (Fig. 7).

The informational value of this method was limited only by artifacts turning up in places with extensive bridgework, which occasionally impaired the reconstruction of vessels located near the base of the skull.

When one also considers the extremely short examination time and minimal invasive nature of SCTA, which can be easily performed on an outpatient basis, it becomes clear, that SCTA of extracranial cerebral vessels is indeed a highly promising alternative to conventional angiography.

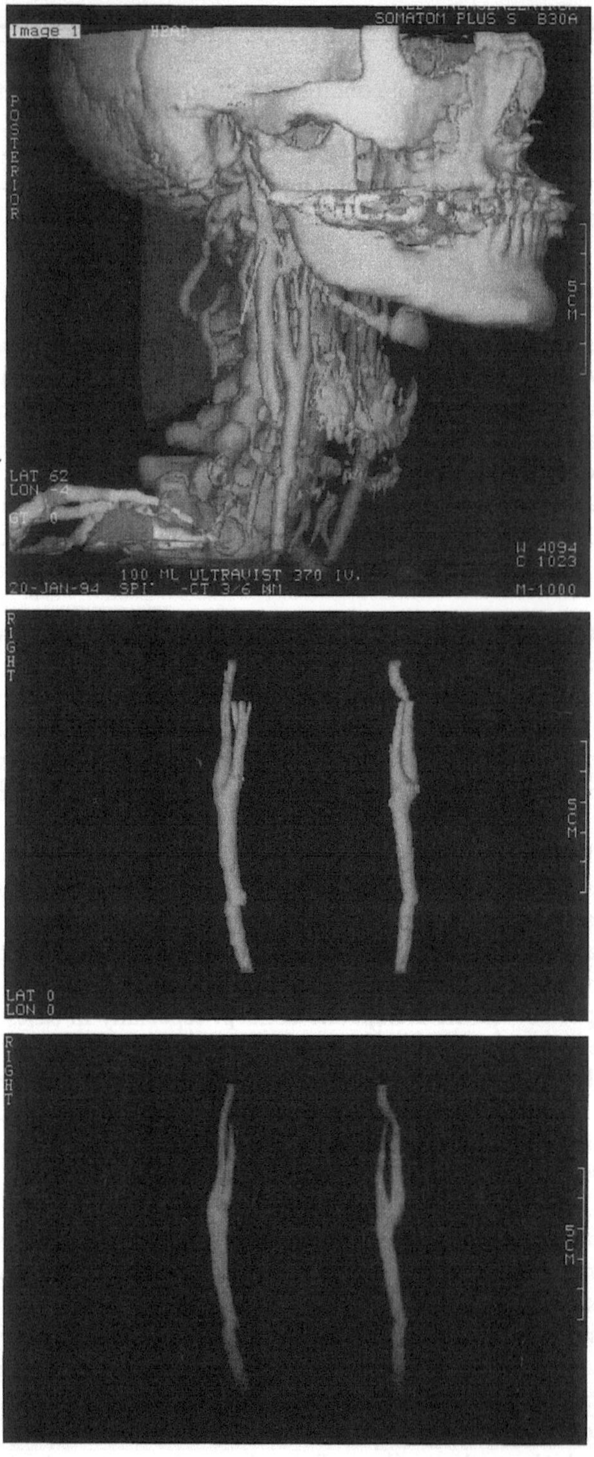

a
b
c

Fig. 2 a–c. Circumscribed compression of both common carotid arteries by the transverse processes of sixth vertebral body

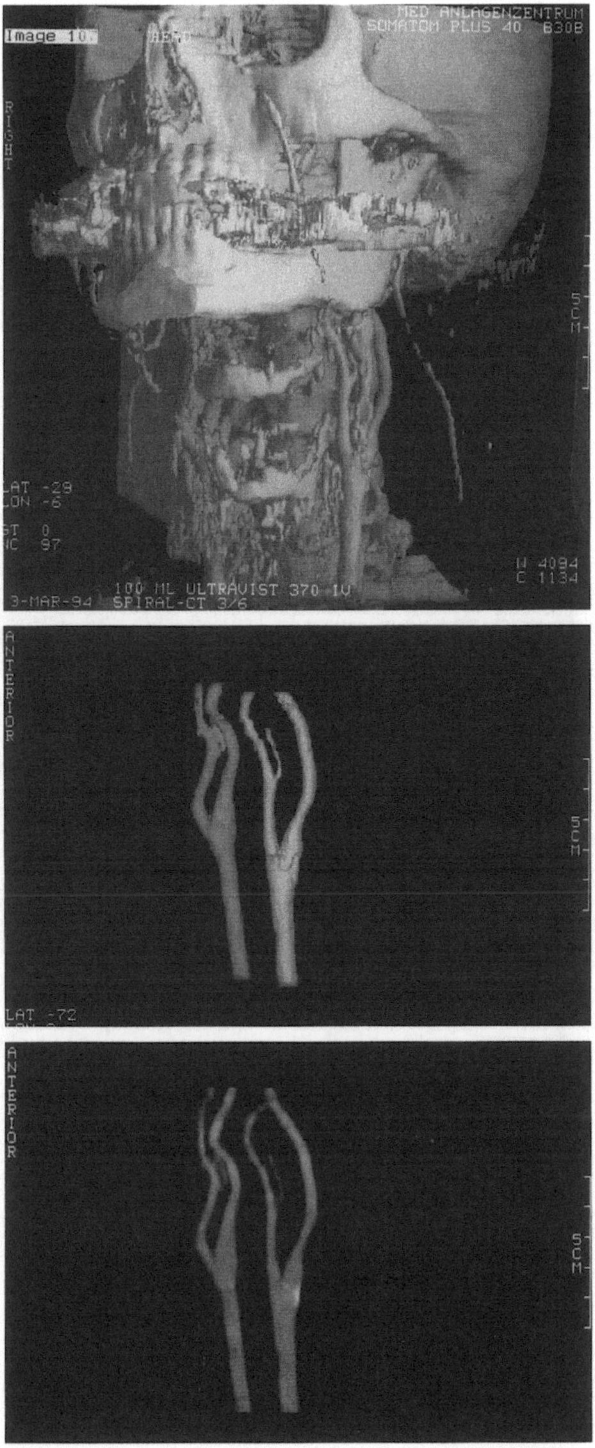

a

b

c

Fig. 3 a – e. Stenosis of left internal carotid artery of 51 %. 3D display using Shaded-surface-display und Maximum-intensity-projection (**a – c**). Stenosis was measured planimetrically from the 2D axial images (**d, e**) by comparing the area of the constricted lumen (0.18 cm^2) with the area of the artery distal to the region of the stenosis (0.39 cm^2)

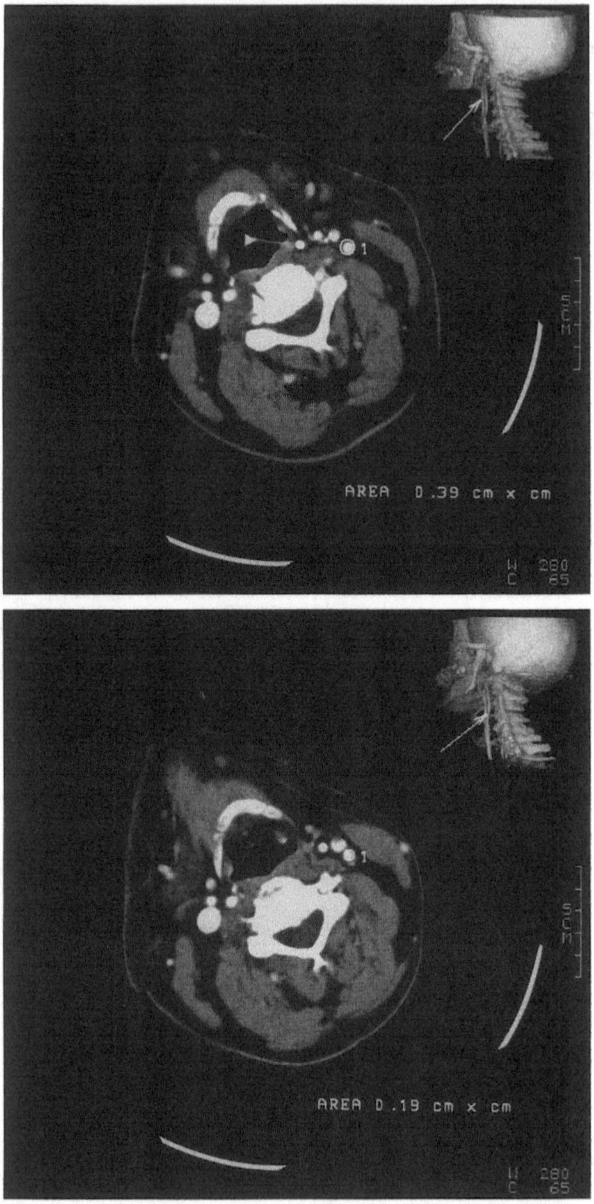

d

e

Fig. 3 d, e

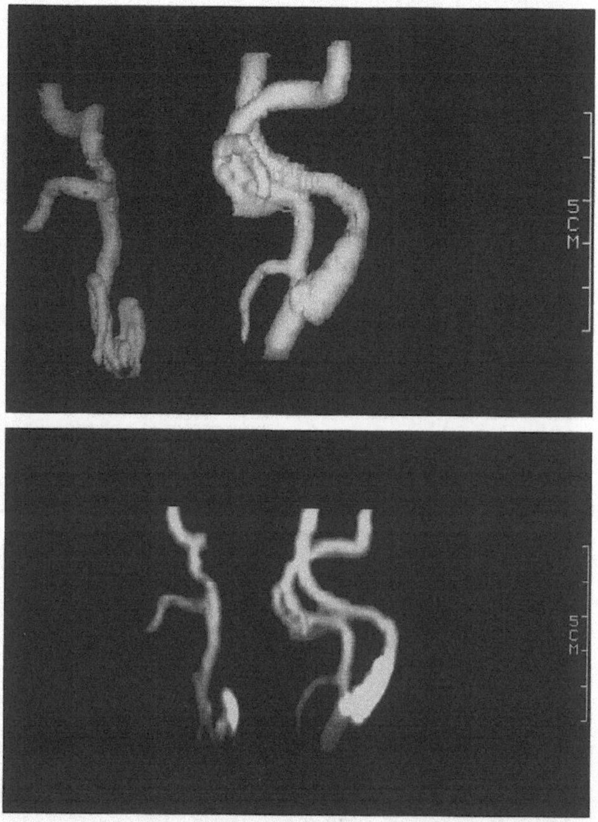

a

b

Fig. 4 a, b. Carotid artery bifurcation in a 78-year-old woman with occlusion of right internal carotid artery. 3D angiogram: Large irregularities of the vascular wall of left internal carotid artery, just beyond bifurcation (**a**). Maximum intensity projection shows nearly circumferential calcification (**b**)

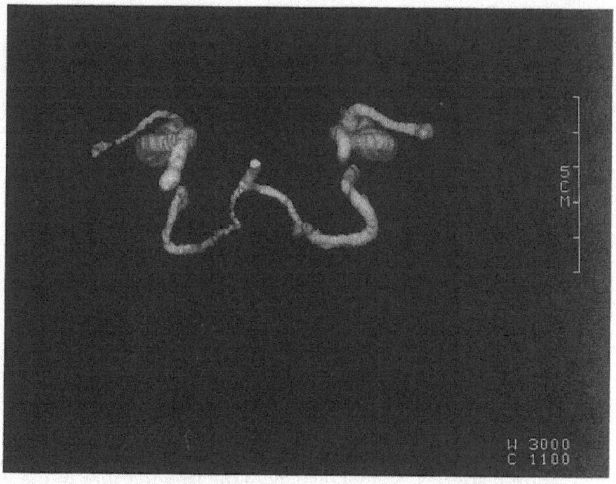

Fig. 5. SCTA of the vascular network

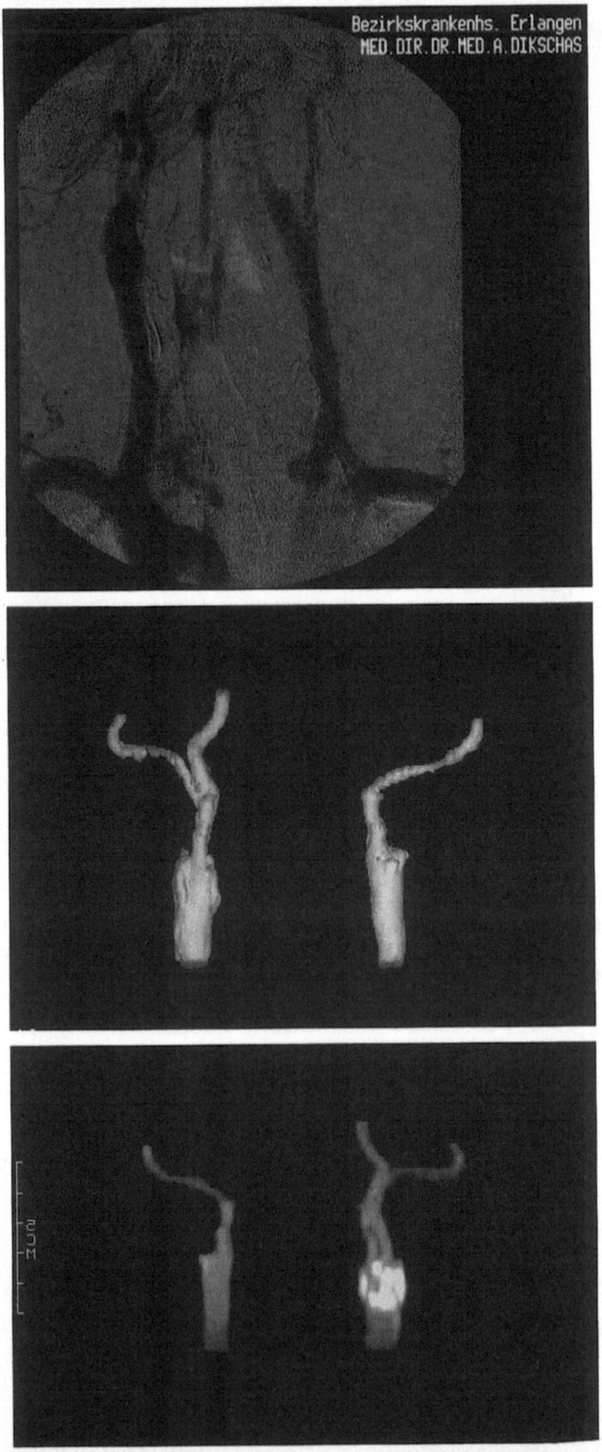

a

b

c

Fig. 6 a–c. Occlusion of left internal carotid artery. **a** Digital subtraction angiogram of both carotid arteries. Spatial display of the irregularities of the vascular walls by shaded surface display (**b**). Maximum intensity projection (**c**) shows multiple signal intensities within circumferential calcified plaques through this area

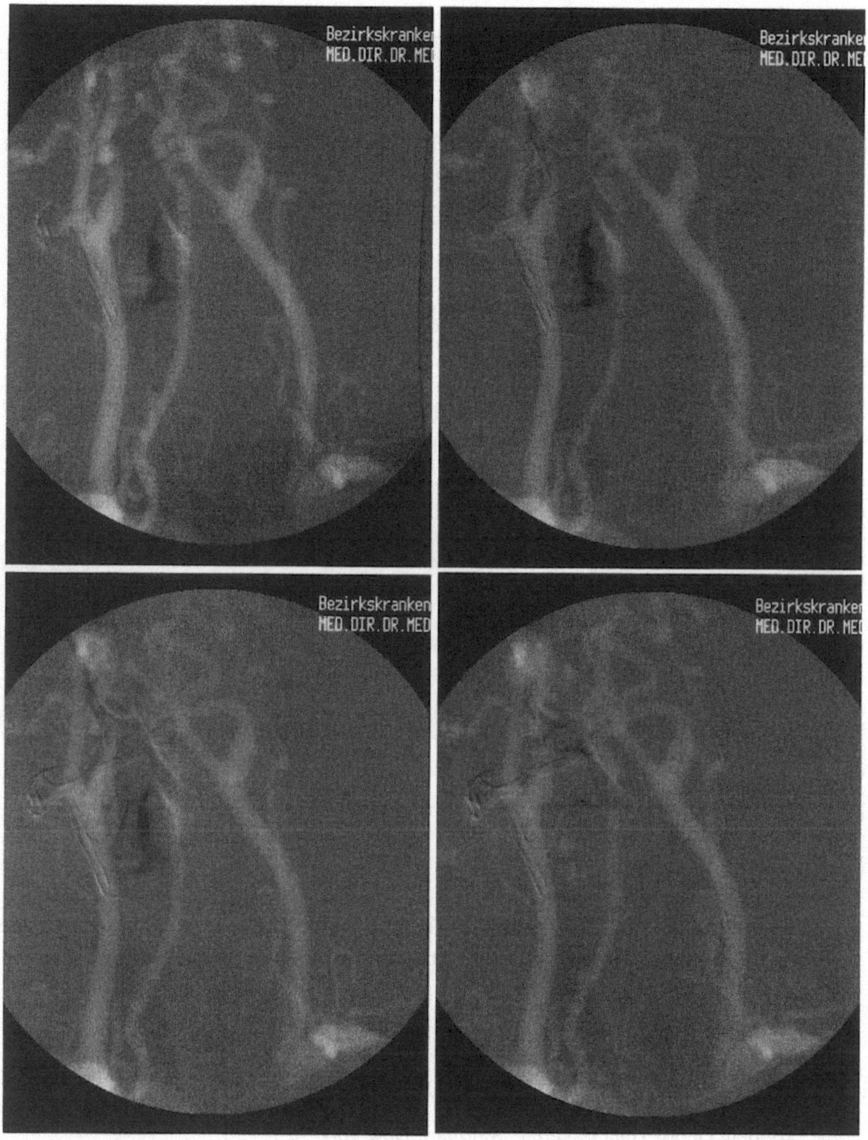

a

Fig. 7a–c. Vascular convolutions in digital subtraction angiogram can be broken down through rotation of the reconstructed vessels

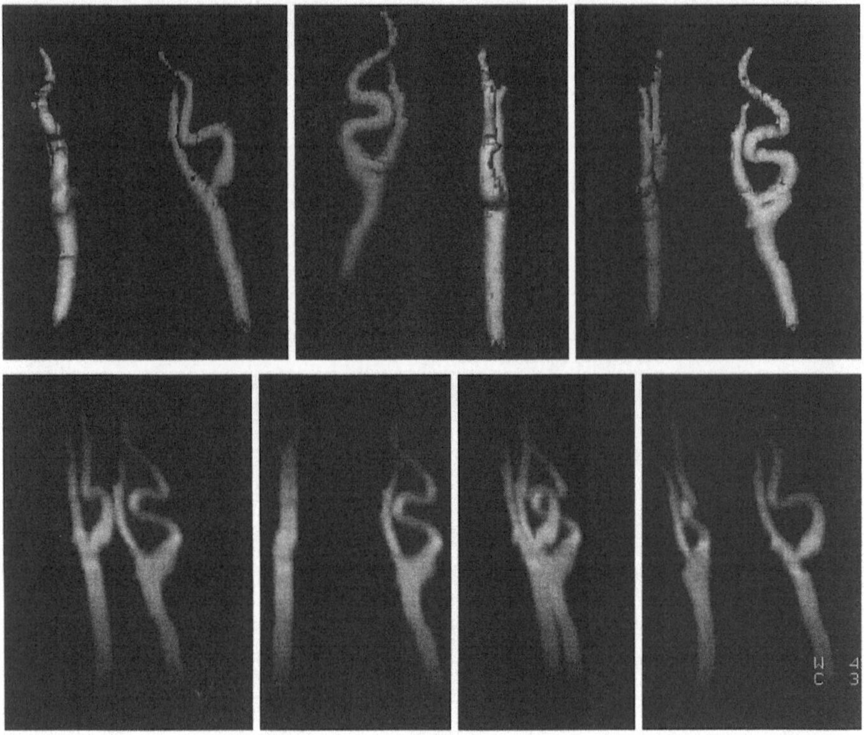

b

c

Fig. 7b, c

Due to increasing experience with this method in our department extracranial cerebrovascular conventional angiographies are now only performed very rarely.

References

Büdingen HJ, von Reutern GM, Freund HJ (1982) Dopplersonographie der extracraniellen Hirnarterien. Georg Thieme Verlag, Stuttgart, New York

Dickschas A (1993) CT-Angiography of extracranial cerebral vessels (abstr.) ECR '93 – 8th European congress of Radiology: Scientific Programme and Abstracts (1202) Springer International

Fürst G, Kahn T, Sitzer M, Fischer H, Hofer M, Fehlings T, Aulich A, Steinmetz H (1993) Quantifizierung extracranieller Karotisstenosen-Magnetresonanzangiographie und Dopplersonographie versus intraarterielle Angiographie. Fortschr. Röntgenstr. 159,4 : 368 – 374, Georg Thieme Verlag Stuttgart – New York

Magnusson M, Lenz R, Danielson PE (1991) Evaluation of methods for shaded surface display of CT volumes. Comput Med Imaging Graph, 15 : 247 – 256

Moran CJ, Vannier MW, Erickson KK, et al. (1991): Diagnosing extracranial atherosclerotic disease with spiral CT (abstr.) Radiology; 181 (P): 162

Napel SA, Marks MA, Rubin GD, et al. (1992): CT angiography with spiral CT and maximum intensity projection.

Abdominal Aortic Aneurysms: Evaluation by CT Angiography

R. Braunschweig, P. E. Huppert, S. Duda, H. Seboldt, C. D. Claussen

Introduction

For the evaluation of thoracical and abdominal aortic aneurysms digital subtraction angiography (DSA) and conventional computed tomography (CT) have been developed to standardized methods. On one hand the DSA shows the flow phenomenas in the aorta and the connective vessels, particularly iliacal and femoral arteries and the size of the aneurysms itself. In cases of thrombosis in the aneurysms DSA does not reveal the total volume of the that. On the other hand CT gives information about the aortic wall, side branches and the surrounding soft tissue of the aneurysms. For taking all these informations we still need two methods. Every investigation has its own risks, advantages and disadvantages.

The spiral CT has the one big advantage of combining 1-second tube rotation with continuous patient transport. More than 30 scans can be obtained during the vascular phase of a contrast-enhanced study in a single breath hold. In order to the choice of thick sections (1, 2, 4, 8 and 10 mm) data of a volume of more than 30 cm are available. The recent development of multiplanar reconstructions, particularly the maximum intensity projection (MIP) as volume rendering and surface rendering as 3-D-display, combines volume scanning in small sections and multiplanar reconstructions for the CT angiography.

However, the technique has some limitation and the aim of reporting our preliminary results is to show the investigation procedure, some clinical examples and to carry out the advantages and disadvantages of CT angiography with MIP and 3-D display, particularly in the diagnostic procedure of aortic aneurysms.

Material and Methods

To date, we have investigated 10 patients (seven male, three female, age range from 23 – 81 years). We used the Siemens Somatom Plus-S scanner (Siemens AG; Erlangen/Germany). A total of 100 ml of nonionic contrast medium (Solutrast 370; Byk Gulden; Konstanz/Germany) was injected in all cases by a power injector (SIMTRAC;Siemens AG; Erlangen/Germany). We used a flow of 3 – 4 ml/s. A 19-gauge infusion set was placed in an antecubital vein. All patients were instructed to hyperventilate before starting the volume scanning and suspended ventilation for the complete acquisition of data. The doctor were standing by during the procedure.

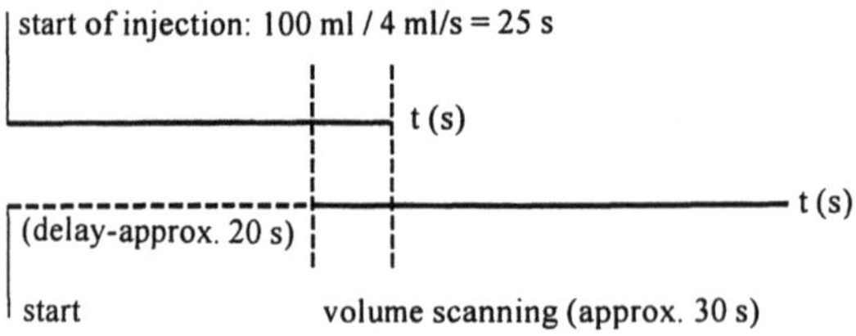

Fig. 1. Time relation between injection of contrast medium and volume scanning. Volume: 100 ml; flow: 3–4 ml/s; single-breath-hold. 30 s; delay for spiral CT: approx 20–25 s

After a topogram we obtained a conventional CT from the diaphragm to the bifurcation in a 1-cm collimation and a table feed of 3 cm. In order to the length of the aneurysm a 12 or 24-cm-long scan volume was determined. A Serio-CT was performed to take the right delay time. Ten scans with a cycle time of 3 s and a delay of 10 s have been taken at the top of the aneurysm. The time for increasing the contrast in the aorta (Hounsfield units) was added to the time of delay of the Serio-CT (Fig. 1).

For the spiral CT 3 examinations were performed with 120 kV and 165 mA and for 7 examinations we changed to 210 mA. A table speed of 8 (three cases) or 4 mm/s was combined with a collimation of 4 mm. All images were reconstructed by using standard axial view with an increment of 4 or 2 and volume (MIP) and surface rendering. For using the MIP regions of interest (ROIs) were selected to suppress as much bone as possible and emphasizing the vessels of interest. Threshold values ranged from 110 to 150 Hounsfield units (Hu). Multiplanar images were reconstructed in different views and as a surface rendering 3-D images displayed. Maximum intensitiy projections were compared with angiograms (Fig. 2 a) in respect to the vascular branches and pathologic signs such as stenoses, aneurysms and wall calcifications. In one case we could compare the abdominal CT angiography with a magnetic resonance (MR) angiogram.

Results

Procedure

Figure 3 shows the conclusion of our experiences and from the literature [5, 6, 8, 9, 10] for managing the spiral CT as a CT angiography. Its a matter of fact that we can only acquire a approximately 30 s volume scanning in a single medium breath. The other fact is the length of aneurysm which we have to examined. As an example, to cover a 12-cm-long aneurysm in a 30-s spiral scan we have to use a table feed of 4 mm/s. In order to the multiplanar reconstructions collimation should be in proportion to table feed as 1 : 1 or in maximum 1 : 2 (Fig. 3). That means, in our example, there is the choice of collimation between 4 or 2 mm. However, as far as the increment is concerned the same rule is recommendable: The proportion to collimation is 1 : 0.5. In that way we get expressive pictures and examination results, particularly the MIP technique is very reliable.

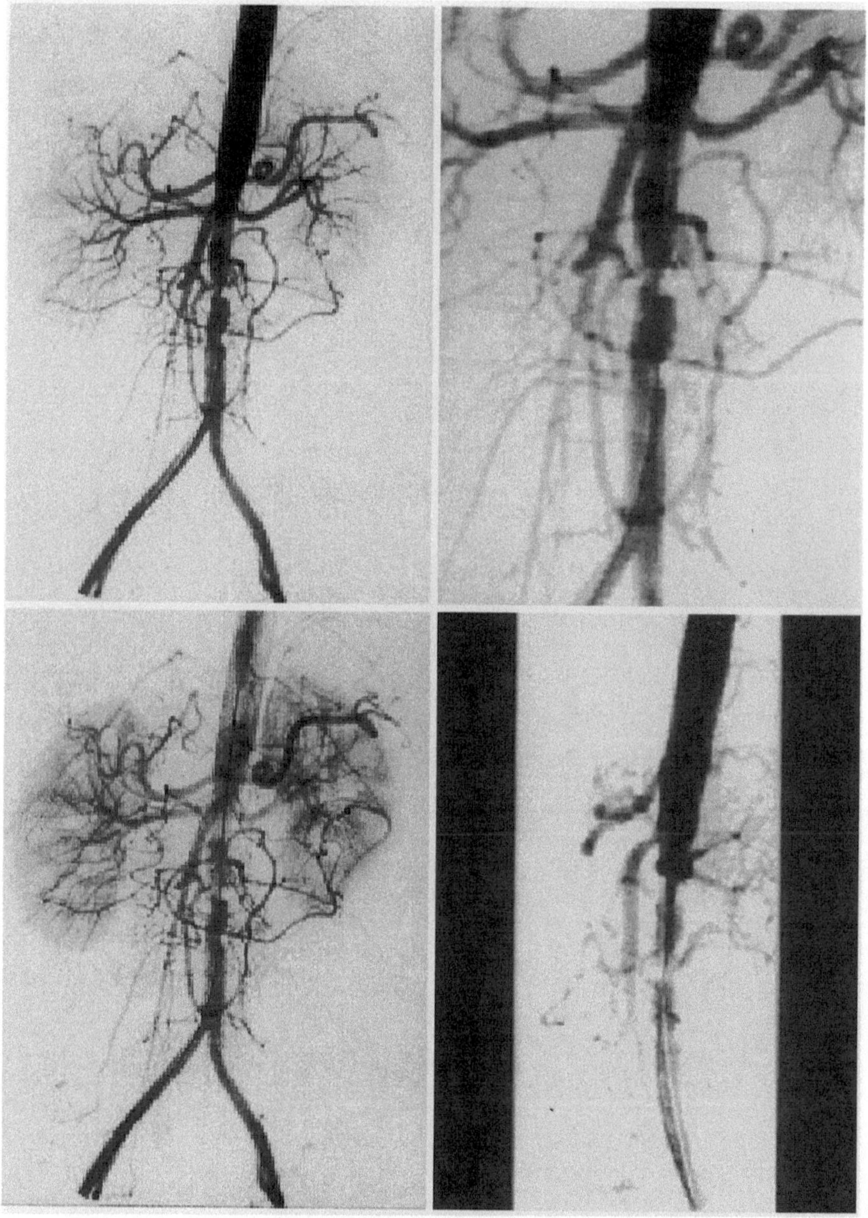

a

Fig. 2 a/b. Comparison of DSA and CT Angiography in a 23-year-old female patient with premature artherosclerosis. DSA and CT angiography show the signs and vessels

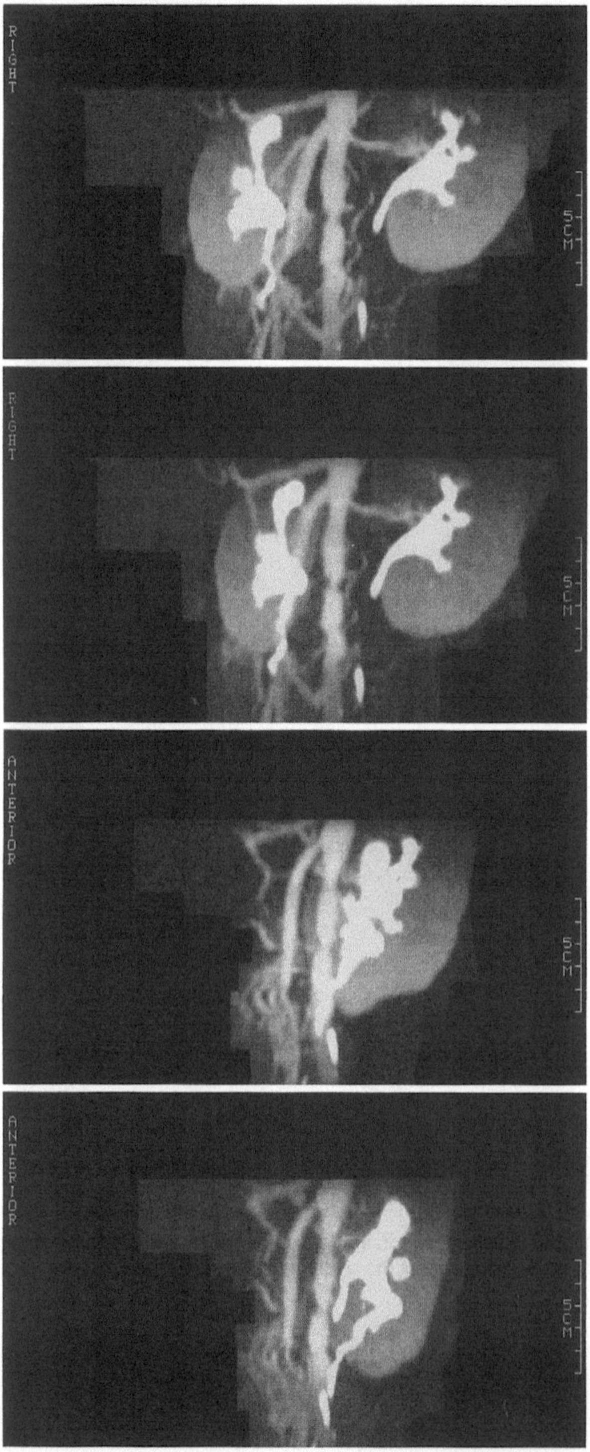

Fig. 2b

acquisition: (table feed = length : time)

table feed	:	slice	:	increment
2 / 1	:	1	:	0.5

Fig. 3. Proportion of table feed, collimation (slice) and increment. There are two factors: length of aneurysm and single breath-hold. The table feed is according from that

Using the correct delay time for injection of contrast medium and the right volume and flow is very important. In all cases we determined the delay time with a Serio-CT. That gives the ability to start the injection of contrast medium and the volume scanning coincidential and makes the investigation easier. Figure 1 shows the relationsship of injection and spiral CT. For a good opacification of the aorta throughout the scanning-procedure at least a volume of 100 ml of contrast media is necessary. A flow of 3–4 ml/s increases the aortic opacification to about 200 HE (Hounsfield units). This is relatively diminuished in comparison with higher volumes and flow rates. However, there is no venous opacification still at the same phase of the examination, which makes better arterial reconstructions.

Display

For the reconstructions we use the MIP and sometimes the surface rendering as a 3-D display. Figures 4 and 5 show examples for the volume rendering as the CT angiography and 3-D display. Aorta and side branches are clearly evident, particularly with associated aneurysms or calcifications. On the other side, without any calcification of the aneurysm documentation of a thrombosed aneurysm is really difficult. However, there is a excellent reveal for the anatomical topography of the superior mesenteric and renal artery. Different views show the correct distance between the aneurysm and the superior mesenteric and renal artery. In another case (Fig. 2b) DSA corroborated to the results of CT angiography, particularly the aortic and iliacal stenoses.

Discussion

CT angiography is dependent on adequate acquisition procedure of data and concentration of intravascular contrast medium while scanning. The length of aneurysm and the 30-s single breath hold determined the table feed (Fig. 1). For a good reconstruction in multiplanar volume rendering images thin collimation and increment is obligatory. So far, for a long coverage table travel should be increased. For that, particularly collimation width should be constant, section sensitivity profile will be degraded. In conclusion, table feed and collimation have to be not more than 2:1 (Fig. 3). The limitation for the imaging volume is the recommendable collimation of

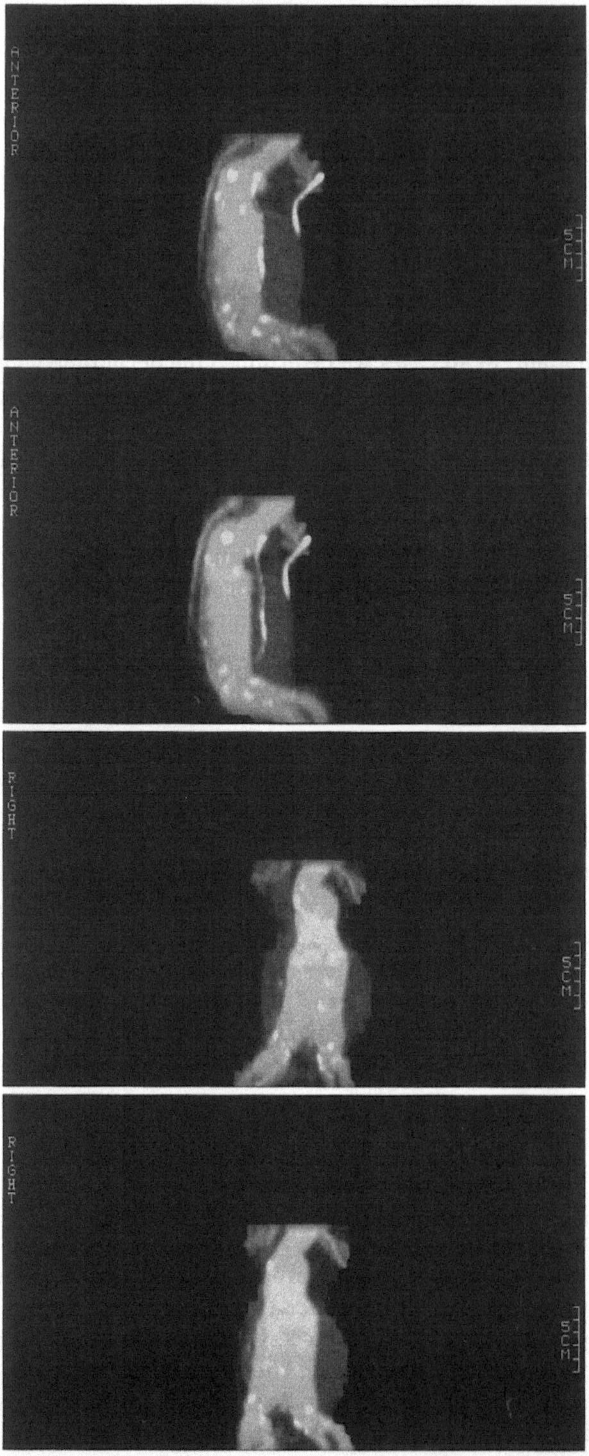

Fig. 4. MIP of an abdominal thrombosed aneurysm in a 67-year-old male patient. Without any calcification of aneurysm the evaluation is very difficult by MIP

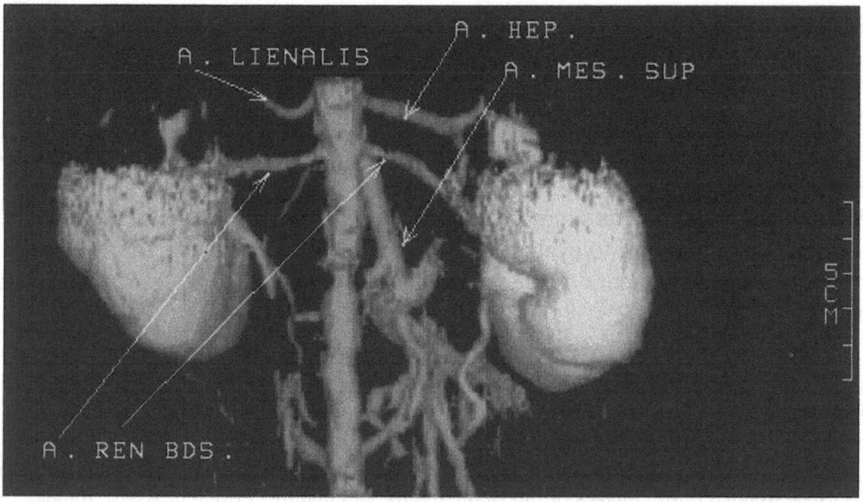

Fig. 5. Surface rendering as 3-D reconstruction in same patient as Fig. 3, back view. Side branches of the aorta are well documented. Renal arteries, *small arrow*; superior mesenteric artery, *long arrow*

2–4 mm. This result in a total of 12 cm for the scanning volume as a compromise of all influences. Is there a larger imaging colume a second run is necessary.

For a good opacification of the vessels timing, volume and flow of the injection of the contrast medium are very important. MIP requires a increased density about 200 HU and a threshold value at least 110 HU [10]. For that, we take always a Serio-CT on top of the aneurysm determining the individual delaytime (Fig. 1). For the volume scanning the volume of contrast medium should be at least 100 ml. A flow of 3–4 ml/s is obligatory. Under those conditions bolus profile could be a long plateau and ROIs for MIP may be selected.

For the display two mathematical models are available. As we know from MR angiography [1, 2], MIP is a volume rendering method. A two-dimensional image is showing the vessels and perpendicular and rectangular side branches like the DSA. Moreover, MIPs are generated from different view angles and can be displayed in a cine loop for a 3-D impression. In contrast to the DSA MIP is able to reveal intramural calcifications. Otherwise, in cases of thrombosed aneurysms without marginally calcifications MIP has not the correct discernibility of grey values (HU) to show the aneurysm itself (Fig. 4). Spatial resolution of DSA is superior, but CT angiography offers a rapid examination with lower radiation dose [8], without any arterial punction and gives an excellent anatomical overview with correct distances to renal and superior mesenteric arteries.

As a 3-D display shaded surface rendering is available. In connection with a predetermined threshold pictures result in clear imagination of vessel morphology. This calls the attention to the anatomical structures beside the aneurysms.

Last but not least, volume scanning by spiral CT with axial reconstructions gives all useful information by a cross-section examination method. Surrounding soft tissue and other intraabdominal organs are well described.

Conclusion

CT angiography by spiral CT is a non-invasive-method for rapid examination intra-abdominal vessels, particularly the aorta. The method is less expensive and is able to demonstrate cross-sections, angiographical-like pictures with anatomical features and 3-D images.

We recommend the CT angiography using volume scanning by spiral CT after the sonographic examination to evaluate abdominal aneurysms before DSA. In cases there are questions for more details, particularly by the surgeons, the DSA can be added.

References

1. Cline HE, Lorensen WE, Souza SP, Jolesz FA, Kikinis R, Gerig G, Kennedy ThE (1991) 3D Surface Rendered MR Images of the Brain and its Vasculature. J Comput Assist Tomogr 15 (2):344–351
2. Keller PJ, Drayer BP, Fram EK, Williams KD, Dumoulin ChL, Souza StP (1989) MR Angiography with Two-dimensional Acquisition and Three-dimensional Display. Radiology 173:527–532
3. Heisermann JE, Drayer BP, Fram EK, Keller PJ, Bird CR, Hodak JA, Flom RA (1992) Carotid Artera Stenosis: Clinical Efficacy of Two-dimensional Time-of-Flight MR Angiography. Radiology 182:761–768
4. Kim D, Edelmann RR, Kent KC, Porter DH, Skillman JJ (1990) Abdominal Aorta and Renal Artery Stenosis: Evaluation with MR Angiography. Radiology 174:727–731
5. Kalender WA, Seissler W, Klotz E, Vock P (1990) Spiral Volumetric CT with Single-Breath-Hold Technique, Continuos Transport, and Continuos Scanner Rotation. Radiology 176:181–183
6. Marks MP, Napel S, Jordan JE, Enzmann DR (1993) Diagnosis of Carotid Artery Disease: Preliminary Experience with Maximum-Intensitiy-Projection Spiral CT Angiography. AJR 160:1267–1271
7. Masaryk AM, Ross JS, DiCello MC, Modic MT, Paranandi L, Masaryk ThJ (1991) 3DFT MR Angiography of the Carotid Bifurcation: Potential and Limitations as a Screening Examination. Radiology 179:797–804
8. Napel S, Marks MP, Rubin GD, Dake MD, McDonnell ChH, Song SM, Enzmann DR, Jeffrey RB (1992) CT Angiography with Spiral CT and Maximum Intensitiy Projection. Radiology 185:607–610
9. Prokop M, Schaefer C, Kalender WA, Polacin A, Galanski M (1993) Gefäßdarstellungen mit Spiral-CT. Radiologe 33:694–704
10. Rubin GD, Dake MD, Napel SA, McDonell ChH, Jeffrey RB (1993) Three-dimensional Spiral CT Angiography of the Abdomen: Initial Clinical Experience. Radiology 186:147–152

Acute and Chronic Aortic Dissections: Evaluation with Spiral CT Angiography

A. KOEHLER[1], M. PROKOP[1], M. HEINEMANN[2], M. GALANSKI[1]

Introduction

Aortic dissection is caused by an intimal tear (entry) of various location and extension. The media as a result is divided lengthwise with development of two channels: the false channel burrowing into the media and the original intima-lined true channel. The most commonly used classification system is the one proposed by the Stanford group [1]: dissections with extension to the ascending part of the aorta (type A) are distinguished from those involving only the descending part (type B). Spiral computed tomography (CT) allows continuous acquisition of data from a large scan volume [2] and has proved to be an ideal diagnostic tool for imaging the aorta and its large branching arteries [4].

Materials and Methods

Seventy-two patients with aortic dissections (15 women and 57 men; mean age 52.6 years, range 20–76 years) underwent 136 spiral CT examinations (87 thoracic and 49 abdominal studies). Twenty-three patients initially presented with acute dissections (12 type A, 11 type B) and 20 patients with subacute or chronic non-operated dissections (8 type A, 12 type B). Twenty-nine patients initially presented after operative repair of aortic dissection (24 type A, 5 type B). Section thickness was chosen between 2 and 5 mm and table feed between 2 and 9 mm depending on patient size and clinical question. Start delay was determined from a test bolus of 10 ml contrast medium. It varied from 10 to 34 s (mean 18 s) in thoracic studies and from 14 to 46 s (mean 23 s) in abdominal studies. In thoracic studies, the venous approach was cubital in 60 cases and femoral in 27 cases. A power injector was used to inject up to 160 ml of contrast medium with a flow of 3–4 ml/s. The scan length varied from 10.5 to 30.6 cm (mean 19.1 cm) in thoracic studies and from 11.4 to 33.6 cm (mean 22.8 cm) in abdominal studies, excluding two examinations performed because of suspected renal artery stenosis (6.6 and 7.0 cm). The reconstruction interval usually was set to 2 mm. Cine mode, multiplanar reformations (MPRs) and – where warranted – maximum intensity projections (MIPs) and three-dimensional surface shaded displays (3D SSDs) were used for evaluation.

[1] Department of Diagnostic Radiology I, Hannover Medical School
[2] Department of Thoracic and Cardiovascular Surgery, Hannover Medical School

Results

With respect to the presence of dissection, the supraaortic arteries could be assessed in 80/87 thoracic examinations (92%). Failure was either due to improper timing of the contrast bolus or a too narrow scan range in three cases (3%) each, but diminished considerably with increasing experience of the investigators. In one case (1%) the scan was prematurely aborted. In 8/69 patients (12%) variants of the origin of the supraaortic arteries were found: a short common origin of the brachiocephalic trunc and left common carotid artery was seen in five patients, an aortic origin of the left vertebral artery and a retrooesophageal right subclavian artery could be demonstrated in one patient each.

In 41/47 abdominal studies (87%) the origin of visceral and iliac arteries and the relation of the true and false chanel could be fully assessed. In five patients (11%) the scan was terminated above the aortic bifurcation and only one patient (2%) showed no sufficient vascular opacification. No case of improper timing of the contrast bolus occured.

Two abdominal studies were carried out because of suspected renal artery stenosis. One patient had normal renal arteries whereas the other had a re-stenosis after percutaneous transluminal angioplasty (PTA) of the left renal artery and chronic iatrogenic dissection limited to the abdominal aorta (Fig. 1). Multiple renal arteries (up to four on each side) were found in 9/39 patients with abdominal sudies (23%). Multiple channels and aortic cobwebs were demonstrated in 5/72 (7%) and 4/72 (6%) patients, respectively. Table 1 shows the frequency of aneurysms and detected entries in 43 patients with acute or non-operated chronic aortic dissections (Figs. 2–4). After reconstruction or replacement of the ascending aorta, spiral CT demonstrated remaining entries in 16/26 patients (62%) with persistent dissection.

Artifacts due to highly contrasted veins in the scan field frequently occured in thoracic studies with cubital approach. A mixture of 80 ml contrast medium (300 mg J/ml) diluted with 80 ml 0.9% NaCl provided sufficient arterial contrast (34 patients, average maximum arterial opacification 198 HU) and reduction of artifacts. Streak artifacts in many cases considerably disturbed image quality, especially quality of three-dimensional reconstructions. Using a femoral venous approach and 120–150 ml of undiluted contrast medium vascular opacification was high and no artifacts occured (27 patients, average maximum arterial opacification 310 HU).

Viewing of axial slices (interactive cine mode) was best suited for evaluation of vessel diameters, extension of the dissection, location of entry sites and separation of motion artifacts of the aortic wall from intraluminal membranes. MPRs were mainly used for evaluation of the configuration of the thoracic aorta (Fig. 3) and the course of the membrane within the aortic arch. The 3D SSDs improved spatial orientation in cases of thoracic aneurysms or complex vascular anatomy, but needed absence of marked thrombus (Fig. 4a). For thoracic studies MIPs were time-consuming and yielded no additional information (Fig. 4b). MIPs along the x- and z-axis were helpful for documentation in selected abdominal studies, especially in presence of renal artery pathology (Fig. 1). As a conclusion from our study we

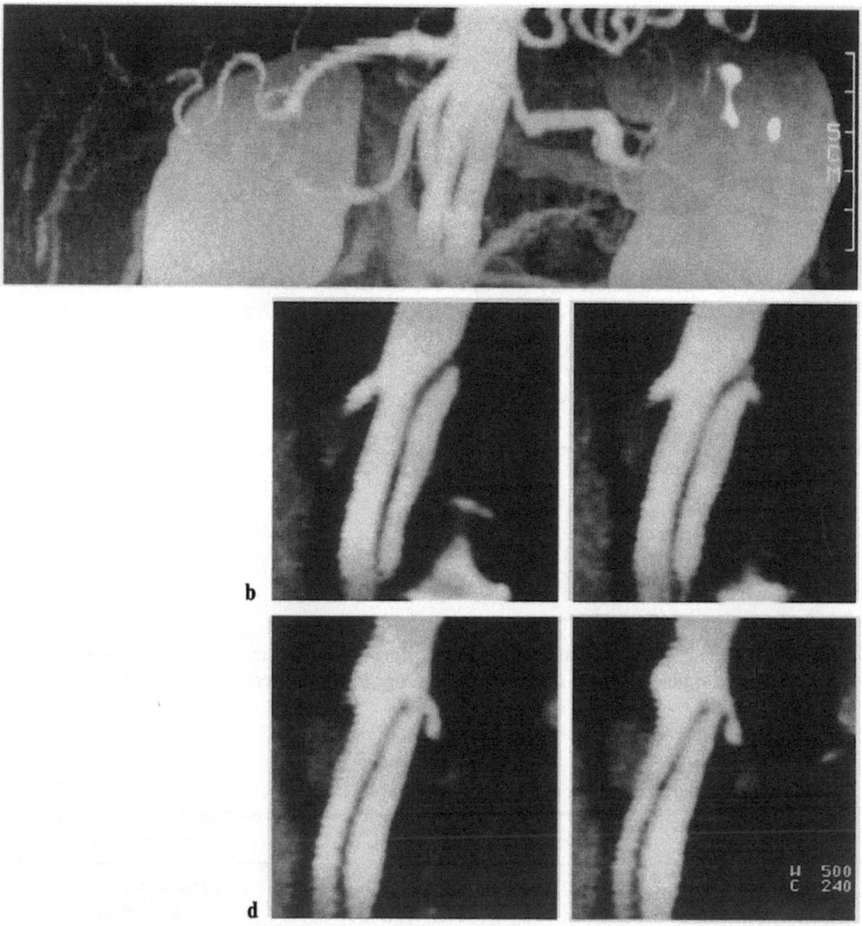

a b c d e

Fig. 1a–e. Maximum intensity projection (**a**) and multiplanar reformations (**b–e**) in a patient with restenosis after percutaneous transluminal angioplasty of the left renal artery. Iatrogenic chronic abdominal dissection with proximal entry

Table 1. CT findings in 43 patients with non-operated aortic dissections

	AADA ($n = 12$)	AADB ($n = 11$)	CADA ($n = 8$)	CADB ($n = 12$)
Thoracic CT	12 (12 pat.)	12 (11 pat.)	9 (8 pat.)	12 (10 pat.)
Entry	5/9[a]	2/11	7/8	5/9[b]
Aneurysm	8/12	2/11	7/8	7/10
Abdominal CT	2 (2 pat.)	6 (6 pat.)	2 (2 pat.)	8 (8 pat.)
Entry	0/2	1/6	2/2	4/8
Aneurysm	1/2	0/6	1/2	2/8

AADA/AADB, acute aortic dissection type A/B; CADA/CADB, chronic aortic dissection type A/B.
[a] Three patients with intramural hematoma.
[b] One patient with intramural hematoma.

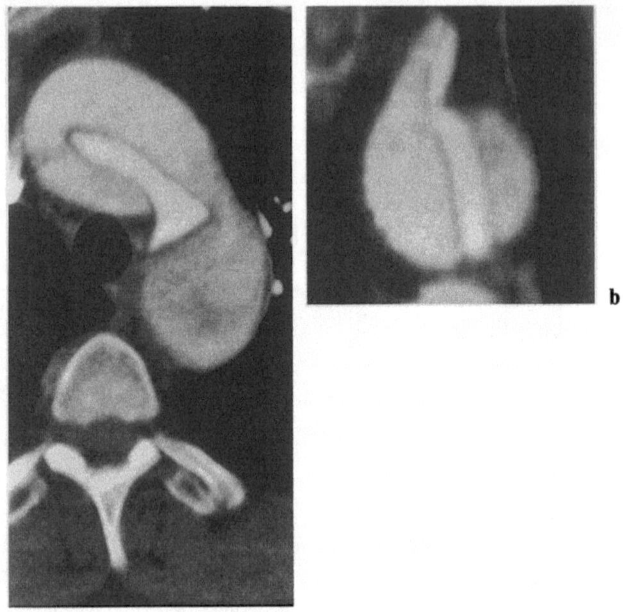

Fig. 2 a, b. Axial image (a) and multiplanar reformations (b) in a patient with chronic dissection type A. Membrane extending into the left common carotid artery

Table 2. Scan parameters for spiral CT angiography

	Thoracic CT	Abdominal CT
Approach[a]	Femoral	Cubital
Contrast medium[a]	120–150 ml	120–150 ml
Flow	4 ml/s	4 ml/s
Start delay	Test bolus	Test bolus
Section thickness	3 mm	3 or 5 mm
Table feed	5–6 mm	6–9 mm
Reconstruction interval	2 mm	2 mm
Scan direction	In/out	In

[a] In studies of the entire aorta or patients with anticoagulation, a cubital approach is chosen and the amount of contrast medoum for thoracic studies is reduced to 80 ml diluted 1 : 1 with 80 ml 0.9% NaCl.

Table 3. Suggested viewing and display modes of spiral CT slices

	Thoracic CT	Abdominal CT
Axial slices	standard	standard
MPR	standard	optional
3D SSD	optional	selected cases
MIP	impracticable	selected cases

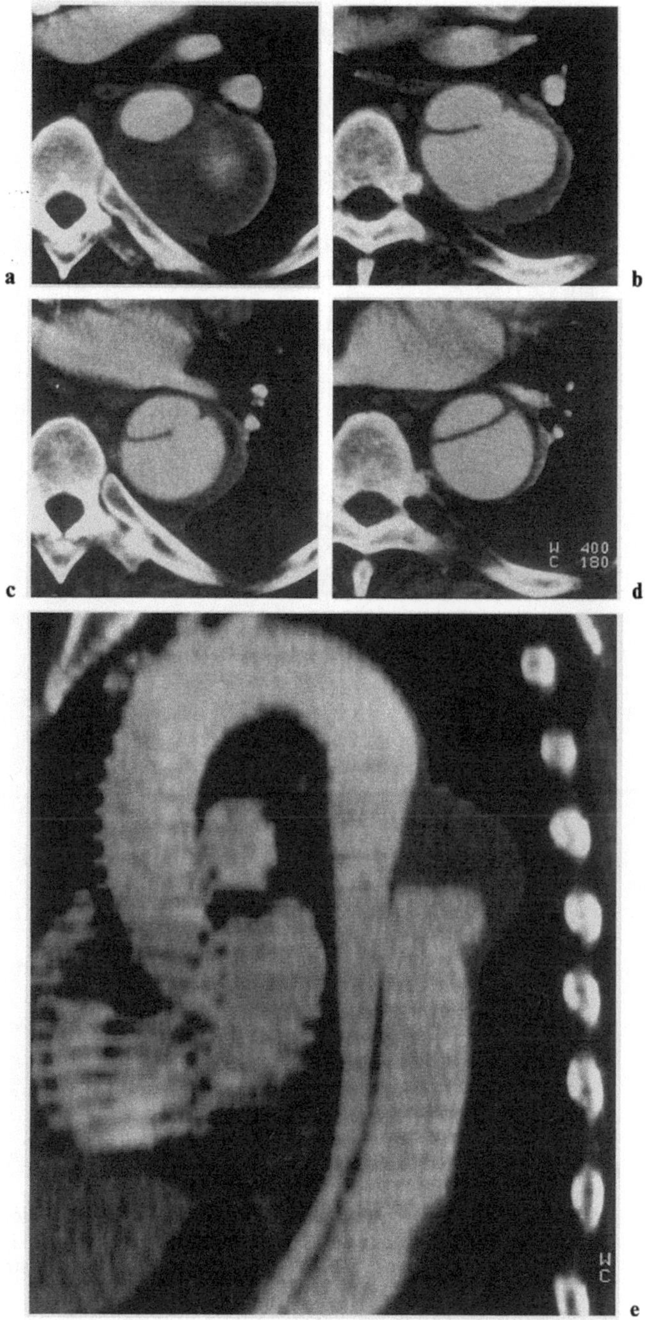

Fig. 3a–e. Axial images (**a–d**) and multiplanar reformations (**e**) in a patient with chronic dissection type B. Large entry in a partly thrombosed aneurysm of the descending aorta

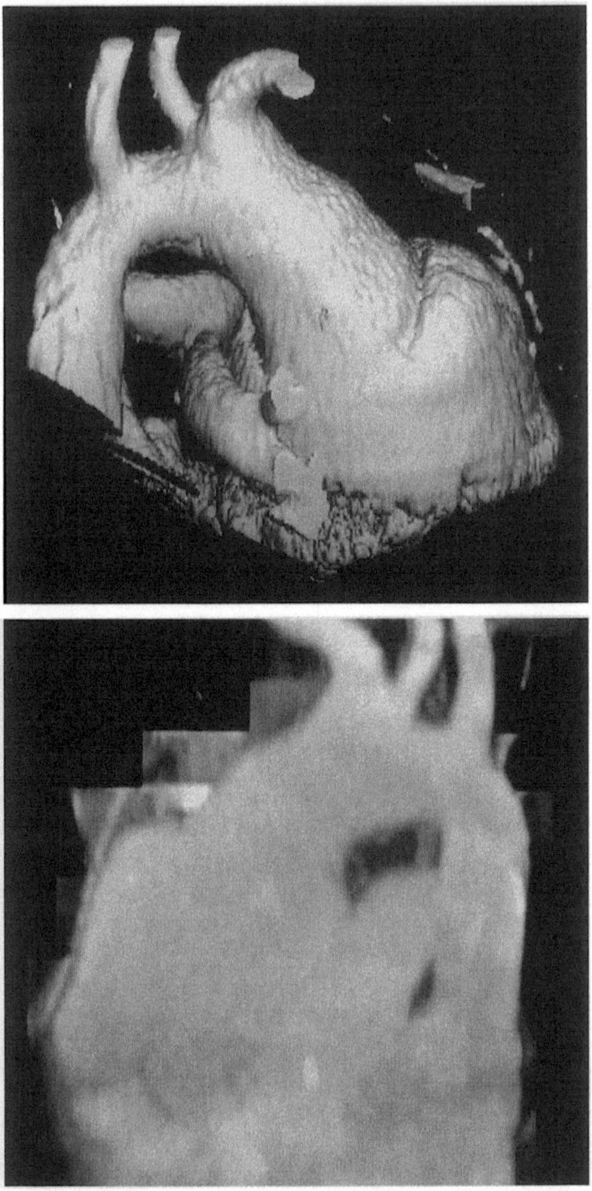

a

b

Fig. 4 a, b. Aneurysm of the ascending aorta in chronic dissection type A. Short common origin of the brachiocephalic trunc and the left common carotid artery. Three-dimensional surface shaded display (**a**) and maximum intensity projections (**b**) both demonstrate the partly widened aortic arch suggest the scan and evaluation parameters of spiral CT angiography given in Tables 2 and 3.

Discussion

Evaluation of patients with acute or chronic aortic dissections in general should include classification of dissection (type A and type B), assessment of major branching arteries, vessel diameters and presence of thrombus, location of entries, exclusion of perforation and – in selected cases – assessment of cerebral or spiral cord blood supply. We consider only the last item as the remaining indication for primary arterial angiography in these patients. Compared to angiography, spiral CT allows arbitrary projections of the opacified vessels and assessment of arterial wall structures such as thrombus, intramural hematoma and plaque calcification.

Interactive viewing of axial images and multiplanar reformations provides the necessary information in a short time. MIPs require editing for complete removal of bony structures and therefore are very time-consuming especially in the chest. In thoracic studies veins and pulmonary vessels are superimposed on the aorta and often negatively affect image quality. Therefore, MIPs should mainly be used in abdominal studies. In 3D SSDs bony structures do not have to be completely removed ("cut" function). Except for 3D displays of the thoracic aorta, which may provide additional information for the surgeon, both display modes are useful only for documentation of findings and should not be carried out routinely.

To obtain a high quality of spiral CT images, some basic aspects have to be considered. The 180° LI interpolation algorithm ("slim", Somatom Plus S) allows doubling of table feed without deterioration of slice profile [3]; the pitch factor (table feed/nominal section thickness) should be chosen between 1 and 2 [4]. Section thickness in general should not exceed 5 mm because of increasing object distortion along the z-axis [5]. For evaluation of the aortic arch and the supraaortic arteries a section thickness of 3 mm should be preferred. In abdominal studies due to the perpendicular course of the aorta (z-axis) and the larger scan volume section thickness may be increased to 5 mm.

Spiral CT is an ideal tool in evaluation of patients with chronic aortic dissections. In acute type A dissection, complete assessment of the aorta and its major branching arteries is often unnecessary but spiral CT should be considered in stable patients with equivocal echocardiographic findings.

References

1. Daily PO, Trueblood HW, Stinson EB, Wuerflein RD, Shumway NE (1970) Management of acute aortic dissections. Ann Thorac Surg 10:237–247
2. Kalender WA, Seissler W, Klotz E, Vock P (1990) Spiral volumetric CT with single-breath-hold technique, continuous transport, and continuous scanner rotation. Radiology 176: 181–183
3. Polacin A, Kalender WA, Marchal G (1992) Evaluation of section sensitivity profiles and image noise in spiral CT. Radiology 185:29–35
4. Prokop M, Schaefer C, Kalender WA, Polacin A, Galanski M (1993) Gefäßdarstellungen mit Spiral-CT: Der Weg zur CT-Angiographie. Radiologe 33:694–704
5. Schaefer C, Prokop M, Nischelsky J, Reimer P, Bonk K, Galanski M (1992) Vascular imaging with spiral CT. In: Felix R, Langer M (eds.). Advances in CT II. Springer, Berlin Heidelberg New York, pp 109–115

The Somatom Plus for Aortic Dissection: A 4-Year Review

A.K. Dixon, J.H. Small, R.A. Coulden, C.D. Flower

Introduction

The first reports of the use of computed tomography (CT) for the diagnosis of aortic dissection were announced in the early 1980s. A milestone paper at that time was by Thorsen et al. (1983) who reported excellent results using a technique which evaluated the aorta during a bolus enhanced sequence of images obtained at three separate anatomical levels. However, data acquisition times were then in the region of 5 s and were limited by an inherent 5 s interscan delay in order to allow tube cooling. Various artefacts were reported and became recognised as potential pitfalls. The value of close scrutiny of unenhanced images was emphasised: around 50% of acute dissections can be predicted before enhancement because of high attenuation material within the false lumen (Heiberg et al. 1985). This knowledge can assist the choice of anatomical sites for subsequent enhancement. There followed occasional reports of very thin dissection flaps being obscured by a combination of the dense contrast medium and their extreme mobility during the 5 s data acquisition. CT for the detection of dissection then started to be applied in non-specialist centres, which often had to struggle with less than ideal equipment. The inevitable (although occasional) misleading resuls led to some anxiety on the part of clinicians. Some centres still insist on a second test before definitive surgery. The second test has historically been aortography, on the grounds that the aortic valve, the coronary arteries and the longitudinal extent of the dissection can be readily evaluated. Much depends on the working practice of the surgeons at individual centres.

During this period, there were also rapid developments in oesophageal ultrasound (both transthoracic and transoesophageal) and magnetic resonance imaging (MRI).

Transoesophageal ultrasound (TOE), in experienced hands, is an extremely accurate technique in the diagnosis of aortic dissection (Khandheria 1992). The flap can be demonstrated in real-time and there are few confusing artefacts. In particular the all important relationship between the flap and the aortic root can be well demonstrated. The only drawbacks are blind sports related to interposition of the trachea for the anterior aortic arch and that not all centres have experienced operators available on a 24-h basis.

MRI is now probably the optimal technique for aortic dissection (Nienaber et al. 1992). Not only can the diagnosis be made, but the longitudinal extent can be shown. With the advent of modern phase contrast techniques, aortic valve function can also be assessed. However, MRI is still not widely available and out of hours access may be limited. MRI may prove problematical for the acutely ill patient who is in severe pain and requires close monitoring.

With all these techniques to choose from, different centres have adopted different policies (Naidich and Crystal 1994; Petasnik 1991). In the UK, CT is the most widely available test for the acute problem and is generally recommended (Clague et al. 1992). Hence continued interest in CT techniques.

During the late 1980s two new CT developments occurred which have had substantial impact on the CT evaluation of aortic dissection. The first was that of ultrafast (electron gun) CT (Hamada et al. 1992). During sequential 50 ms data acquisitions the mobile intimal flap can be evaluated with much the same real time clarity as TOE. However its expense means that ultrafast CT is limited to a small number of specialist hospitals.

The second development, continuous CT data acquisition, has much more general applications. During Kalendar's (1990), development of spiral CT the need for tubes with better heat dissipation became evident; the result has been a continuing improvement in tube design. Quite apart from allowing their intended task (spiral CT), these tubes have opened up a whole new concept of dynamic CT. On the Somatom Plus, the dynamic multisequence mode offers numerous applications, including a robust technique for the evaluation of aortic dissection.

Technique

Since acquiring a Somatom Plus system in 1989, a standard protocol for the evaluation of aortic dissection has been adopted in Addenbrooke's Hospital, Cambridge. The protocol is based on the three level technique proposed by Thorsen et al. (1983). Following an AP topogram (scanogram), a limited series of unenhanced images of the thoracic aorta is obtained at 2 cm increments from just above the aortic arch to below the aortic valve to include the pericardium. Then an appropriate anatomical level through the mid-ascending aorta is chosen for the first enhanced run. The Dynamic Multisequence mode is chosen and a 12-s continuous acquisition is obtained, immediately after a rapid (10 s) hand injection of 33 ml of standard (300 mg/ml) non-ionic contrast medium. Ideally the patient should maintain suspended inspiration during the data acquisition but this is not always possible when pain is severe or cooperation otherwise limited. The data is reconstructed so that images are displayed at 1 s intervals. Close attention to viewing parameters is needed (see Fig. 1). Should artefacts be troublesome, it is worth performing further reconstructions at 100 ms intervals for a limited portion of the data. This can reveal changes in position of an intimal flap (see Fig. 2) or prove the cause of the artefact (e.g. translocation, Fig. 3). If the initial enhanced run shows no evidence of dissection, second and third runs are obtained, one at the level of the aortic arch and one just above the aortic valve, each with another 33 ml of contrast medium (100 ml in total).

If the initial run shows a definite dissection, the second sequence of images is often a spiral run from the great vessels to the pericardium to show the full extent of the dissection, after injecting the remaining 66 ml of contrast medium. There are

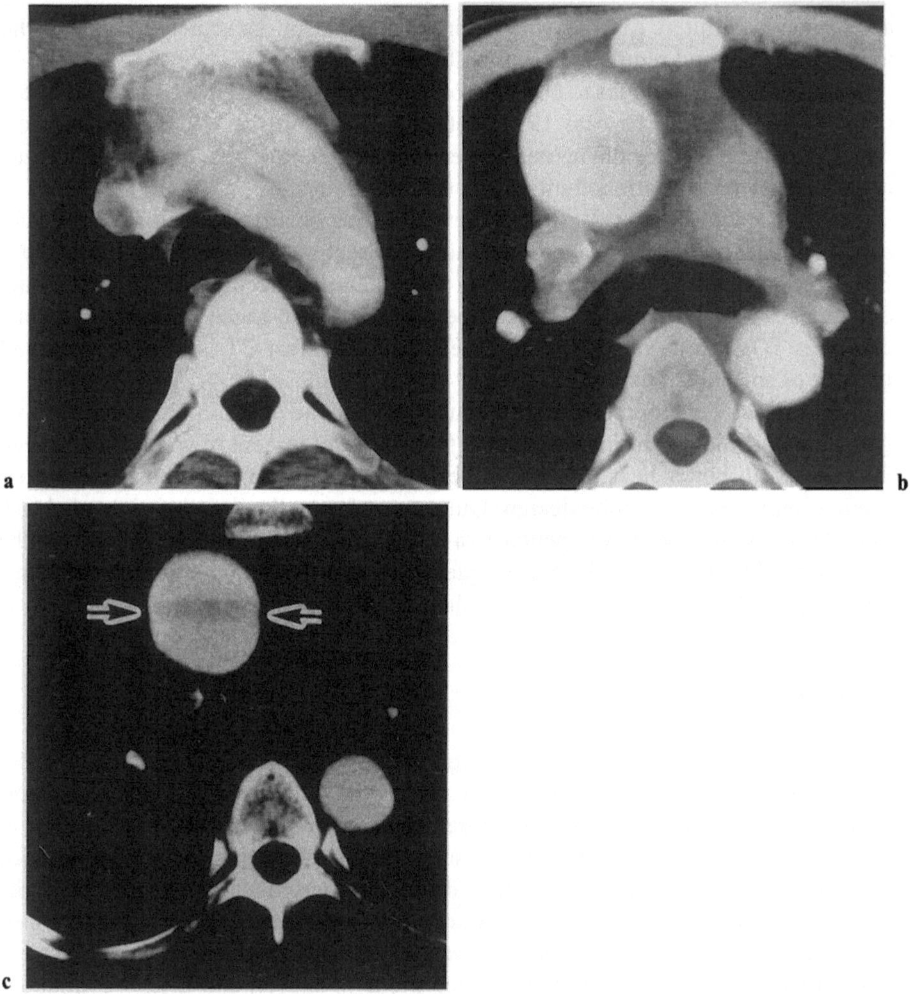

Fig. 1 a – c. A patient with a classical type A aortic dissection. **a** The flap is easily seen within the arch. **b** At conventional window settings (W 400, L +20 HU) the intimal flap in the ascending aorta is obscured by dense contrast medium. **c** At different window settings (W 200, L +200 HU) the intimal flap in the ascending aorta can be seen as a broad band of reduced attenuation (*arrows*). The flap appears thick because of obliquity within the plane (partial volume) and movement

obvious advantages in limiting the volume of contrast medium to 100 ml in total, just in case aortography is still required.

Whether a dissection is demonstrated or not, it is worthwhile to obtain a few images through the distal thoracic, proximal and mid abdominal aorta, particularly to assess the kidneys – even though this rarely influences management. Some claim that it is worth assessing the heart too, as a few patients referred with possible aortic dissection prove to have a myocardial infarction which can be shown by enhanced CT.

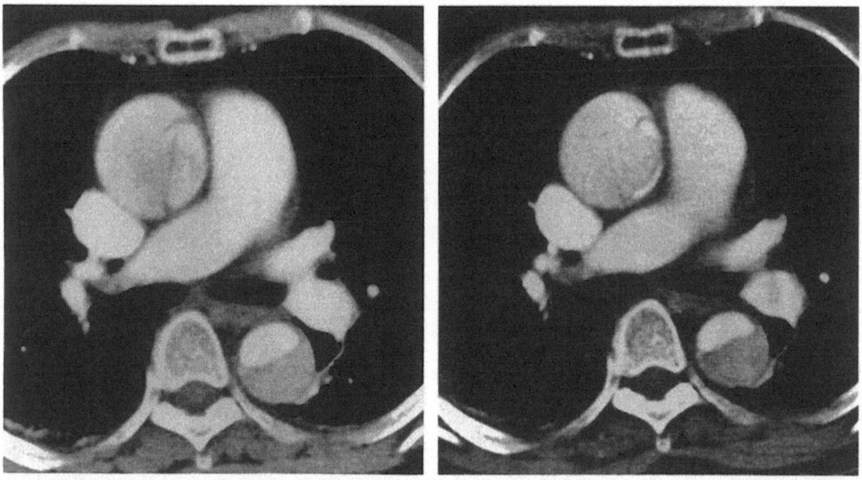

a b

Fig. 2 a, b. A middle-aged female patient with a type A dissection. Note the different appearances of the intimal flap during different phases of the cardiac cycle. **a** The intimal flap lies about one third of the way across the ascending aorta. **b** Now the intimal flap is almost compressed against the left lateral ascending aortic wall. Note also the change in shape of the intimal flap within the descending aorta

Subsequent Management

Much depends on the clinical situation, the policy of the referring clinician, the quality of the CT images and the confidence of the radiological report.

If the radiologist is entirely confident about the diagnosis of an ascending (Type A) aortic dissection, the patient will be urgently referred to a surgical unit without further imaging. Most patients with definite (Type B) descending aorta (dissections) will be treated by medical rather than surgical means. For those patients in whom the radiologist is entirely confident that the aorta is normal at CT, no further imaging should be performed unless the clinical case is very convincing.

It was considered of interest to audit the use of CT for aortic dissection on the Somatom Plus at Addenbrooke's Hospital, Cambridge.

Setting

Addenbrooke's Hospital is a large (800 bed) teaching Hospital attached to the University of Cambridge. It serves a local population of over 300000 people and receives referrals from further afield. During a 4-year period (1990–1993 inclusive), 54 patients were referred on account of possible acute aortic dissection. Eight patients (15%) were referred straight from the admitting room; 12 (22%) were referred directly from the coronary care unit having been initially admitted with suspected myocardial infarction.

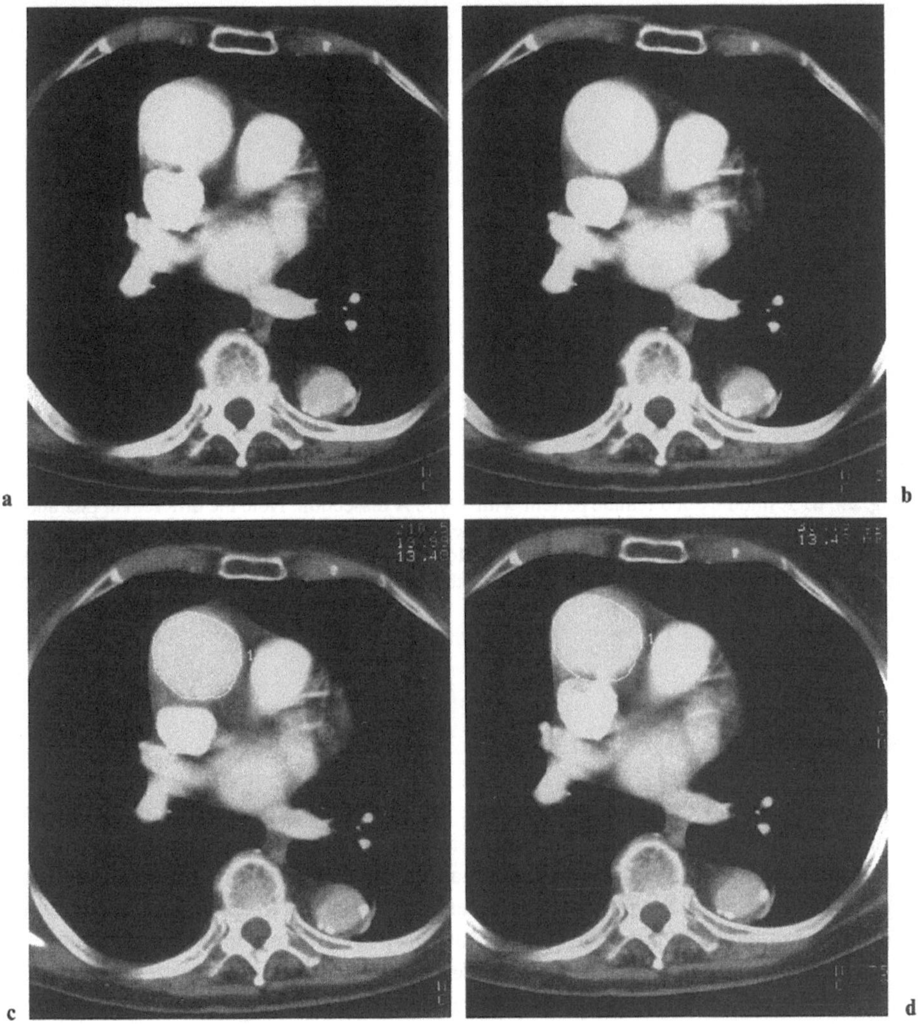

Fig. 3 a–d. Another manifestation of movement artefact in a patient without dissection. **a** There is a rind of poor enhancement on the left anterior aspect of the aorta which could possibly be due to an unenhanced false lumen. **b** However, this rind cannot be seen on an image reconstructed 200 ms earlier. **c** The aorta in **b** is outlined by a region of interest. **d** Superimposition of the region of interest on **a** shows that the aorta has moved within the xy plane and thus the poor "enhancement" can be accounted for by partial volume effect

Results

Of the 54 patients referred, CT demonstrated definite aortic dissection in 22 (type A: 12, Type B: 10). In two patients the CT report of the ascending aorta was equivocal and further imaging was advised. In one aortography confirmed dissection within the aortic root. In the other, both CT and TOE were equivocal about a subtle type A dissection in a very elderly patient.

a 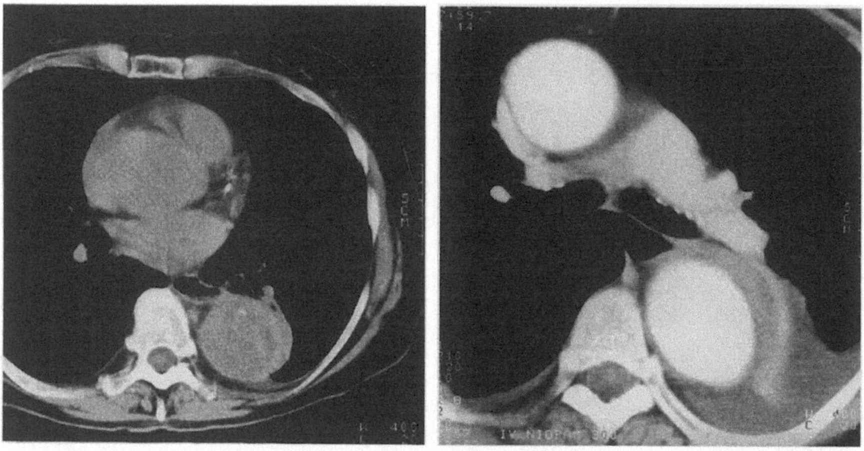 b

Fig. 4 a, b. A 68-year-old women with giant cell arthritis who experienced sudden chest pain. **a** Unenhanced image just above the aortic valve. Proximal aorta dilated; some calcification in L. A. D. coronary artery. Calcification internal to margin of ectatic descending aorta with high attenuation rind peripheral to the calcification indicating a dissecting haematoma. **b** Enhanced image at the level of the mid-ascending aorta showing a type B aortic dissection. Ascending aorta normal (as at other levels too). Descending aorta shows prompt opacification of the presumed true lumen; no opacification of false lumen. Some enhancement of adventitia/parietal pleura surrounded by pleural fluid. This patient was treated conservatively but experienced further chest pain. Echocardiography raised the possibility of a flap in the ascending aorta. Repeat CT and subsequent MR both showed a normal (although ectatic) ascending aorta. She remains well on conservative therapy

In those 52 patients with confident reports of the ascending aorta (positive for dissection: 12; negative: 42), no new features have emerged to suggest that the CT reports were erroneous and all of these type A dissections have either had surgical proof or radiological follow-up.

In the descending aorta there were 10 definite type B dissections (e.g. Fig. 4). In nine of the 12 type A dissections the flap extended into the descending aorta. In the remaining 35 patients, the descending aorta was confidently reported as normal in 28. In seven patients the descending aorta showed subtle CT abnormalities of uncertain cause and significance. However, in none of these patients did circumstances develop to suggest that the initial CT study had missed a frank type B dissection.

Problems

Motion Artefact

In the early days of CT, streak artefacts from beam hardening or motion were quickly recognised (Gallagher and Dixon 1985) although technical improvements helped to reduce them. However, the advent of 1s data acquisition times created a new type of motion artefact (Burns et al. 1991). This artefact tends to be maximal in the

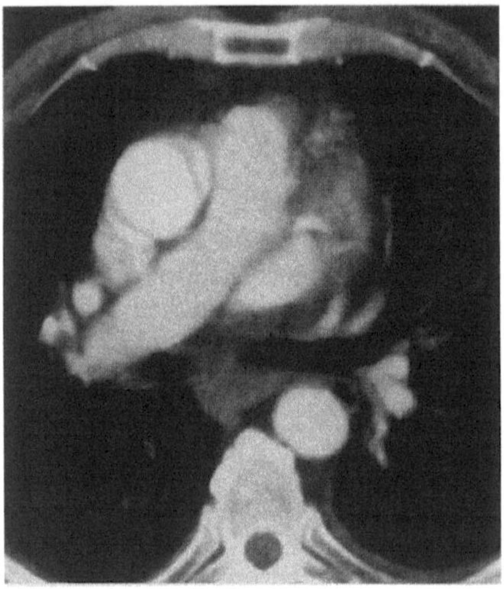

Fig. 5. Typical movement artefacts associated with 1s data acquisition in the healthy ascending aorta in this patient with lymphoma. Note the way that the artefacts are maximal on the left anterior and right posterior aspect of the aorta (at right angles to the plane of the aortic arch)

proximal ascending aorta and at lie at 90° to the plane of the aortic arch (Fig. 5). Some at the artefact is due to movement of the aorta within the thorax (translocation) and images reconstructed at 100 ms intervals can prove this (see Fig. 3). It also seems likely that relative expansion of the aorta during systole (compliance) may be a contributing factor. Indeed there is some evidence that these artefacts are more evident in those patients with healthy aortas, which have most compliance (Set et al. 1993).

Local Haematoma

The distinction between an acute dissection with no flow in the false lumen and a mural haematoma is one of semantics; indeed some now favour the term "dissecting haematoma" for all such lesions (Naidich and Crystal 1994). Exactly where the term "penetrating atherosclerotic ulcer" (Kazerooni et al. 1992) fits in, is less clear, but these lesions occur most commonly in the descending aorta. Mural thrombus is yet another pitfall in the distal aorta (it is relatively rare in the ascending aorta). All these pathological entities with little or no flow within the lesion create difficulty. CT, aortography and MRI may be inconclusive and, as there is no mobile flap, TOE may be unhelpful. At least unenhanced CT and MRI will provide some clues that the haematoma is acute rather than chronic.

References

1. Burns MA, Molina PL, Gutierrez FR, Sagel SS (1991) Motion artefact simulating aortic dissection on CT. AJR 155:465–467
2. Clague J, Magee P, Mills P (1992) Diagnostic techniques in suspected thoracic aortic dissection. Br Heart J 67:428–429

3. Gallagher S, Dixon AK (1984) Streak artefacts of the thoracic aorta: pseudodissection. J Comput Assist Tomogr 8 : 688 – 693
4. Hamada CT, Takamiya M, Kimura K, Imakita S, Nakajima N, Naito H (1992) Tye A aortic dissection: evaluation with ultrafast CT. Radiology 183 : 155
5. Heiberg E, Wolverson MK, Sundaram M, Shields JB (1985) CT characteristics of aortic atherosclerotic aneurysm versus dissection. J Comput Assist Tomogr 9 : 78 – 83
6. Kalendar WA, Seissler W, Klotz E, Vock P (1990) Spiral Volumetric CT with single-breath-hold technique. Radiology 176 : 864 – 867
7. Kazerooni EA, Bree RL, Williams DM (1992) Penetrating atherosclerotic ulcers of the descending thoracic aorta: evaluation with CT and distinction from aortic dissection. Radiology 183 : 759
8. Khandheria B (1992) Aortic dissection: the diagnostic dilemma resolved. Chest 101 : 303 – 304
9. Naidich JB, Crystal KS (1994) Diagnosis of dissecting haematoma of the aorta: a choice between good and better. Radiology 190 : 16 – 17
10. Nienaber CA, Spielman RP, von Kodolitsch Y et al. (1992) Diagnosis of thoracic aortic dissection: magnetic resonance imaging versus transesophageal echocardiography. Circulation 85 : 434 – 447
11. Petasnick JP (1991) Radiologic evaluation of aortic dissection. Radiology 180 : 297 – 305
12. Set PA, Lomas DJ, Maskell GF, Flower CDR, Dixon AK (1993) Artefacts in the ascending aorta on computed tomography: another measure of aortic distensibility? EJR 16 : 107 – 111
13. Thorsen MK, San Dretto MA, Lawson TL, Foley WD, Smith DF, Berland LL (1983) Dissecting aortic aneurysms: accuracy of computed tomographic diagnosis. Radiology 148 : 773 – 777

Digital spiral CT Angiography of the Aorta and Its Main Branches

M. Oldendorf, E. Zeitler, K. Maatsch, P. Weber

Computed tomographic angiography (CTA) is a new minimally invasive method for displaying vessels. Planar images are processed from the images of a spiral CT examination, delivering results comparable with an angiography.

The sofware we used for this purpose works according to the same principle used in magnetic resonance (MR) angiography. A multiplicity of possibilities of improved imaging, primarily in the abdominal region, are shown in the application in computed tomography. Angiograms with selective vascular display can be reconstructed from the existing CT images parallel to the CT image without additional catheterization.

A prerequisite for this is a spiral CT scan with contrast medium bolus application. Projections are produced in all three spatial axes from the images of the scan. These projections can in turn be rotated as desired about their axes. After previous subtraction of disturbing image data such as bones, etc., one obtains CT angiograms which are comparable with DSA images because of their two dimensional character.

In contrast to the previous customary 3D display, in which solely the surface condition of the organ or of the vessel could be seen, images revealing the pathological changed vascular lumen are obtained. Anneurysmatic widening or higher grade vascular stenoses can be displayed by this new technique.

The present paper shows by reference to 61 case the applicability of spiral CT angiography in the abdomen for the diagnosis of anatomical deviations from the norm, for preoperative planning in the case of pancreatic tumors, the display of abdominal aortic aneurysms and the acquisition and assessment of renal artery stenoses.

Material and Method

The examinations were performed on a Somatom Plus S. Sixty-one patients were examined, 23 with a tumor in the epigastric region, 24 patients with a renovascular hypertension and 14 patients with an infrarenal aortic aneurysm. The gold standard to check the results was in all cases the arterial angiography. To guarantee high spatial resolution, a slice thickness of 2 or 3 mm and a table feed of 3 – 6 mm/s were selected. In this way a vascular region up to 240 mm in size in the cranio-caudal direction can be acquired. Slice thicknesses of more than 3 mm proved to be unsuitable because of too intensive step formation in the image reconstruction.

The stored raw data enable overlapping image reconstruction: 1 mm slice overlap proves to be suitable. The number of transaxial slices is so kept within acceptable limits. The axial tomograms are now processed further with the maximum intensity projection (MIP) software by which the maximum CT values in one direction are displayed. Since bone structures would be superimposed on vessel details because of their high radiation absorption, these density values must be erased by editing the pictures.

If a selective display is wanted, the individual images can be changed in addition: subtraction of the aorta or erasing the renal profile for display of the vessels free of superimposition. Any venous structures that may be disturbing can also be erased easily in this way.

The angiograms are then reconstructed from this new image data. They can be reconstruced in all three spatial axes; up to 360 single projections can be displayed in each axis. The coronal image plane proves to be suitable, as it corresponds to the customary angiographic image. The axes should not be rotated beyond 90° in order to avoid errors in image interpretation, in particular confusion between sides. Image angles up to 45°, corresponding to the RAO or LAO projection in the angiogram, are suitable for displaying images free of superimpositions. Image displays in the other two spatial planes (x-axis, y-axis) are diagnostically of little use in the abdominal region.

Contrast was administered as bolus injection in two steps:

- First, 120 ml of contrast medium (Ultravist 300) at a flow rate of 4 ml/s.
- Second, 60 ml of NaCl solution also at a flow rate of 4 ml/s to push the contrast bolus towards the peripheral parts of the vessels by saving contrast medium. For that we used a special computer controlled automatic injector (Ulrich, Germany).

In all examinations the spiral scan was started 15 s after beginning of the injection of contrast medium.

It must be borne in mind additionally that slight spatial distortion occurs in all CT angiograms: the vessels appear to be somewhat extended in the cranio-caudal direction. This effect is visible primarily with large slice thickness and high table feed (Figs. 1–5).

Epigastrium

Patients with tentative diagnosis of pancreatic tumor or tumor in the region of the papilla or gall bladder always require a contrast CT scan to clarify suitabilty for surgery: If surgery is possible because of size and localisation, the surgeon requires for surgical planing for each of this patients a preoperative arteriography with display of the celic artery and the superior mesenteric artery. Detecting deviations from the norm, primarily atypical origins of the superior mesenteric artery and of the hepatic artery with their main branches are of decisive importance. In 5% of all patients, the right hepatic artery originates from the superior mesenteric artery.

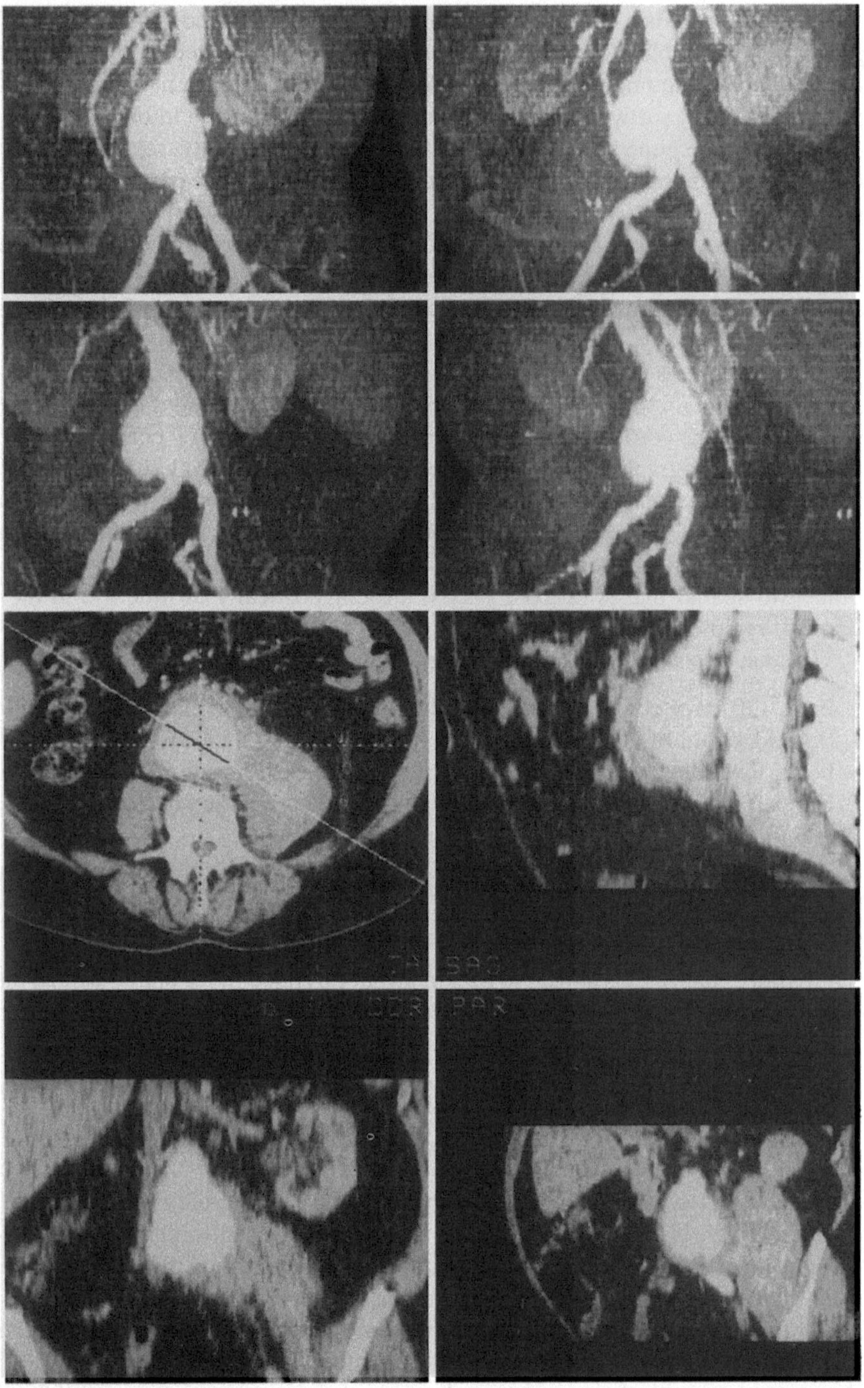

a

b

Fig. 1 a, b. Infrarenal aortic aneurysm in a 77-year-old patient. Thrombosed wall; no dissection; no renal artery involvement

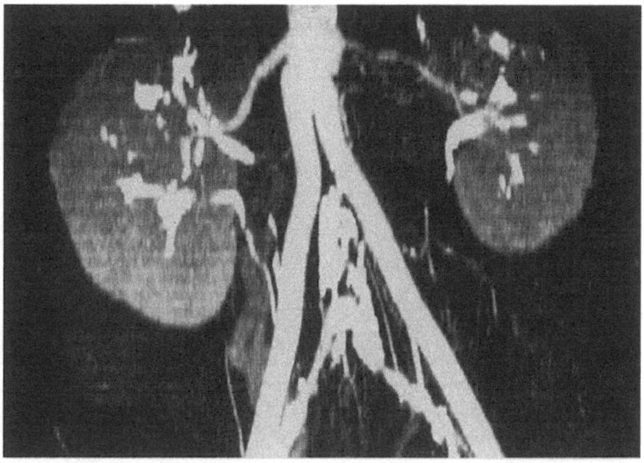

Fig. 2. Renal artery stenosis in small left kidney. Implantation of Y-prosthesis after occlusion of distal aorta in a 59-year-old woman

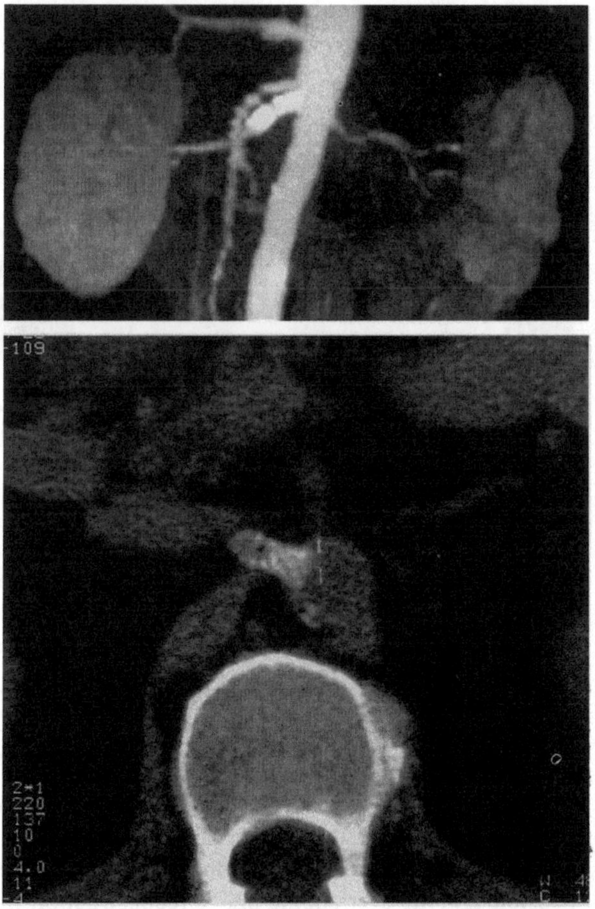

a

b

Fig. 3 a, b. Stent implantation right renal artery after percutaneous transluminal angioplasty for stenosis in known diabetic nephropatia in left kidney of a 46-year-old woman

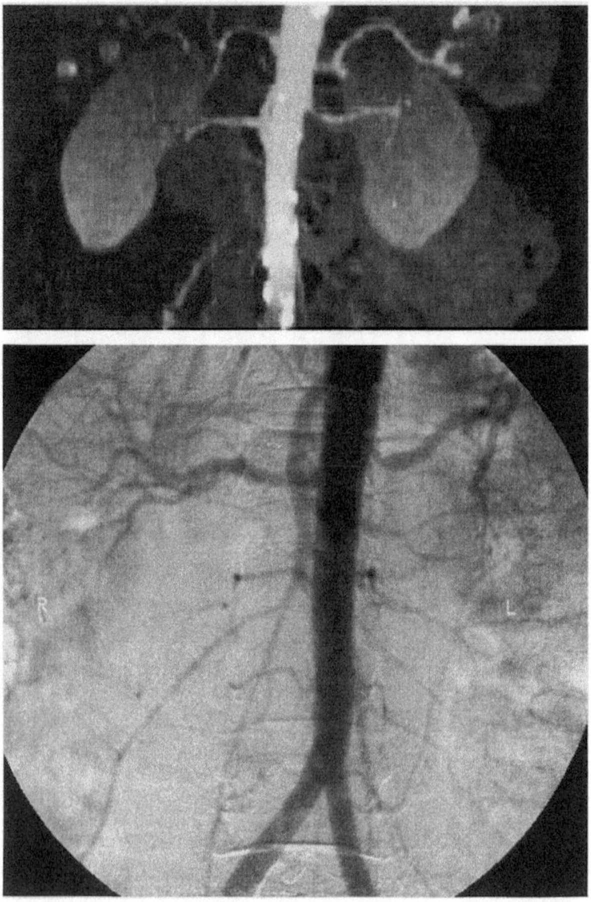

a

b

Fig. 4 a, b. Renal artery stenosis left side. Hemodynamically effective and no vascular calcification. Successful percutaneous transluminal angioplasty in a 65-year-old man

The second piece of information contains the display of the portal vein system in the region of the tumor. If there is an occlusion of the large venous system, surgery is not possible.

We used the following examination parameters to answer these questions:

- Precontrast scan: 10-mm slice thickness, 10-mm table feed
- Spiral scan: 2-mm slice thickness, 4-mm table feed, 32-s scan time and 10-mm slice thickness and table feed after that up to the end of the abdomen.

To achieve display of the vessels free of superimposition, we used water as oral contrast medium: 500–1000 ml distributed over 30 min. This provides sufficient contrasting of the stomach and duodenum. The slice thickness was kept as low as possible and the overlapping image reconstruction was held at 1 mm.

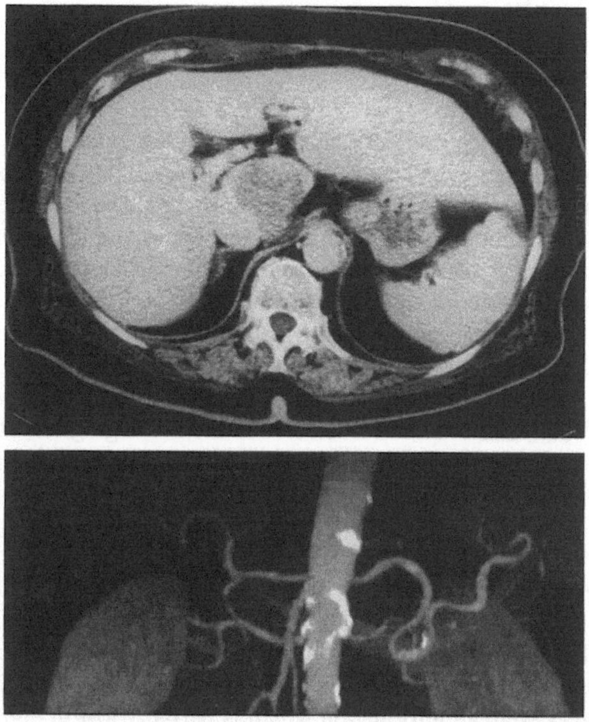

a

b

Fig. 5 a, b. Solitary metastasis of a colonic carcinoma in the right lobe of the liver. No anatomic abnormalities

Aortic Aneurysms

In the clinical diagnosis of an aortic aneurysm, CT with contrast medium is always performed to confirm the finding. Thrombi, calcifications and dissections and the cranio-caudal extend including the renal vessels and aortic bifurcation must be visualized. We selected the following examination parameters: Spiral scan, 3-mm slice thickness, 6-mm table feed and 32-s scan time.

Renovascular Hypertension

In the case of renal artery stenoses, vascular calcifications are of great clinical importance. They decide on the therapeutic procedure, vascular calcifications usually necessitating surgery, while in other cases, percutaneous transluminal dilatation (PTA) is possible. For our patients we selected as examination parameters: Spiral scan, 3-mm slice thickness, 5-mm table feed and 32-s scan time.

Results

Epigastrium

CT of the epigastric organs showed in the axial single images the accurate tumor localisation with size and relation to the neighbouring organs in all cases. Vascular anatomy and deviations from the norm could be identified in 22 of 23 patients clearly from the angiograms in the celiac artery and the superior mesenteric artery. I All larger vessels up to the arteries of the segment of the liver could be displayed, smaller arteries could not be identified.

In one patient the identification was not possible because of heavy respiration artifacts – he was in a very poor health.

Portal vein occlusion can be detected in the axial tomogram. Portocaval collateral circulations can be detected in the CT angiogram as faint contrast. Intrahepatic vascular processes, in particular cavernous haemangiomas, are delineated poorly in the CT angiogram.

Aortic Aneurysms

The CT angiograms showed the remaining blood supplied lumen of the aneurysm in the angiographic image in all 14 patients. All wall calcifications could be detected very well,. an information which is partially lost in digital subtraction angiography (DSA). The axial images provide information as customary on thrombus size, size of the remaining lumen and dissection or perforation. However, in cases of high seated aneurysms, involvement of the renal arteries could not be clarified sufficiently in two patients and arteriography was necessary.

Renovascular Hypertension

High-grade stenoses of the renal vessels can be acquired well. It is ot possible to determine the degree: three patients showed in the CT angiography an occlusion, the arteriography revealed a high graded stenosis. Any vascular calcifications could always be diagnosed very well.

Summary

Spiral CT angiography is a less invasive method for the detection and documentation of vascular anomalies in the epigastrium. It permits clear diagnosis of atypical vascular paths of the celic artery and the superior mesenteric artery. It is well accepted by surgeons and is in these cases comparable with angiography for properative planning. Collateral circulations in the protal vein region do not achieve the quality of indirect splenoportography.

Infrarenal abdominal aortic aneurysms are diagnosed completely with CT angiography in a single examination. An additional arteriography should always be performed if there is suspicion of involvement of the renal arteries.

Renal arterial stenoses can be diagnosed reliably in CT angiography but it is not possible to distinguish between high-grade stenoses and vascular occlusion. No statement can be made on haemodynamic effectiveness. Vascular calcifications can be acquired well -important for the therapeutic concept: surgery or PTA.

The advantages compared with other non invasive vascular examinations as MR angiography can be summarized as follows:

- Short examination time
- No respiratory artifacts
- High information density with one spiral scan
- Display of vessels in all three spatial axes
- Elimination of overlapping neighbouring organs and veins
- High spatial resolution
- Image display independent of blood flow velocity

The radiation exposure and the need for a contrast medium containing iodine with the possibilty of intolerance can be named as disadvantages.

References

Bautz W, Strotzer M, Lenz M, Dittler HJ, Kalender WA (1991) Preoperative Evaluation of the Vessels of the Upper Abdomen with Spiral CT: Comparison with conventional CT and Arterial DSA. Radiology 188 (P): 261

Kalender WA, Seissler W, Klotz E, Vock P (1990) Spiral Volumetric CT with single Breath-Hold Technique, Cotinuous Transport and Continuous Scanner Rotation. Radiology 176 : 181–183

Rubin GD, Dake MD, Napel SA, et al. (1993) Three-dimensional Spiral CT Angiography of the Abdomen: Initial Clinical Experience. Radiology 186 : 147–152

Napel SA, Marks MP, et al. (1992) CT Angiography with Spiral CT and Maximum Intensity Projection. Radiology 185 : 607–610

CT Angiography with Maximum Intensity Projection in the Assessment of Pelvic Arterial Disease

F. J. FERSTL, P. UHRMEISTER, P. FLÜGEL, U. BLUM, A. BARKE, G. LANDES, M. LANGER

Introduction

Stenosis or occlusion of iliac arteries are primarily investigated by noninvasive methods like doppler ultrasound and duplex sonography followed by diagnostic angiography with interventional procedures. The aim of this ongoing study is to determine whether computed tomographic (CT) angiography with maximum intensity projection can demonstrate pelvic arterial disease before and after interventional procedures and, in case of stent implantation, the patency and position of the stent in comparison with digital subtraction angiography (DSA).

Material and Method

Fifteen patients with clinically sonographically suspected pelvic arterial disease underwent spiral CT of the pelvis. Data were acquired with a Somatom Plus S CT scanner (Siemens, Erlangen). The following scan parameters were used: 120 KV, 210 mA, 5-mm slice thickness and table feed for a total of 40 s scanning time. Some 120 ml nonionic contrast material was administered by a power injector at a flow rate of 4 ml/s. Images were obtained after a 20-s start delay. Spiral CT scanning began 2 cm above the aortic bifurcation, resulting in a 19-cm length of the scan volume.

The data were reconstructed at 4-mm intervals with a 360° linear interpolation algorithm.

Maximum intensity projection (MIP) images were generated in two steps:

1. Elimination of bony and other interfering contrast filled structures (e.g. ureters) by using a specialized prototype 3D edit programme of the CT scanner.
2. Reconstruction of MIP images from these edited CT sections by applying a prototype MIP programme.

Thirty images were reconstructed for each patient about the z-axis at 4° intervals with a 512 × 512 matrix. Additional MIP images were performed about the x- and y-axis. The cine mode was used for demonstration of three dimensional vascular anatomy.

Results

On pre-interventional angiography obstructions of the iliac arteries were found in seven patients. The common iliac artery was occluded in four patients, the external iliac artery in one patient, and both common and external iliac arteries on one side were occluded in two patients.

High grade stenoses of the common iliac artery ($n = 6$) and the external iliac artery ($n = 4$) were diagnosed in ten patients (Table 1).

In each case, MIP images were of diagnostic quality compared to DSA. All stenoses and occlusions were detected and localized on MIP images (Fig. 1).

The grading of stenoses with MIP corresponded to DSA in 12 patients. The severity of the stenoses was underestimated on MIP in two patients and overestimated in one patient, primarily due to extensive wall calcifications.

The quality of MIP images was closely related to contrast filling of pelvic arteries and the degree of mural wall calcifications. In those three patients with falsely estimated stenoses the reduced diagnostic quality of the MIP images was due to decreased vessel enhancement because of dilating arteriopathy with reduced arterial flow velocity and extensive calcifications which prevented accurate assessment of the perfused residual vessel lumen.

The MIP images after interventional procedures correctly localized the position of the stents implanted in all 11 patients compared to angiography.

The evaluation of the stent patency on MIP was merely dependent on the type of stent implanted. While Palmaz stents produced streak artefacts resulting in marked blurring, MIP images after implantation of wallstents allowed reliable assessment of the stent patency (Table 2). MIP images about the x-axis are less affected by blurring

Table 1. Differentiation of severity of iliac artery stenosis by DSA and MIP

Method	Degree of arterial stenosis			
	<50%	50%–75%	75%–99%	Occlusion
DSA	–	1	9	7
MIP	–	2	8	7

DSA, digital subtraction angiography; MIP, maximum intensity projection

Table 2. Identification and patency of stents[a]

Method	Located (*n*)	Patency
DSA	11	11
MIP	11	4[a]

[a] Stents implanted ($n = 11$): four Wallstents*, seven Palmaz stents
DSA, digital subtraction angiography; MIP, maximum intensity projection

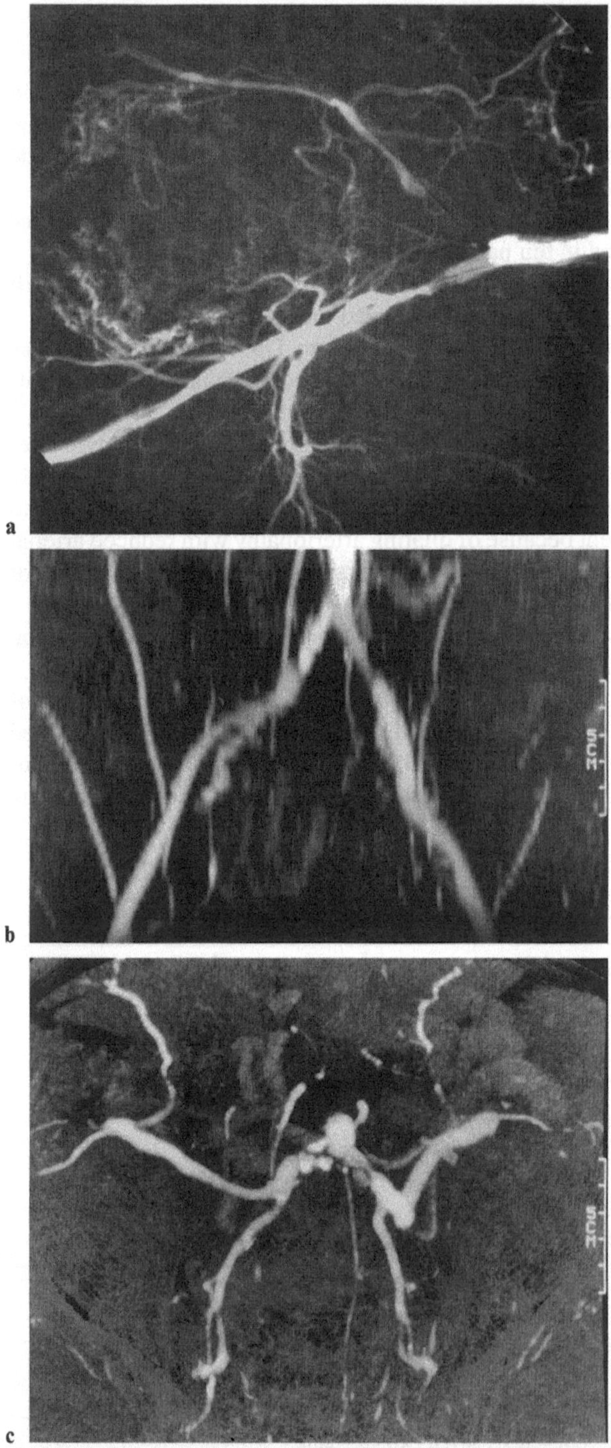
a
b
5CM
c
5CM

and have, therefore, proven to be superior to MIP images about the z-axis for visualization of stent patency.

Conclusions

1. MIP seems to be a promising method for diagnostic assessment of pelvic arterial disease and can probably generate additional information for routine pelvic CT examinations for different reasons.
2. The value of MIP is closely related to vascular enhancement and the amount of vessel wall calcification which can overlay the luminal contrast medium and interfere with the grading of stenoses.
3. As partial volume effects lead to vessel blurring, particularly on MIP images about the z-axis, multiple MIP's must be produced about the z- and x-axis to depict both vessel stenosis and stent patency.
4. The accurate evaluation of the vessel lumen after stent implantation depends on the type of stent used which causes streak artefacts of various severity. Reliable control of stent patency can be best accomplished by MIP images about the x- and y-axis.

Fig. 1 a–c. Arterial digital subtraction angiography (DSA) and maximum intensity projection (MIP) images about z- and x-axis in a patient with occlusion of the right common iliac artery and stenosis of the left common iliac artery. **a** Diagnostic angiogram shows occlusion of the right common iliac artery and concentric, high grade stenosis of the left common iliac artery. **b** MIP image about z-axis shows marked mural calcifications in the region of the occluded right common iliac artery which prevent reliable grading of vessel stenosis. The demonstration of the concentric stenosis of the left common iliac artery is approximately equal to DSA. **c** MIP image about x-axis reveals occlusion of the right common iliac artery, whereas the length of the occluded vessel segment seems to be shorter on MIP compared to DSA. Clear depiction of concentric, high grade stenosis of left common iliac artery

CT Angiographie II

Chairmen: M. Heller, J. Lammer

CT Angiography of the Pelvic Arteries

C. S. Richter, K. Maatsch, G. Biamino, C. Ragg, R. Felix

Introduction

Besides invasive methods such as digital subtraction angiography (DSA) non-invasive methods as color Doppler sonography and magnetic resonance angiography are able to depict pelvic artery stenosis. Spiral computed tomographic (CT) angiography [1–7] represents a further minimally invasive angiographic method which has recently been developed on the basis of digital, reconstructed, sectional imaging techniques. The goal of this study was to compare the value of CT angiography with angiography in the DSA technique for examining the distal aorta and pelvic arteries.

Patients and Method

We used a SOMATOM PLUS S CT (Siemens) system. Technical parameters: spiral CT [2], intravenous injection of 150 ml of non-ionic contrast medium (Ultravist 370), flow rate 3 ml/s, interval between the start of the injection and the initial radiation exposure 25 s, voltage 120 kV, current 210 mA, slice thickness 5 mm, table feed 8 mm/s, time of investigation 30 s, increment of reconstruction 3 mm, "slim profile" algorithm, reconstruction of threedimensional images with maximum intensity projection (MIP) [4] and 3-D display technique [6].

Patients

In all 55 patients were studied (47 men and 8 women; 42–85 years of age, mean 62): 30 patients prior to intravascular intervention, 18 patients after interventional therapy or surgery, seven patients without relevant pelvic artery stenoses were considered as control group. An angiography in DSA technique was available from each of the patients for comparison.

Results

Patients with Stenoses or Occlusions of the Pelvic Arteries

MIP

Common Iliac Artery. Twelve of 16 occlusions were evaluated correctly as occlusions using the MIP method, although they were evaluated as being shorter than in the DSA images (Fig. 1 a, b). Four of the occlusions were underestimated by MIP. In comparison to DSA, 14 of 16 stenoses were evaluated correctly. The other two stenoses were slightly underevaluated by MIP.

External Iliac Artery. Eight of the 10 occlusions were evaluated correctly as occlusions and 2 were underevaluated as stenoses. Regarding the stenoses, the results of the evaluation were comparable with MIP and DSA in 7 of the 13 cases, three stenoses were underevaluated and three were overevaluated with MIP.

The MIP technique was the only procedure which could provide an excellent display of calcifications of the vascular walls (Figs. 2, 3 a). Non-calcified plaques could be differenciated from thrombi (Figs. 2, 3 a).

Whereas all stenoses and occlusions consisting of thrombotic plaques were correctly assessed, stenoses and occlusions with massive calcification throughout the vessel wall were underevaluated on MIP images.

a 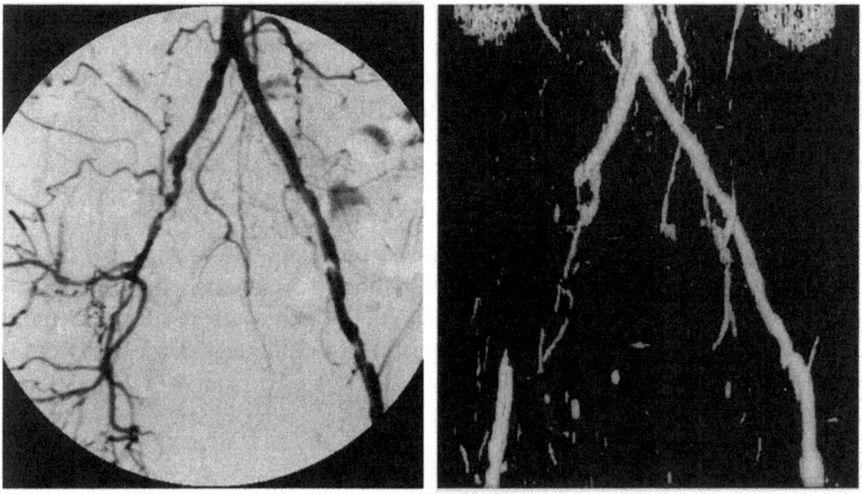 b

Fig. 1 a. A 53-year-old man with occlusion of the right iliac artery. The digital subtraction angiography (DSA) image demonstrates a long occlusion but does not show the artery distal the obstruction

Fig. 1 b. 3D-display of the iliac arteries in the same patient as shown in **a**. The computed tomographic angiography visualizes a shorter occlusion as the DSA image. The patient was succesfully treated by interventional therapy (balloon dilatation)

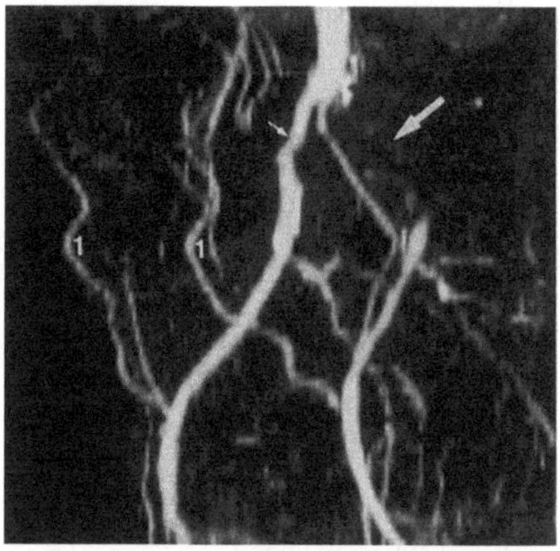

Fig. 2. A 43-year-old male patient with occlusion of the left common iliac artery (*arrow*). Maximum intensity projection display, left anterior view. No calcification is seen in the region of the occlusion. There is a slight to moderate stenosis of the right common iliac artery (*small arrow*). The inferior epigastric arteries (*1*) as sign of collateral circulation are easily recognisable an both sides

Three-Dimensional Display

Common Iliac Artery. Eleven of the 16 occlusions were diagnosed correctly with the three-dimensional (3-D) display technique. Three of the remaining occlusions were incorrectly identified as short stenoses and the other two were incorrectly identified as normal vessels. Eight of the 16 stenoses were evaluated correctly and 6 were underevaluated. A stenosis in one patient was not recognized.

External Iliac Artery. Eight of ten occlusions were diagnosed correctly and two were interpreted incorrectly as being stenoses. Nine of the 13 stenoses were evaluated correctly, two were underevaluated and two were overevaluated.

As shown by MIP all non calcified stenoses and occlusions could be correctly assessed on 3-D images. Calcified stenosis was present in all cases of underevaluation or false negative findings. While massive calcification caused underevaluation of stenoses on MIP images slight calcification of the vessel wall could already mask the stenoses on 3-D images. No relationship to the calcification of a vascular process was found in the overevaluated stenoses.

Both MIP and the 3-D display techniques were able to provide an image of the collateral arteries in 5 patients with stenoses of the pelvic arteries. These collaterals were the inferior epigastric arteries (Fig. 2) and the deep iliac circumflex arteries.

Patients Following Intervention

All stenoses and occlusions being identified as non calcified and thrombotic on MIP images could be treated successfully by laser assisted angioplasty and/or stent implantation. In two patients with calcified stenoses a slight residual stenosis

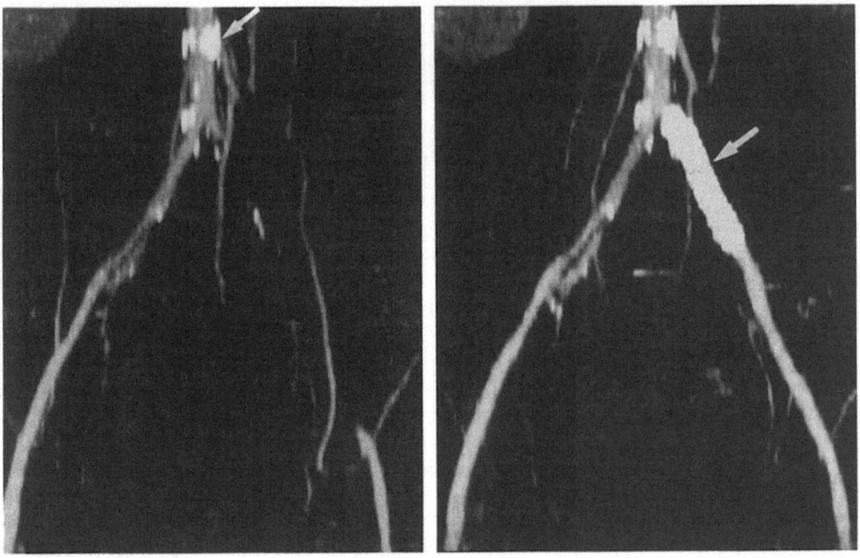
a b

Fig. 3 a. A 53-year-old male patient with occlusion of the left common and external iliac artery before undergoing interventional therapy. Maximum intensity projection (MIP) display demonstrates a "soft" occlusion. Calcified plaques in the distal aorta and right iliac artery (*arrow*)

Fig. 3 b. MIP display of the iliac arteries in the same patient as in **a** after implantation of an intervascular stent (Strecker). The position of the stent (*arrow*) is clearly recognisable

remained after intervention. In all cases STRECKER intravascular stents were recognized accurately by MIP (Fig. 3 b) In contrast, none of these stents was detected using the 3-D display technique. Whereas the CT angiography in seven cases was performed only a few days after implantation of the stent, one patient was examined 9 months after stent implantation and was correctly diagnosed as having a renewed stenosis of the distal external iliac artery with both MIP and the 3-D display technique.

Both aortobifemoral bypasses were displayed and evaluated as being patent with the MIP and DSA techniques as well as with the 3-D display technique. MIP images could show that there was no calcification of the implant.

Patients Without Stenotic or Occlusive Vascular Processes

Stenoses or occlusions of the pelvic arteries could be excluded in seven cases. In five of seven patients MIP reconstructions revealed an initial vascular calcification without affecting the caliber of the vessel.

Discussion

The MIP method [4] displays the voxel of the maximal density value seen in every projectional plane. Since calcifications are more CT dense than contrast medium, they can even be seen in vessels filled with contrast medium. Thus MIP provides valuable information about the nature of the stenosis, information which may be decisive in selecting the proper therapeutic procedure. However, assessment of the degree of stenosis on MIP images, could not always be performed reliably. Severe calcified stenoses were underevaluated by MIP. The contrast medium column was superimposed by massive calcification of the vessel walls, making a correct assessment of the stenosis impossible.

Controlling the position of intravascular stents is, in our opinion, a further practical site of application for MIP. Since stronger radiation absorption is seen by contrast medium than by the stents, stents are often impossible to display with DSA. As with calcifications, the higher CT density of metal stents in comparison to that of contrast medium seen in MIP reconstructions permits an accurate determination of their position (Fig. 3 b).

Through the selection of a threshold value, the contrast medium column in vessels as well as the vessel calcifications viewed with the 3-D display technique depict images which are equivalent. In contrast to imaging with MIP, a differentiation of contrast medium and calcification with this method is impossible. This explains the relatively high underevaluation errors seen in calcified vascular processes when using the 3-D method. On the other hand, the 3-D method proved to be effective in the evaluation of stenoses which were not calcified (Fig. 3 a). The thrombotic material in these stenoses had substantially lower density values than the threshold value used and no erroneous assessments occurred.

In patients with vascular stents, the high CT density values of the stents, like those of the contrast medium, are above those of the selected threshold value so that no differentiation of the stents from the contrast medium-filled vascular lumen was possible.

Primarily two factors are responsible for the fact that occlusions seen with 3-D reconstruction methods (MIP and 3-D display techniques) are frequently shorter than those visualized with DSA (Fig. 1 a, b) and that the stenoses are underevaluated. First of all, the duration of passage of the contrast medium bolus differs in the two methods. The contrast medium bolus in the CT angiography is injected intravenously with a delay of 25 s. After these 25 s, the CT examination is performed for a period of 32 s so that a period of nearly one minute is assessed. Therefore, the contrast medium passage is followed for a substantially longer period of time than with the DSA where the scan duration lasts only a few seconds. We were able to conclude that this temporal delay enabled the display of collateral arteries which could not be fulfilled with the DSA scanning series (Fig. 2).

As a second factor, the mode of contrast medium application (intravenous for the CT and intra-arterial for the DSA) certainly plays a decisive role in the tendency to underevaluate stenoses and occlusions with the 3-D CT reconstructions. Intra-arterial contrast medium administration, as used in DSA, causes the contrast medium to be pressed through the stenosis with a higher velocity. This pressure stream does not immediately follow the vessel walls distal to the stenosis, but continues to travel in the middle of the vessel lumen for a certain distance. It is feasible that this could be a reason for the evident overevaluation of stenoses with DSA. Because of the different mode of contrast medium application, the intravenous contrast medium in the CT does not result in a rapidly moving pressure stream but rather in a slower contrast medium passage. For this reason, certain limitations are seen in the use of DSA as a reference method for stenoses and occlusions.

According to our current experience, the clinical value of the MIP method is clearly superior to that of the 3-D display technique. This value is based on information attained concerning the nature of the stenosis and the subsequent selection of an interventional procedure. The MIP method can therefore be seen as a valuable supplement to DSA, both prior to the interventions as well as in post-interventional follow-up.

References

1. Eikelboom BC, Mali WPThM (1993) Changing perspectives in vascular diagnosis and surgery. Medica Mundi 37:115–123
2. Kalender WA, Vock P, Polacin A, Coucek M (1990) Spiral-CT: Eine Technik für Volumenaufnahmen. I. Grundlagen und Methodik. Röntgenpraxis 43:323–330
3. Lenz M, Gmeinweiser J, Wunderlich A, Bautz W, Kersting-Sommerhoff B, Gerhardt P (1992) Three-dimensional imaging of thoracic and abdominal organs and vessels from spiral CT data sets. In: Felix R, Langer M, ed. Advances in CT II. 2nd European Scientific User Conference Somatom Plus. Berlin: Springer: 163–172
4. Napel S, Marks MP, Rubin GD, Dake MD, McDonnell CH, Song SM, Enzmann DR, Jeffrey RB Jr (1992) CT angiography with spiral CT and maximum intensity projection. Radiology 185:607–610
5. Rubin GD, Dake MD, Napel SA, McDonnell CH, Jeffrey RB (1993) Three dimensional spiral CT angiography of the abdomen: initial clinical experience. Radiology 186:147–152
6. Strunk H, Schweden F, Schild H, Thelen M (1993) Spiral-CT mit dreidimensionaler (3D) Oberflächendarstellung zur Beurteilung solitärer Lungenherde. Fortschr. Röngenstr. 158:26–30
7. Wunderlich AP, Lenz M, Gerhardt P, Helmberger H, Groß M (1993) 3D Rekonstruktionen aus CT-Datensätzen. Röntgenpraxis 46:57–65

CT Angiography of the Renal Arteries

M. Galanski, M. Prokop, A. Chavan, C. Schaefer-Prokop

Introduction

Renal arterial stenoses are clinically important due to two reasons. Firstly, they may cause arterial hypertension which can be cured by successful renal angioplasty and secondly, they may progress to complete arterial occlusion with resultant renal insufficiency. When the primary diagnostic tests strongly suggest renal arterial stenosis or when a strong clinical suspicion exists despite inconclusive or negative preliminary examinations, a suitable diagnostic modality becomes necessary to confirm the diagnosis. Arterial angiography is still considered the gold standard for definitive diagnosis although color doppler sonography, magnetic resonance (MR) angiography and of late computed tomographic angiography (CTA) as invasive or semi-invasive investigations have gained considerably in significance as competitive modalities to angiography (Prokop et al. 1993).

The purpose of the study was to establish the role of CTA in the diagnosis of renal arterial stenosis.

Materials and Methods

CTA followed by i.a. digital subtraction angiography (DSA) was carried out in 52 patients with suspected renovascular hypertension. Of the patients, 34 were male and 18 female between the ages of 20 and 72 years (mean age 52 years). Findings in CTA and angiography were compared.

Examination Technique

The CT examinations were carried out on a Somatom Plus S (SIEMENS/Erlangen). Plain sections were first taken through the upper abdomen for localization of the upper limit of the scan volume at the level of the origin of the superior mesenteric artery. A test bolus of 15 ml contrast medium was injected intravenously and a dynamic series of scans was carried out at the level of the kidneys in order to determine the transit time of the contrast medium from the site of injection of the abdominal aorta. In order to scan the renal arteries in the plateau phase of opacification, 2 – 5 s were added to the transit time and this time was taken as the start delay for the subsequent spiral scan. Contrast medium was injected with an automatic injector at a rate of 3–5 ml/s. Depending upon the scan length and the patient constitution, the total contrast medium volume varied between 100 and 150 ml (Ultravist 300 Schering/Berlin). Slice thickness, table translation (2 or 3 mm) and the scan time were tailored to suit the individual patients. If on the basis of the plain scan multiple arterial supply was suspected, maximum scan time and thus the maximum scan length were used. The reconstruction interval at the level of the renal arteries was 1 mm and at other levels 2 mm.

Angiographies were performed in DSA technique via a transfemoral access using 5-F catheter material. Aortic flush angiography and selective catheterization of the renal arteries was performed. In patients with significant stenosis, PTA was attempted in the same session.

Image Evaluation

Evaluation of angiograms and CTA was performed independently. Both examinations were assessed with respect to vascular anatomy (single or multiple renal arteries), grading of stenosis (grade 0 = no stenosis, grade I = mild stenosis < 50%, grade II = 50–75% stenosis, grade III = > 75% stenosis, grade IV = occlusion), localization of stenosis (proximal/intermediate/distal segment) and kind of stenosis (arteriosclerosis, fibromuscular dyplasia). Pathology of the vessel wall (calcification, thrombotic plaques) was also noted. Analysis of CTA always included all display modes, i.e. axial sections, multiplanar reformats, 3D surface shaded displays and maximum intensity projections (MIP). Goal of this extensive use of display modes was to find an optimized protocol for evaluation of renal artery stenosis with CTA.

Results

All CTA examinations were diagnostic. Of 52 patients studied, 15 had multiple renal arteries and two had a single artery after renal transplantation. In all, 124 renal arteries were included in the evaluation.

All accessory or multiple arteries were correctly diagnosed with CTA.

In 42 of the 52 patients, a renal artery stenosis could be proven angiographically, with involvement of 76 of 124 renal arteries. In 23 of the 76 arteries, a grade I stenosis was seen, in 11 arteries a grade II stenosis and in 36 arteries a grade II stenosis was found. Six arteries were completely occluded. In 72 of 76 vessels, the stenosis was localized close to the ostium or in the proximal segment. In addition, two cases with fibromuscular dysplasia, one anastomotic stenosis after transplantation and one stenosis at the site of an arterial bifurcation were detected.

With the exception of four cases, all 76 stenoses or occlusions were detected with CTA and localized correctly. The CTA grading was identical to that from DSA in 104 of 124 arteries. Differences ccurred in 20 cases, with 10 over- and 10 underestimations of the stenoses by one grade. Four normal renal arteries were diagnosed as grade I stenosis, 6 grade I stenoses were classified as grade II. Four grade I stenoses were diagnosed as normal, 4 grade III stenoses were classified as grade II, and 2 occlusions were seen as grade III stenoses.

Sensitivity of CTA was 95% with respect to the differentiation between normal and stenosed vessels. With respect to the differentiation between hemodynamically significant stenoses (grade II–IV) that require angioplasty and those that do not (grade 0–I), the sensitivity was 100% in our patient group. The specificity in both situations was 92%. The positive predictive value, i.e. the probability with which a positive result actually corresponded to a stenosis requiring PTA, was 85%. The negative predictive value, i.e. the probability with which a negative result really corresponded to a not hemodynamically relevant stenosis was 100% in our group. Thus, no patient was excluded from a possibly curative therapy (angioplasty) when CTA was applied for screening.

Discussion

Renovascular disease accounts for less than 5% of arterial hypertension. As only those patients can undergo potentially curative therapy, diagnosis or exclusion of a hemodynamically significant stenosis (>50%) is necessary. Due to the low prevalence of renal artery stenosis in patients with hypertension, diagnostic screening procedures are important. Angiography as the most sensitive diagnostic procedure is not suited for screening because of its invasiveness, effort and expense. On the other hand, there was so far no screening procedure with sufficiently high sensitivity *and* specificity. High sensitivity is necessary to assign all patients with a hemodynamically significant stenosis to a curative therapy. A sufficiently high specificity is necessary to reduce the number of invasive diagnostic procedures based on false positive screening results. For these reasons a careful pre-selection of patients is important to improve the positive predictive value of a screening procedure by increasing the prevalence of disease in the screened patient group (Davidson and Wilcox 1992). A careful clinical examination appears to fulfil this requirement. Based on this selection it is the task of the consecutively performed imaging methods to find the final diagnosis. Objective of our study was to evaluate the value of CTA as a diagnostic tool for hemodynamically significant renal artery stenosis.

Given an adequate examination technique, CTA of the renal arteries was found to be highly suited for diagnosis, localization and quantification of renal artery stenosis. The examination parameters that were most important for a good image quality were a slice thickness of 2–3 mm (in adipose patients image noise could be reduced by using the larger slice thickness), a small reconstruction interval of 1 mm, a high vascular enhancement and an optimum timing of contrast application and spiral scan.

In our experience, a sufficiently high vascular enhancement can be reached by injecting 100–150 ml contrast medium with a flow of 3–5 ml/s into a cubital vein using a power injector. The higher flow should be used in young patients and in patients with high cardial output to reduce dilution effects. An exact timing of contrast application and delay time is necessary for three reasons: (1) to achieve a

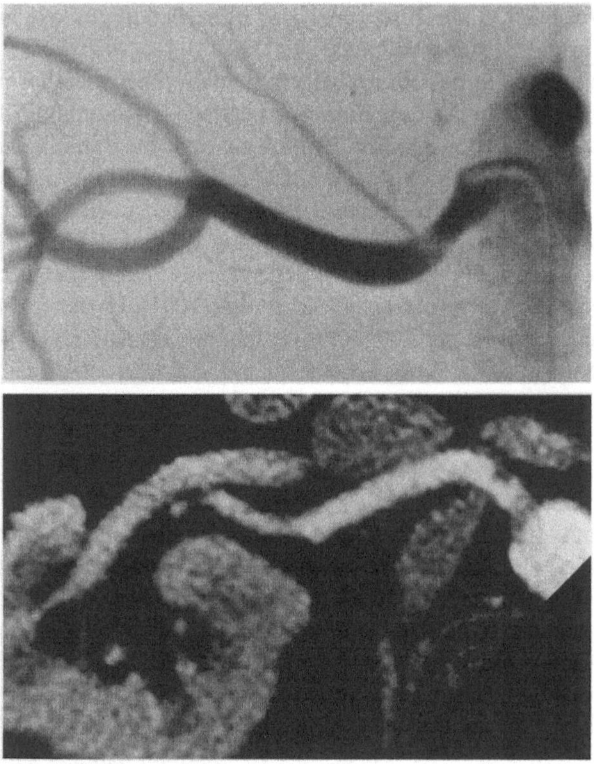

a

b

Fig. 1a, b. Patient with a circumscribed stenosis due to a plaque at the anterior wall of the right renal artery. This subtle finding on digital subtraction angiography (**a**) is well visualized on the axial spiral computed tomographic image (**b**)

sufficiently long and constant enhancement in the perirenal aortic segment, (2) to minimize superposition by the renal veins and (3) to keep the volume of contrast as small as possible.

Evaluation of CTA scans usually starts with the axial sections. They are used to determine the presence of single or multiple renal arteries. Interactive viewing of axial images in the "cine mode" is most helpful since renal arteries often have an undulating course and may frequently cross the scan plane especially in their distal segment. It is mandatory to view the renal arteries in a second plane in order not to miss a craniocaudal stenosis. Interactive multiplanar reformats were best suited for this purpose. Together, axial images and multiplanar reformats provide the full diagnostic information and are sufficient for evaluation of the renal arteries in almost all cases (Fig. 1).

MIPs produce angiographic images from various viewing angles and thus provide a god visualization of the anatomic situation (Fig. 2). Osseous structures that have higher CT numbers than surrounding tissues have to be removed prior to reconstruction using the VRT edit software option on the Somatom Plus. An advantage of MIP images is that contrast-enhanced vessels and calcified wall plaques can be dif-

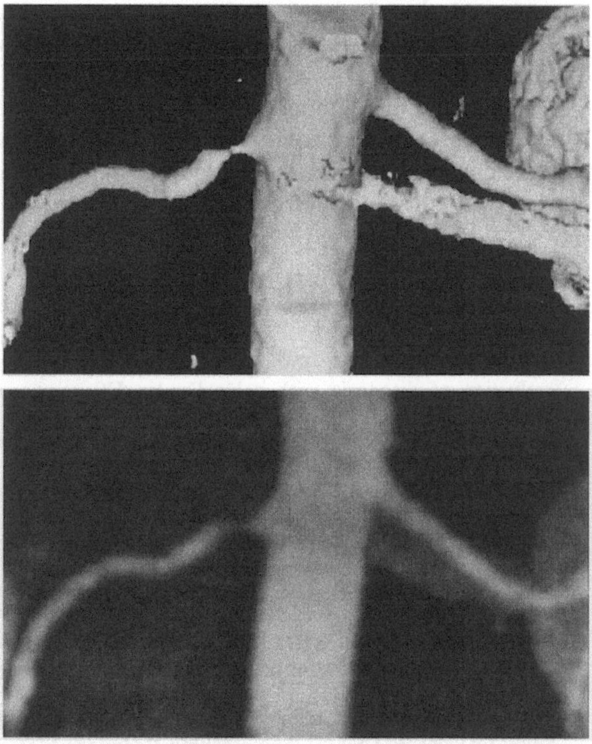

a

b

Fig. 2 a, b. Proximal stenosis of the right renal artery: comparison of 3D surface display (**a**) and maximum intensity projection image (**b**)

ferentiated due to different CT values. Small vascular structures can be visualized as long as their CT numbers are higher than those of surrounding tissues. On the other hand, renal arteries with little enhancement will be suppressed by overlying renal veins of similar enhancement (Napel et al. 1992; Galanski et al. 1993).

Similarly to a MIP, the 3D surface display is well suited for visualization of the anatomic situation (Fig. 2). There are, however, important drawbacks of 3D surface displays: the vascular diameter and thus the diameter of the stenosis are dependent on the threshold used for segmentation; the grade of the stenosis can only be estimated and cannot be measured; very small vessels, e.g. in patients with multiple renal arteries, can be totally missed if the threshold was chosen too high.; high-grade stenoses may appear as pseudo-occlusions (Schaefer et al. 1992).

Advantages of CTA over i.a. angiography are the improved visualization of the anatomy and the simultaneous availability of information about the vascular lumen and the vessel wall. As compared to MR angiography CTA detects accessory renal arteries with higher accuracy and shows a considerably lower rate of overestimation of stenoses Richter et al. 1993; Rubin et al. 1994). Disadvantages of color Doppler ultrasound are the bad visualization of the peripheral artery segment and of accessory arteries, the larger time requirements and especially the dependence of the diagnostic accuracy on the examiner's skills (Berland et al. 1990; Hillman 1989; Middleton 1992).

Yet, there are also limitations of CTA. These include imaging of peripherally located stenoses of segmental arteries and the dependence on patient compliance. Another drawback of CTA is the requirement of a relatively large contrast volume that may limit the indication for patients with impaired renal function.

References

1. Berland LL, Koslin DB, Roth WD, Keller FS (1990) Renal artery stenosis: Prospective evaluation of diagnosis with color Duplex US compared with angiography. Radiology 174 : 421 – 423
2. Davidson RA, Wilcox CS (1992) Newer tests for diagnosis of renovascular disease. JAMA 268 : 3353 – 3358
3. Galanski M, Prokop M, Chavan A, Schaefer C, Jandeleit K, Nischelsky JE (1993) Renal artery stenosis: Spiral CT angiography. Radiology 189 : 185 – 192
4. Hillman BJ (1989) Imaging advances in the diagnosis of renovascular hypertension. Am. J. Roentgenol. 153 : 5 – 14
5. Middleton WD (1992) Doppler US evaluation of renal artery stenosis: Past, present and future. Radiology 184 : 307 – 308
6. Napel S, Marks MP, Rubin GD, Dake MD, McDonnell CH, Song SM, Enzman DR, Jeffrey RB (1992) CT-angiography with spiral CT and maximum intensity projection. Radiology 185 : 607 – 610
7. Prokop M, Schaefer C, Kalender WA, Polacin A, Galanski M (1993) Gefäßdarstellung mittels Spiral-CT: Der Weg zur CT-Angiographie. Radiologe 33 : 694 – 704
8. Richter CS, Krestin GP, Eichenberger AC, Schöpke W, Fuchs WA (1993) Assessment of renal artery stenosis by phase contrast magnetic resonance angiography. Eur. Radiol. 3 : 493 – 498
9. Rubin GD, Dake MD, Napel SA, Jeffrey RB, McDonnelle CH, Sommer FG, Wexler L, Williams DM (1994) Spiral CT angiography of renal artery stenosis: Comparison of three-dimensional rendering techniques. Radiology 190 : 181 – 189
10. Schaefer C, Prokop M, Nischelsky JE, Reimer P, Bonk K, Galanski M (1992) Vascular imaging with spiral CT. In: Felix R, Langer M (ed.) Advances in CT II. Springer, Berlin Heidelberg New York, 109 – 115

Evaluation of Vascular Stent Patency with Spiral CT Angiography, Doppler Ultrasound and Clinical Findings: A Comparative Study

M. Freund, J. Link, J. Brossmann, E. Schweizer, M. Heller

Introduction

Computed tomographic angiography (CTA) has evolved as a less invasive diagnostic tool rendering 3-D images of arteries after intravenous contrast agent application.

CTA allows visualization of surface, lumen, calcified plaques, occasionally thrombi as well as topographic relation to surrounding structures (Napel et al. 1992; Rubin et al. 1993, 1994). In comparison with arteriography this can be achieved less invasive using CT after intravenous contrast administration.

Purpose

The purpose of the study is to develop additional objective criteria for the success of stent placement, and to evaluate the capability of CTA to determine the patency of vascular stents in comparison to clinical findings and Doppler ultrasound.

Material and Methods

Patients

CTA of the iliac arteries was performed in 11 patients (six men, five women; age range: 53 – 76 years; mean age: 64 years).

All patients had proven peripheral arterial occlusive disease. Before treatment (percutaneous transluminal angioplasty, PTA, and stent placement) nine patients had a limited walking distance of less than 200 m (stage IIb), one patient more than 200 m (stage IIa) and one patient had pain at rest (stage III).

After treatment, at the time of CTA eight patients had no limitations of their walking distance, one patient could walk more than 200 m (IIa) and one patient less than 200 m (IIb).

The arm-ankle index was determined before treatment and before CTA. Before treatment two patients had a good (0.9 – 0.75) quotient, four patients had a medium (0.74 – 0.5) and seven patients had a poor (less than 0.5).

At the time of CTA, after treatment 11 patients had a good and two patients had a poor quotient.

The time between treatment (PTA and stent placement) and CTA ranged from 2 days up to 20 months.

All patients were provided with Wallstents (Schneider), eight patients with one stent, two patients with two stents and one patient was treated with three stents.

Five stents were placed in the left common iliac artery, four stents were inserted in the right common iliac artery, four in the right external iliac artery and two stents in the left external iliac artery.

Stent

The Wallstent is a self-expanding, elastic, macroporous tubular prosthesis, woven from stainless steel.

Wallstents can be implanted in peripheral arterial vessels, coronary arteries, veines and the biliary tract (Friedrich et al. 1992; Günther and Vorwerk 1991, 1992; Strunk et al. 1992; Triller et al. 1990).

CTA Technique

Spiral CTA (SCTA) was performed using a Somatom Plus-S CT scanner (Siemens).

An 18-gauge intravenous cannula was placed in an antecubital vein and an injection of 150 ml contrast material with a flow of 4 ml/s was initiated using a power injector (CT-Injector XD 5500, Ulrich). After a delay of 30 s, a SCTA scan of 30 s was started with a table feed of 6 mm and a slice thickness of 3 mm (120 kV, 210 mA), increment: 2.

Shaded surface display (SSD) and maximum intensity projection (MIP) images were generated and density measurements in the aortic lumen and behind the stent were performed. For correlation purposes additional measurements were obtained in the corresponding iliac artery at the opposite side (Fig. 1).

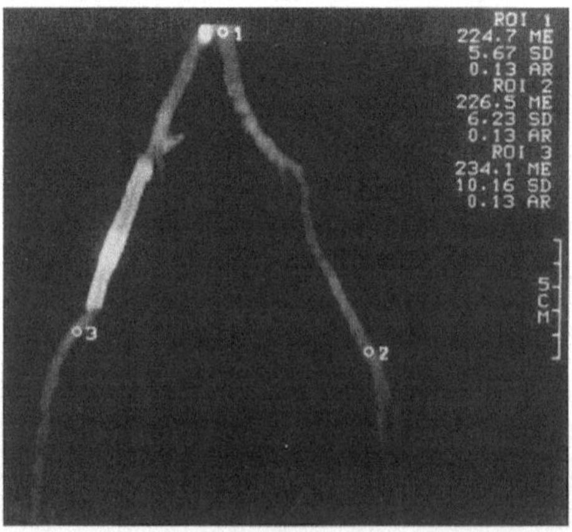

Fig. 1. Density measurement in the aortic lumen (*1*), behind the stent (*3*) and in the correspondent opposite artery (*2*). Maximum intensity projection

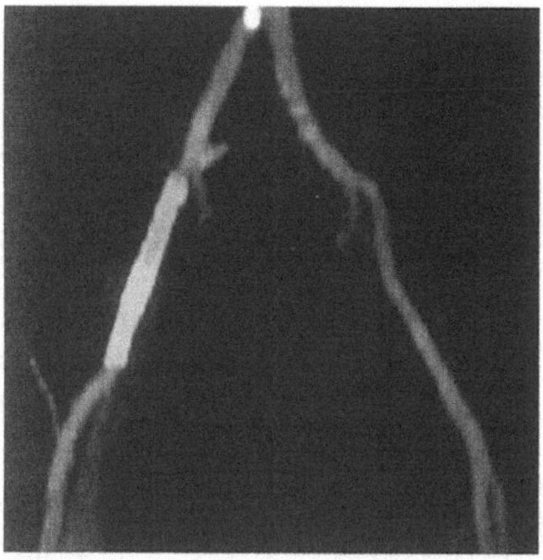

Fig. 2

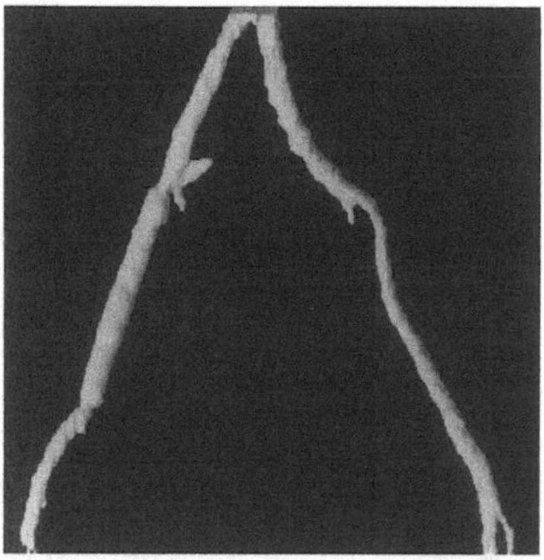

Fig. 3

Fig. 2. Patent Wallstent in the right common iliac artery. Mural calcification. Maximum intenstiy projection

Fig. 3. Patent Wallstent in the right common iliac artery, shaded surface display

Table 1. Density Measurement

Patient no	Aorta (HU)	Post-stent (HU)	Opposite side (HU)
1	459	166	170
2	309	290	304
3	491	382	351
4	270	190	215
5	NM	263	239
6	270	NM	NM
7	202	212	186
8	NM	309	275
9	226	NM	NM
10	328	302	310
11	339	369	NM
Mean	321	276	256

HU, Hounsfield units; NM, no measurement

Results

All 15 stents were visible (Fig. 2). No stent showed signs of stenosis or occlusion (Fig. 3). The density measurements showed no significant difference between the treated artery and the opposite artery (Table 1).

Good correlation was obtained between CTA results, clinical findings and Doppler ultrasound.

In addition to the purpose of the study CTA detected 15 stenoses of the other visualized arteries, eight were low-grade, five were middle-grade and two were high grade stenoses. Calcified plaques of the iliac arteries were found in nine patients.

Discussion and Conclusion

CTA is able to visualize patency after PTA and stent placement and seems to have a good correlation to clinical findings, if the stent is patent. All stents appeared as patent and all patients expanded their walking distance after PTA and stent placement. Except two patients all others had a better arm-ankle index after treatment, and at the time of CTA.

Another advantage of CTA is the possibility of detecting mural calcifications, which cannot be adressed by arteriography (Rubin et al. 1994). Mural calcification was noted in the MIP projections in nine patients (Fig. 2), but no mural calcification was detected in the SSD projections (Fig. 3).

Density measurement showed no significant difference between the treated artery and the corresponding opposite artery, which can be a hint for stent patency.

To determine whether CTA is able to detect stenosed or occluded stents further research is necessary.

References

1. Friedrich JM, Hutschenreiter S, Mickley V, Rilinger N, Häberle J, Goldmann A (1992) Stentgestützte Therapie bei Beckenvenenstenosen nach operativer Thrombektomie und Shuntanlage. Fortschr. Röntgenstr. 157, 6
2. Günther RW, Vorwerk D (1991) Indikationen zur Implantation von vaskulären Endoprothesen (Stents). Radiologe, 31:108–113
3. Günther RW, Vorwerk D (1992) Stents: intravasculär, endoluminal und transparenchymatös. Dtsch. med. Wschr. 117:272–275
4. Napel S, Marks MP, Rubin GD, Dake MD, McDonnell ChH, Song SM, Enzmann DR, Jeffrey RB (1992) CT Angiography with Spiral CT and Maximum Intensity Projection. Radiology, 185:607–610
5. Rubin GD, Dake MD, Napel SA, McDonnell ChH, Jeffrey RB (1993) Three dimensional Spiral CT Angiography of the Abdomen: Initial Clinical Experience. Radiology 186:147–152
6. Rubin GD, Dake MD, Napel S, Jeffrey RB, McDonnell ChH, Sommer FG, Wexler L, Williams DM (1994) Spiral CT of Renal Artery Stenosis: Comparison of Three-dimensional Rendering Techniques. Radiology 190:181–189
7. Serruys PW, Strauss BH, de Feyter P, Urban Ph (1991) The Wallstent: A Self-Expanding Stent. J Inv Cardiol: 3, 3:127–134
8. Sigwart U, Puel J, Mirkovitch MD, Joffre F, Kappenberger L (1987) Intravascular Stents to prevent Occlusion and Restenosis after transluminal Angioplasty. N Engl J Med 316
9. Strunk HM, Schild HH, Dahm M (1992) Beckenarterienverschluß: antegrade Sondierung zur Stentplazierung. Fortschr Röntgenstr. 157, 3:279–281
10. Triller J, Looser Ch, Schweizer W, Blumgart LH (1990) Erste Erfahrungen mit einer selbstexpandierenden Endoprothese (Wallstent) zur palliativen Behandlung der biliären Obstruktion. Schnetztor-Verlag Konstanz: 106–111

Advanced Techniques for Editing and Visualizing CTA Data

D. Hentschel, J. Ezrielev, R. Fisler, C. Flanders, A. Bani-Hashemi,
C.-C. Liang, S.-P. Liou, S. Samaddar, A. Singh, D. Ney

Introduction

Spiral computed tomography (CT) allows for fast acquisition of a truly volumetric data set (Kalender et al. 1990). If contrast material is injected during scanning, the vasculature can be assessed in three dimensions. This procedure is named CT Angiography (CTA) and provides an excellent visualization of vessel lumina, stenoses and lesions (Napel et al. 1992). Contrast filled vessels share a common range of Hounsfield units with bone. Therefore, it is necessary to eliminate bone structures prior to 3D visualization. As interactive editing of bones, especially on a slice by slice basis, can be very time-consuming, we have developed a semi-automated technique (Slab-Editor) and various automatic methods for specific parts of the body, which minimize user interaction or even make it obsolete.

CTA data are typically visualized with maximum intensity projection (MIP) or suface shaded display (SSD). The lumen is very well displayed with MIP, however, it might be obscured by calcifications. We are evaluating the volumetric rendering technique VRT; (Debrin et al. 1988; Levoy 1988) to overcome these deficiencies. Each visualization method provides different information which is often complimentary.

Slab Editor

The basic idea of editing is to remove certain structues such as bone from the data set for the subsequent use of the modified images in the visualization of vessels. A reliable but time consuming approach is manual outlining of these structures. To speed up the manual interaction, the outlining is not done slice by slice but on a subset or slab of the stack of slices. This method is called slab editor (Ezrielev et al. 1994).

The selection of the slabs is done graphically by displaying a side view MIP of the entire image stack. The selection of the borders of the slabs is done by pointing to their locations in the image stack. For each slab, a MIP image is calculated. This image has a characteristic of displaying the structures with the highest intensity values, which is useful to identify bone structures. The user makes modifications on the MIP image of every slab. These modifications are applied to every image in the slab. In this way the entire stack is traversed sequentially. Each slab inherits the contours of the previously modified subset. The user can adjust the inherited contours on top of the MIP image instead of having to draw new ones. This method speeds up the bone removal by the ratio of the number of slices to the number of slabs.

Abdominal Bone Removal

For abdominal data sets we have added a tool to the Slab-Editor, which finds the contours of the spine and the ribs without user interaction. This operation is performed on the MIP image of each slab. The MIP image is thresholded by a preset value such that a pixel is set to zero if it is below the value. The pixel with the highest intensity value is then defined as the seed point and a flood filling algorithm (Foley et al. 1990) is performed to define a region which has pixels with zero intensity as its boundary. This flood filling algorithm is repeatedly applied until no more pixels above the threshold can be found. Thresholding and region extraction does not delineate bones reliably as the inner area of bones is not homogeneous and the edges of bones are degraded by partial volume effects. The descending aorta might create difficulties as it can be close to the vertebrae (Napel 1992). Therefore, in a subsequent step the detection of bones is refined by making use of the anatomical location and shape of ribs and spine in the abdomen.

A slice of an abdominal data set is displayed in Fig. 1 before and after the algorithm for abdominal bone removal has been applied. The outer part of the body, which contains the ribs and the spine have been identified by the algorithm and removed. The aorta which is in close proximity to the spine is not affected by the procedure. The method has been successfully applied to 10 data sets.

Selection of the Lung

Spiral CT of the lung using breath-holding techniques provides high quality images of the lung. For subsequent 3D reconstruction of the acquired data, it is necessary to remove the higher density tissue outside of the lung. Manual editing by defining contours is prohibitively tedious and time consuming. We use an automated process which was previously described for conventional CT (Kavuru et al. 1991) to isolate the lung from the rest of the chest. This technique uses a flood fill algorithm with a threshold value in three dimensions to form an approximate shape of the lung. This shape generally has holes and gaps due to larger bronchial structures, so it is then necessary to use morphological operators to fix these deficiencies. This is done by dilating the shape by 10 to 15 millimeters and then eroding it approximately the same amount. The final shape can then be used to mark which voxels in the data are "lung" voxels and which are not. The result of the extraction can be seen in Fig. 2. The algorithm was uniquely identified the contour of the lung and of the trachea.

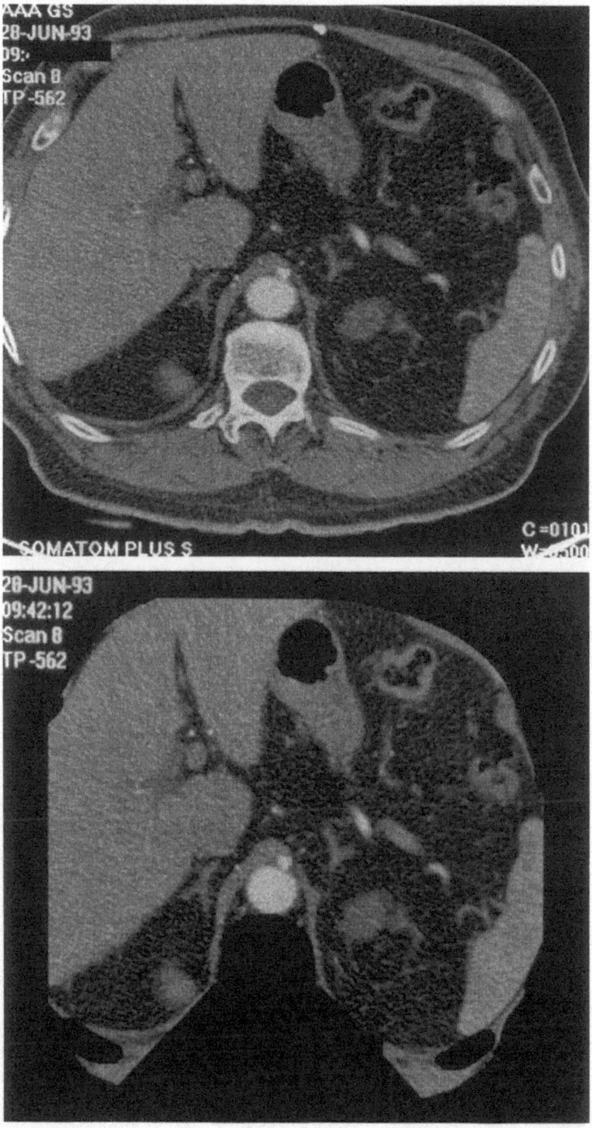

a

b

Fig. 1 a, b. A slice of an abdominal data set before (**a**) and after (**b**) the algorithm for abdominal bone removal has been applied

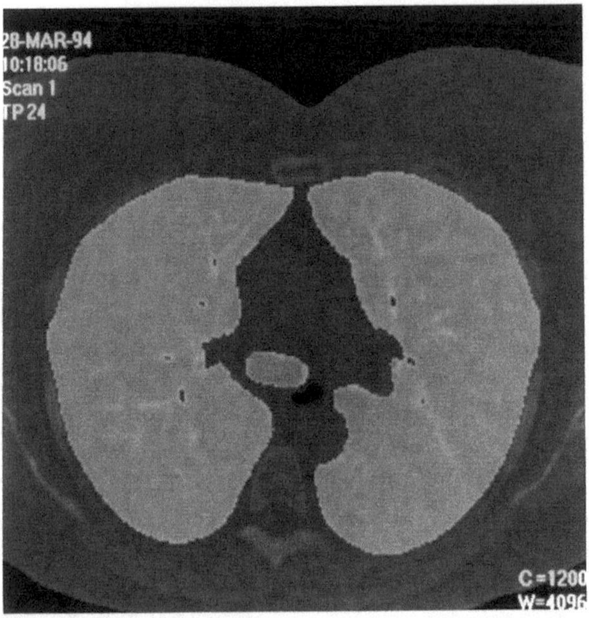

Fig. 2. A slice from a chest data set with the automatically extracted contours of the lungs and the trachea

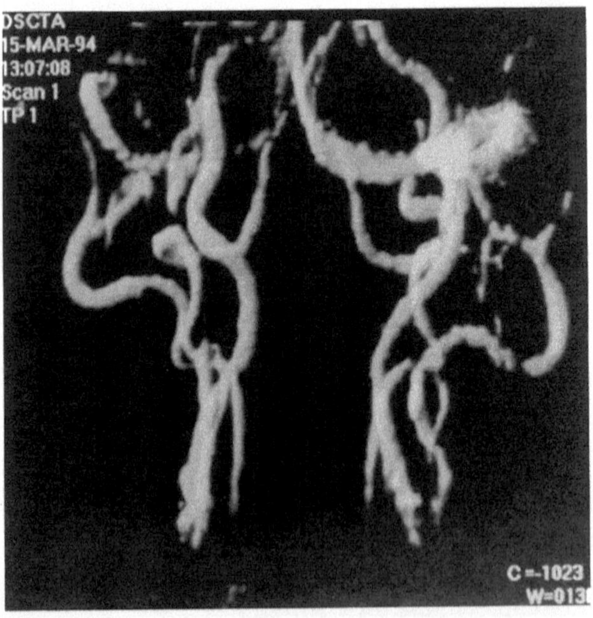

Fig. 3. A very first result of the digital subtraction computed tomographic angiography of the head and neck area above the carotid bifurcations. Data sets have been measured prior and during contrast administration and subtracted after a three-dimensional registration. The resulting data set is volume rendered to display the surface of the vessels

Digital Subtraction CTA

The removal of bones in the head and neck is even more demanding as bone and vessels can be in close proximity, which makes region growing unreliable (Napel et al. 1992; Marks et al. 1992). Therefore, we have extended the well-established method of digital subtraction angiography to CT (DSCTA). One data set is measured prior to contrast material administration and a second one during contrast injection. Ideally, the subtraction of both sets on a slice by slice basis would result in an image displaying only the vasculature. In reality the patient moves between both measurements which results misregistrations between both data sets. Therefore, it is necessary to register the data sets prior to subtraction. Whereas a rigid transformation is sufficient for intracranial vasculature local elastic matching is required for the neck area which is not only affected by complex motion of the neck but also by swallowing in the gullet. The automatic three-dimensional registration procedure is based on anatomy and uses a similarity measure known as deterministic sign change (Venot et al. 1984; Venot and Leclerc 1984) which has been successfully used on two dimensional DSA images. A very first result of these approach is shown in Fig. 3.

Visualization

SSD and MIP are mainly used to display the vasculature. These methods have the advantage of a simple user interface; no parameter has to be set in case of MIP or just one threshold value in the case of SSD. However, these methods do not provide all information the clinician is interested in. SSD depicts the morphology of the vessel tree but not the vessel lumen, calcifications or stents (Napel et al. 1992). The latter two are visible by MIP images but they might obscure the vessel lumen. These deficiencies can be overcome with VRT. The VRT method attributes to each voxel in the data set a gray value or color and a transparency or opacity. Depending on these parameters the resulting images can differ completely.

Figure 4 shows the same data set rendered with SSD, MIP and two different parameter sets for VRT. SSD only shows the outside of the vessels. With the exception of the stent vessel lumina are very well displayed with MIP. As the stent is in a unique range of Hounsfield units parameters can be chosen by the user to include or exclude the stent in the volume rendered image. As calcifications are in the same range Hounsfield units these are also included or excluded. This is especially important for circumferential calcifications. Comparing the VRT images to the MIP image, it can be seen that the visualization of depth is better with VRT. The mesenteric artery is clearly visible in front of the aorta.

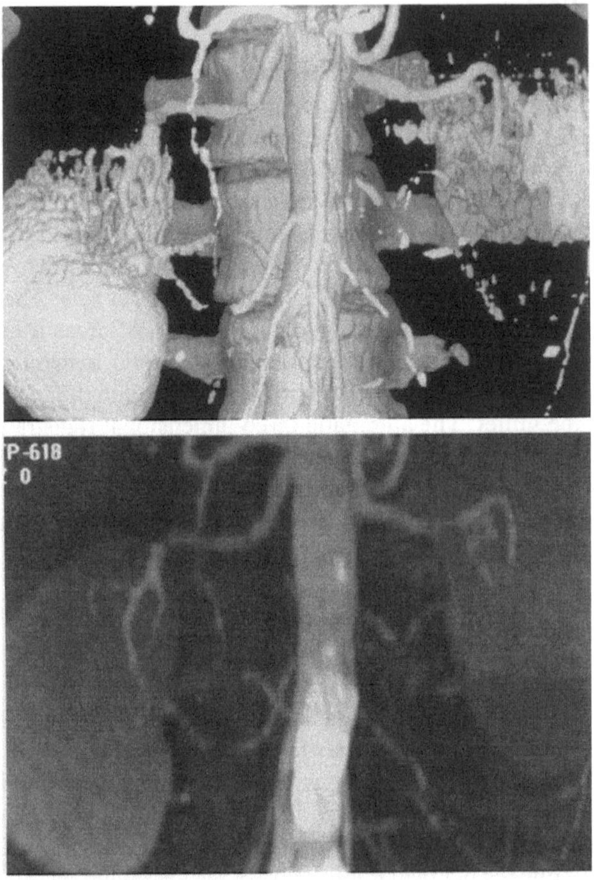

a

b

Fig. 4 a – d. An abdominal data set is visualized with **a** surface shaded display, **b** maximum intensity projection, **c** and **d** volume rendering technique. Besides (**a**) all images are edited. The volume rendering was done with two different parameter sets that suppress the stent and the calcifications (**c**) or include them in the image (**d**)

Conclusion

So far CTA has been hampered by the tedious process of interactively removing bones prior to the visualization. This process can be sped up or even automated using methods which are adapted to specific regions of the body. In the abdomen the removal of bones on a slice by slice basis was in the order of 45 min. With the slab editor this time decreases to 5 min. The current implementation of the abdominal bone removal takes about 1 min which is mainly the time to calculate the MIP images for all slabs. First experience indicates that no user interaction will be needed. The extraction of the lung is completely user independent and takes less than 1 min for a chest data set. The technical feasibility of the concept of removing

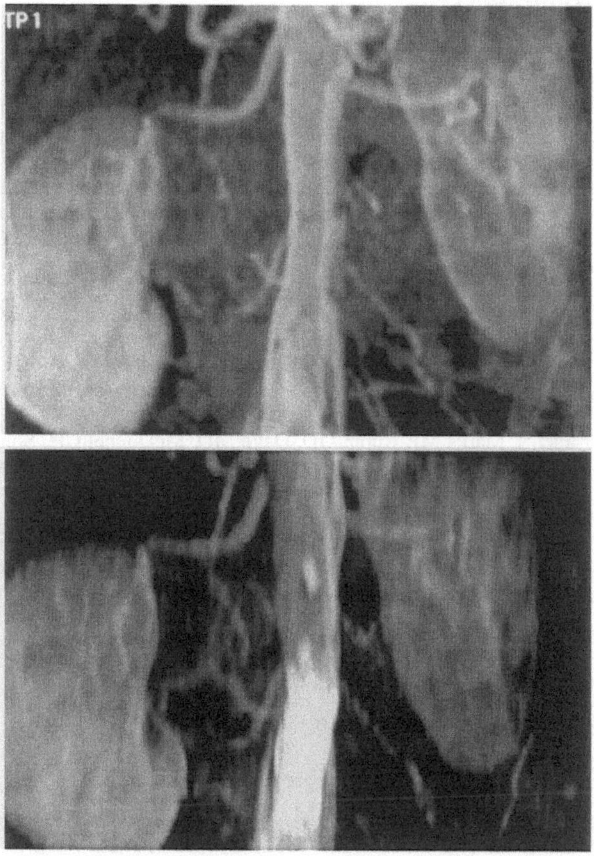

c

d

Fig. 4 c, d

bone in the head and neck with DSCTA has been demonstrated so far. Further research is needed to assess the clinical usefulness of this method. DSCTA is of interest in combination with double spiral CT acquisitions, which minimizes the delay between the acquisition of the mask and contrast data sets.

Three-dimensional data sets can be visualized with various methods. Each method provides specific information. VRT combines the superior depth display of SSD with the display of vessel lumen and calcifications of MIP. Furthermore VRT can also combine soft tissue vasculature and bone in one image. As VRT always works on the complete data set with various user defined parameter settings this visualization method is slower than MIP and SSD. It depends on the clinical application which method provides the best results.

References

Drebin RA, Carpenter L, Hanrahan P (1988) Volume Rendering. Computer Graphics (Proc. SIGGRAPH), 22 (4): 65–77

Ezrielev J, Rubin GD, Hentschel D (1994) Advanced Tools for 3-D Processing of Tomographic Slices. Proceedings S/CAR 94, Winston-Salem, North Carolina, in press

Foley JD, et al. (1990) Computer Graphics. Addison-Wesley

Kalender WA, Seissler W, Klotz E, Vock P (1990) Spiral volumetric CT wtih single -breath-hold technique, continuous transport, and continuous scanner rotation. Radiolog 176:181–190

Kavuru M, Ney DR, Fishman EK, Kuhlman JE, Hruban RH, Hutchins GM: Three-Dimensional Imaging of the Lung in Vivo. Journal of Digital Imaging, Vol 4, No 3 (August), 1991: pp 137–142

Levoy M (1988) Display of Surfaces from Volume Data. IEEE Computer Graphics and Applications 8 (3): 29–37

Marks MP, Napel S, Jordan JE, Enzmann DR (1992) Diagnosis of Carotid Artery Disease: Preliminary Experience with Maximum-Intensity-Projection Spiral CT Angiography. AJR 160:1267–1271

Napel S, Marks MP, Rubin GD, Dake MD, McDonnel CH, Song SM, Enzmann DR, Jeffrey RB (1992) CT Angiography with Spiral CT and aximum Intensity Projection. Radiolog 185 (2):607–610

Venot A, Lebruchec JF and Roucayrol JC (1984) A new class of similarity measures for robust image registration. Computer Vision, Graphics, Image Processing 28:176–184

Venot A and Leclerc V (1984) Automated correction of patient motion and gray values prior to subtraction in digitized angiography. IEEE Transaction on Medical Imaging, MI-3:179–186

Spiral CT and CT-Angiography of Coronary Grafts: Experimental and Clinical Studies

P.E. HUPPERT, S.H. DUDA, R. BRAUNSCHWEIG, H. SEBOLDT, C.D. CLAUSSEN

Introduction

Using conventional and dynamic computed tomography (CT) the rate of correctly demonstrated patent coronary vein grafts (sensitivity) was reported 80–93%. But the rate of suspected graft occlusions confirmed by angiography (specificity) was only 72–78% (Heuser et al. 1982, Godwin et al. 1983, Mühlberger et al. 1990). The lower specificity was mostly caused by confusing occluded grafts with contrasted cardiac structures, coronary arteries, bronchial arteries and graft stumps. Spiral-CT has the potential to improve specificity due to its multislice capability and to improve sensitivity by using peak contrast scanning. However small diameters, curved and wavy courses of grafts and cardiac motions require special imaging conditions.

Purpose

1. Experimental evaluation of acquisition and reconstruction parameters suitable for 2D and 3D imaging of small vessels in Spiral-CT.
2. Comparative clinical study of Spiral-CT and angiography for postoperative patency control in aortocoronary vein grafts (ACVG) and internal mammarian artery grafts (IMAG).
3. Evaluation of CT-Angiography for ACVG and IMAG.

Methods of Experimental Studies

The vascular phantom used consisted of a water-filled cylinder containing plastic tubes with inner diameters of 1 mm, 2 mm, 3 mm and 4 mm. The tubes were filled with diluted contrast material. Spiral-CT acquisition of the phantom was performed with systematic variation and combination of the following parameters using the Somatom Plus S (Siemens, Erlangen):

collimation	2 mm, 4 mm, 8 mm
pitch	0.5, 1.2
angulation of tubes (in relation to z-axis)	0°, 30°, 60°, 90°
reconstruction increment	50% and 100% of collimation
z-profile	linear interpolation 360°, 180°

Table 1. Methods and parameters of Spiral-CT acquisition, CT-postprocessing and intraarterial DSA

Spiral-CT	CT-Postprocessing	i.a. DSA
collimation 5 mm	increment 2 mm	aortic injection: 35 ml/1.4 s.
table feed 5 mm/s	180° linear interpolation	projections: PA, LAO, RAO:
time 12 s	2D editing	
acquisitions 2–3	matrix 256	subcl. art. injection: 12 ml/2 s.
contrast injection:	MIP: 30° interval	projection: PA
100–150 ml, 2 ml/s	3D surface reformations	
delay individual	(threshold 120 HE)	

Spatial resolution and contrast resolution of tube imaging were determined quantitatively by using histogram functions (cross sectional area, mean density) and density profile functions (full width at half maximum, area under full width at half maximum).

Results of Experimental Studies

Parameters of image quality in 2 mm, 3 mm and 4 mm tubes were different using both z-profiles. For 360° linear interpolation acquisitions with 4 mm collimation and 4 mm/s table feed resulted in a superior image quality compared to acquisitions with 4 mm collimation and 8 mm/s table feed. For 180° linear interpolation image quality was comparable for acquisitions with 2 mm collimation and a table feed of 2 mm and 4 mm, respectively. For reconstructions of axial 2D images increment of 100% of collimation was sufficient, whereas the quality of maximum intensity projections (MIP) was improved using 50% increment. These differences were independently on the degree of angulations, but image quality was generally lower for 60° angulations when compared to 30° angulations. Images of the 1 mm-tube showed lower quality.

Patients and Methods of Clinical Studies

Between October 1991 and November 1992 a comparative study of Spiral CT (Somatom Plus) and intraarterial DSA was performed including 57 patients with 113 ACVG and 29 IMAG. CT diagnoses based on axial images whereas the reconstruction of CT-Angiograms was not included in this comparison. The parameters for acquisition and postprocessing in CT and during DSA are summarized in the table. For correct segmentation of coronary grafts very time-consuming 2D slice-by slice editing technique was mandatory (Fig. 1). The time interval between operation and CT was 9–15 days and between CT and DSA 1–3 days.

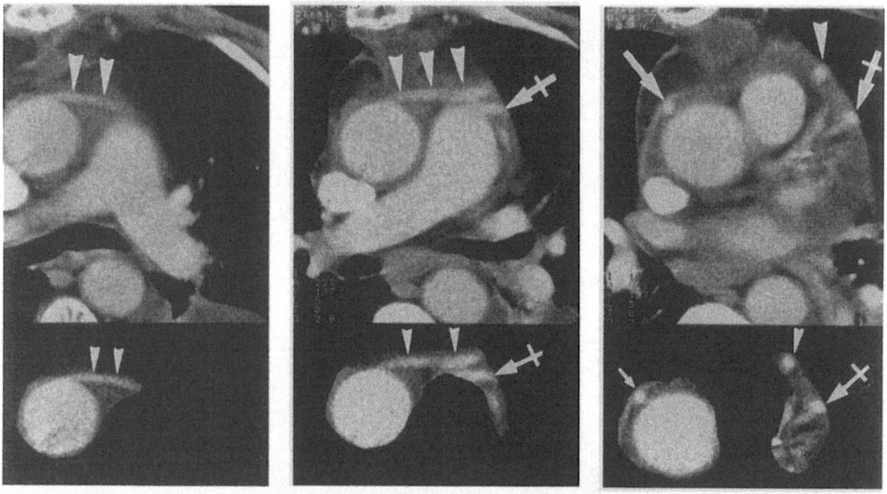

Fig. 1. 65 years old male patient with triple coronary vein graft to the right coronary artery (arrows), left anterior descending artery (arrowheads) and marginal branch (crossed arrows). Corresponding images in the lower pannel demonstrate 2D editing

Results of Clinical Studies

Angiographical patency was 93% in ACVG and 100% in IMAG. In ACVG the sensitivity of Spiral CT was 99% (one graft to the right coronary artery was missed) and the specificity was 100% (8 occlusions). 6 jumped grafts could not be clearly detected. For IMAG the sensitivity was only 69% (20/29). This was probably due to the smaller vessel diameter and to metallic clip artefacts (Fig. 2).

In MIP images complete display resulted in 79% of vein grafts but only in 42% of arterial grafts. In more than 80% of grafts stenoses and occlusios were present without any angiographical correlate (Fig. 2b).

Discussion

Spiral-CT improved the specificity in detection of coronary graft occlusions compared to historical results of conventional CT. Figures are nearly identical to those obtained by electron beam CT (Stanford et al. 1988). Experimental and clinical studies demonstrated, that lower collimations during acquisition and 180° linear interpolation for reconstruction provide better results (Tello et al. 1993, Huppert et al. 1993, Steiner et al. 1994).

Generally CT of coronary grafts should only be performed during the early postoperative period in patients with suspected graft occlusions or with the intention of surgical quality control. Until now neither dynamic CT studies nor Spiral CT and CT-Angiography provide reliable informations in terms of graft stenoses, graft

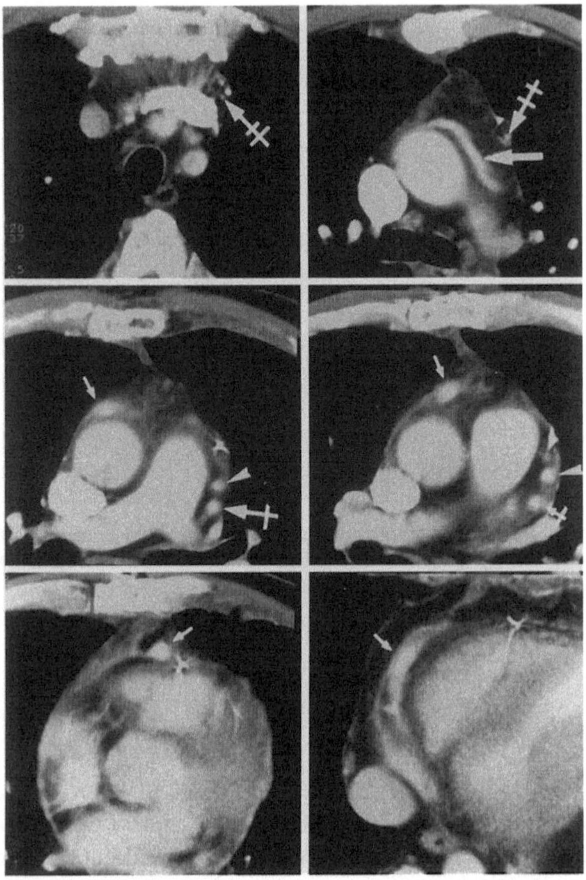

a

Fig. 2 a, b. 62 years old patient with vein grafts to the right coronary artery (arrows), diagonal branch (arrowheads) and marginal branch (crossed arrows). Note several metallic clips near to a small internal mammarian artery graft (double crossed arrows). **a** Cranio-caudal sequence of axial images. **b** Maximum intensity projections: PA (upper left). LAO (upper right). LAP (lower left) and craio-caudal (lower right). Note: Stair step artefacts causing pseudostenoses

quality and coronary arteries. The detection of graft patency is based on the axial images. 3D images are useful for the demonstration of individual anatomical situations. Arteficial graft stenoses in MIP images are probably due to cardiac pulsations causing axial graft motions especially in the lower graft portions.

Conclusions

1. Spiral CT is a reliable method for differentiating aortocoronary vein graft patency and occlusion.

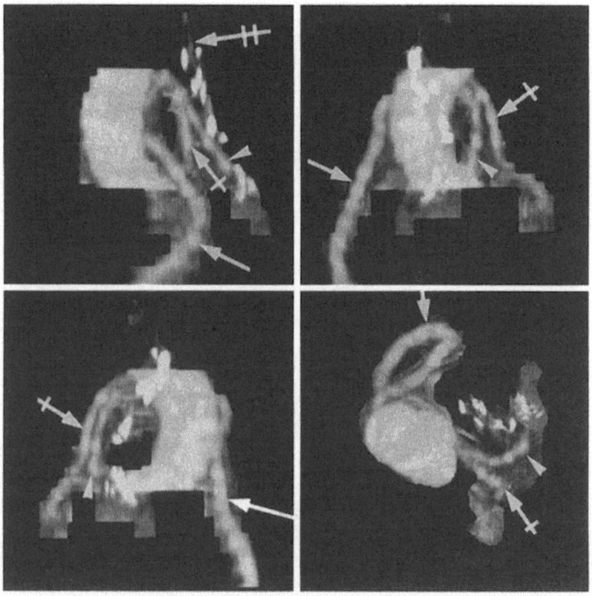

Fig. 2b

2. For clinical applications 2D images basing on 4–5 mm collimation and 2 mm increment are sufficient, however for 3D reconstructions 2 mm collimation and 1 mm increment is recommended.
3. Imaging of arterial grafts with smaller diameters requires further methodical improvements.

References

1. Godwin DJ, Califf RM, Korobkin M, Moore AV, Breiman RS, Kong Y (1983) Clinical value of coronary bypass graft evaluation with CT. AJR 140:649–655
2. Heuser L, Lackner K, Hauser H (1982) Validität der Computertomographie bei der Darstellung offener und verschlossener aortokoronarer Venenbrücken (ACVB). Fortschr. Röntgenstr. 137: 619–626
3. Huppert PE, Seboldt H, Duda SH, Claussen CD (1993) CT-Angiography of aortocoronary vein grafts and internal mammary artery to left anterior descending artery anastomoses. Radiology 189 (P) 112
4. Mühlberger V, Knapp E, z. Nedden D (1990) Predictive value of computed tomographic determination of the patency rate of aortocoronary venous bypasses in relation to angiographic results. Europ. Heart J. 11:380–388
5. Stanford W, Brundage BH, McMillan R, Chomka EV, Bateman TM, Eldredge WJ, Lipton MJ, White CW, Wilson RF, Johnson MR, Marcus ML (1988) Sensitivity and specificity of assessing coronary bypass graft patency with ultrafast computed tomography: Results of a multicenter study. JACC 12:1–7
6. Steiner P, Phillips F, Stiel G, Schuchert A, Rust C, Hauger B, Bücheler E (1994) Validität der Spiral-Computertomographie bei der Darstellung aortokoronarer Bypass-Gefäße. Fortschr Röntgenstr. 160:23–29
7. Tello R, Costello P, Ecker C, Hartnell G (1993) Spiral CT evaluation of coronary artery bypass graft patency. J Comp Assit Tomogr 17:253–259

Special Aspects of Spiral CT

Chairmen: A. K. Dixon, W. I. Dock

Optimisation and Adaptation of Intravenous Administration of Contrast Medium in Spiral Volumetric CT

C. EHRITT-BRAUN, F. J. FERSTL, D. BURGER, M. LANGER

Introduction

Whole-body computed tomography (CT) is a well established method for detection of tumors, pathological lymph nodes and metastases (Carvalho et al. 1991; Steinkamp et al. 1991). To achieve a high accuracy, optimal contrast enhancement of vessels and abdominal organs in required. New technical developments in computed tomography now enable considerable volume reduction of the applied contrast medium.

To determine whether spiral volumetric CT (SVCT) can reduce the amount of contrast media without compromising diagnostic findings, we compared this technique with dynamic incremental CT (DICT) and dynamic screening CT (DSCT).

Material and Methods

Some 132 patients presenting for CT assessment of the neck ($n = 60$), chest ($n = 36$) or abdomen ($n = 36$) were prospectively randomized to either SVCT, DICT or DSCT examination. Patients' ages ranged from 8 to 86 years (mean of 56 years). The patients were examined for different indications using nonionic contrast agent (Ultravist formulated at 300 mg I/ml, Schering).

CT examinations were performed using the following injection protocols:

1. Neck

- DICT, interscan delay 10 s, contrast administration 150 ml, flow 1.5 and 0.5 ml/s
- DSCT, interscan delay 5 s, contrast administration 100 ml, flow 2 and 0.5 ml/s
- SVCT, scanning time 30 s, contrast administration 50 ml, flow 2 and 0.7 ml/s

2. Chest

- DICT, interscan delay 13 s, contrast administration 150 ml, flow 0.7 ml/s
- DSCT, interscan delay 5 s, contrast administration 100 ml, flow 0.7 ml/s
- SVCT, scanning time 30 s, contrast administration 50 ml, flow 2 ad 0.7 ml/s

3. Abdomen

- DICT, interscan delay 13 s, contrast administration 180 ml, flow 0.7 ml/s
- DSCT, interscan delay 5 s, contrast administration 150 ml, flow 2 and 0.5 ml/s
- SVCT, examination time 30 s, contrast administration 50 ml, flow 2 and 0.7 ml/s

All CT studies were performed with a Somatom Plus S CT scanner (Siemens) using 0.7- or 1-s scanning time, slice thickness and table feed were 5 mm for neck studies and 10 mm chest and abdomen examinations. Scanning began 30 s after the of intravenous contrast material (CM) injection. The spiral CT data sets were reconstructed at 10-mm intervals (increment) with an 360° linear interpolation algorithm. For CM administration a power injector (Medrad)) was used enabling delivery of predetermined CM volumes at two different flow rates. Individual patient data were compared in order to evaluate diagnostic accuracy, CM volume, CM enhancement and examination time. Diagnostic accuracy and vessel differentiation were independently scored by three radiologists using a scale from 1–6 (1 = inadequate, 6 = excellent). Visual analysis of image quality for all three CT methods was performed, and time-density-curves plotted.

Contrast enhancement was measured in the internal jugular vein or in the common jugular vein and in the right internal carotid artery or right common carotid artery. In the presenting study of the chest measurements were carried out in the ascending and descending aorta. in the abdominal examination we measured enhancement in the abdominal aorta and the inferior vena cava.

Results

We obtained comparable results with all three methods as it is shown in Table 1. Examination by dynamic incremental CT was very reliable with regard to diagnostic accuracy and differentiation of vessels compared to DSCT and SVCT. In the dynamic screening mode we fund that the breath excursions are not as constant as required for a complete volume scanning to detect all pathological structures such as

Table 1. Analysis of image quality

	Diagnostic accuracy	Differentiation of vascular structures[a]
DICT		
Neck	5.5±0.5	5.3±0.8
Chest	5.3±0.8	5.4±0.8
Abdomen	5.8±0.4	5.5±0.6
DSCT		
Neck	5.5±0.6	5.6±0.4
Chest	5.1±0.9	5.4±0.6
Abdomen	4.8±0.7	5.4±0.7
SVCT		
Neck	5.7±0.6	5.9±0.3
Chest	5.0±0.8	5.3±0.7
Abdomen	4.6±0.7	4.5±0.5

DICT, dynamic incremental computed tomography; DSCT, dynamic screening CT; SVCT, spiral volumetric CT

[a] = inadequate; 6 = excellent.

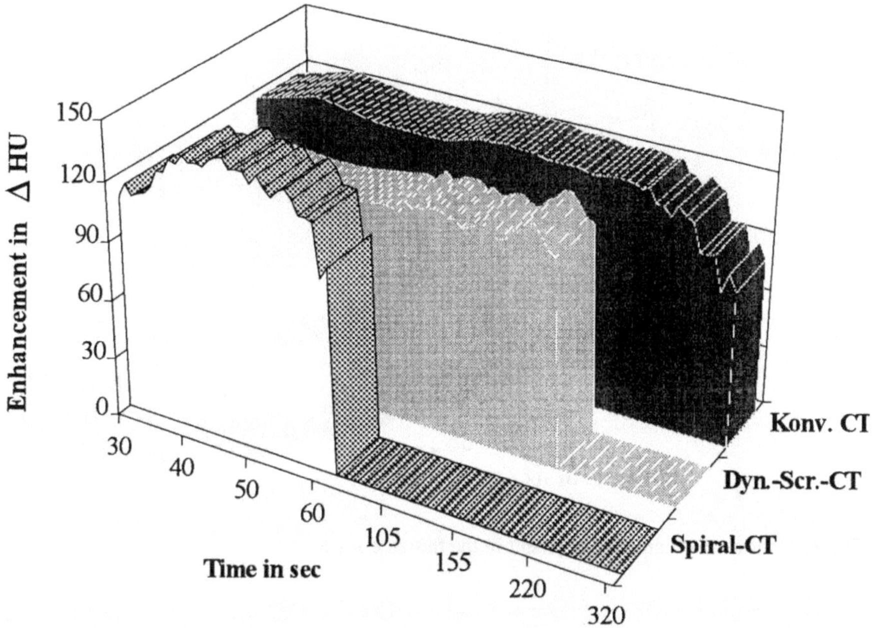

Fig. 1. Right jugular vein enhancement compared with the native scan

lymph node metastases and tumors smaller than 1 cm. In addition, liver and spleen enhancement was not as sufficient in abdominal scanning with SVCT as compared with DICT. On the other hand, SVCT was excellent for detection of small structures, because the whole region could be examined during one inspiration phase (neck and chest) and during one expiration phase (abdomen), both lasting 30 s.

The high contrast enhancement of the vessels of the neck obtained with all three scanning methods is illustrated in Fig. 1. Right jugular vein enhancement is comparable in DICT and DSCT, for former producing slightly higher peak enhancement a few seconds sooner.

The chest examination produced more differences between conventional incremental and spiral volumetric scanning (Fig. 2). The reduced volume of contrast medium (100 ml) in the dynamic screening CT gave a maximum enhancement of 90 HU, compared with 110 HU for conventional incremental scanning. In spiral CT the peak enhancement was around 50 HU, which is sufficient for diagnostic assessment and differentiation of vascular structures.

Contrast enhancement in SVCT peaked at about 50 HU (Δ HU), which enabled the detection of lymph node metastases around the less enhanced vascular structures. In contrast, spiral CT of abdomen did not allow the reliable assessment of liver pathology because of the low contrast enhancement. Table 2 shows the decreased enhancement obtained in liver, spleen, kidneys and abdominal vessels using 50 ml contrast medium in SVCT in comparison to DICT (150/180 ml) and DSCT (100 ml). When CM volume is reduced by 2/3 in SVCT, contrast enhancement is at least halved in comparison with DICT and DSCT. Despite the loss of CM enhance-

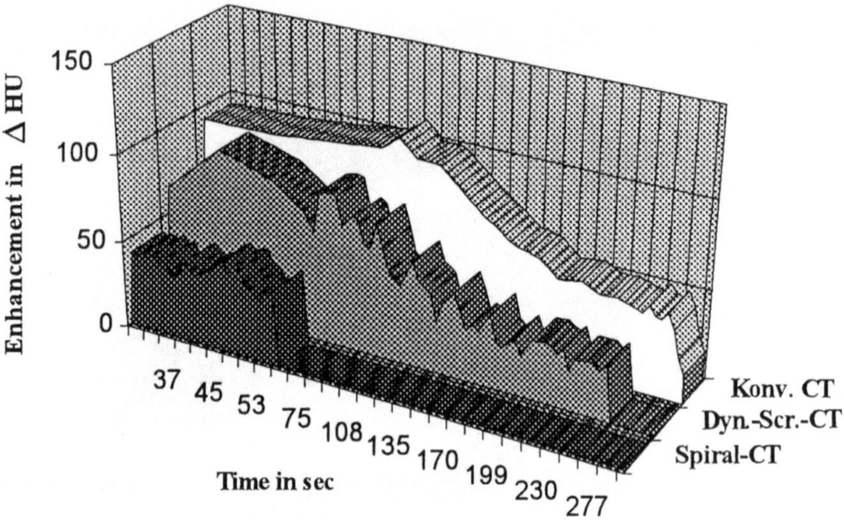

Fig. 2. Contrast medium enhancement in the thoracic aorta

Table 2. Enhancement in parenchymatous organs, abdominal aorta and inferior vena cava

Measured in:	Enhancement in Δ HU		
	DICT	DSCT	SVCT
Liver (right lobe)	52±15	31±8	18±9
Liver (left lobe)	51±18	29±18	21±10
Spleen	57±15	46±9	28±9
Right kidney	142±44	113±39	60±20
Left kidney	137±35	112±34	61±24
Abdominal aorta			
Neck	119±31	113±18	78±28
Chest	122±44	119±26	84±27
Abdomen	120±48	118±26	92±29
Inferior vena cava			
Neck	74±18	54±9	43±20
Chest	77±20	60±15	43±16
Abdomen	78±29	53±17	43±20

DICT, dynamic incremental computed tomography; DSCT, dynamic screening CT; SVCT, spiral volumetric CT ment of abdominal vessels, spiral CT sections were sufficient for diagnostic assessment concerning lymph node metastases. Parenchymal enhancement was insufficient for detection of liver pathology.

Discussion

Spiral CT studies of neck and chest showed that CM volume can be reduced to 50 ml without decreasing image quality, as graded by diagnostic accuracy and vessel imaging enhancement (Hacking and Dixon 1992). Contrary to the findings of Costello et al. (1991) a contrast medium flow of 0.7 to 2 ml/s was well tolerated by nearly all patients.

Our findings confirm that 50 ml CM (SVCT) provides high vascular enhancement in the neck and chest, thus supporting the conclusions of Zwicker et al. (1993) for examination of the upper abdomen. By contrast, the opacification of parenchyma such as the liver, spleen and kidneys in the abdominal examination was not as good as expected in spiral CT (Ditchfield et al. 1993).

Conclusion

Use of SVCT in the examination of the neck and chest enables a reduction of CM from 150 or 180 to 50 ml without loss of diagnostic validity. In abdominal CT scans the amount of contrast media can be decreased by one third without significant diagnostic limitation.

References

Carvalho P, Baldwin D, Carter R, Parsons C (1991) Accuracy of CT in Detecting Squamous Carcinoma in Cervical Lymph Nodes. Clinical Radiology 44 : 79

Costello B, Dupuy DE, Ecker CP (1991) Spiral-CT of the thorax with small volumes of contrast material: a comparative study. Radiology 181 (P): 274

Ditchfield MR, Gibson RN, Australas Fairlie N (1993) Liver CT: A practical approach to dynamic contrast enhancement. Advances in X-Ray Contrast 1 : 24

Hacking JR, Dixon AK (1992) Spiral versus conventional CT in soft tissue diagnosis. EJR 15 (3) : 224

Steinkamp HJ, Zwicker C, Langer M, Mathe F, Uhrmeister P (1991) Halslymphknotenmetastasen: Wertigkeit von Computertomographie und Palpation. RöFo 155, 4 : 305

Zwicker C, Langer M, Langer R, keske U (1993) Bolusapplikation in der Spiral-CT des Oberbauches. Akt. Radiol. 3 : 172

Improved Administration of Contrast Medium in Spiral Computed Tomography

R. Kloeppel, T. Nitzsche, S. Koesling, H. G. Schulz

Introduction

In Spiral computed tomography (CT) single scans separated by interscan pauses are replaced by a continuous data acquisition with continuous table movement (Kalender et al. 1990). This volume scanning that needs less than 1 min requires new modalities of i.v. contrast medium administration. There are many earlier experience on bolus administration of contrast medium in sequential CT (Claussen and Lochner 1983; Foley 1989; Kloeppel and Wittek 1985; Krahe et al. 1985; Partanen et al. 1984) that should be used for spiral CT. There are only few studies on spiral CT (Bautz et al. 1992; Galanski et al. 1992; Heike et al. 1993; Helmberger et al. 1993; Honda et al. 1992; Lenz et al. 1993; Marchal et al. 1991; Marchal and Baert 1992; Zwicker et al. 1993). The present study will be focussed on the transition between the initial and the continuous enhancement in upper abdomen.

Material and Methods

Some 101 abdominal spiral CT examinations on the SOMATOM PLUS S (Siemens) were evaluated retrospectively. The following parameterts were held constant: slice thickness 10 mm, table speed 10 mm/s, increment 8 mm. The i.v. application of contrast medium (Iopamidol 370/Byk Gulden) was made by a computer controlled high pressure injector (XD 5500/Ulrich). Time density curves of the aorta abdominalis, kidneys, spleen, and liver were analyzed in dependence on the following parameters:

1. Age of patients: until 55 years, older than 55 years (without patients with decompensated cardiac insufficiency and liver cirrhosis)
2. Contrast medium Volume: 50 – 150 ml
3. Flow rate: 1 – 6 ml/s
4. Start delay: 14 – 45 s

Table 1. Time-density study in abdominal aorta

Flow (ml/s)	Patient >55 years				Patient ≤55 years			
	n	t* (s)	t̄ (s)	SD	*n*	t* (s)	t̄ (s)	SD
6	4	18–25	21.0	3.55	2	16–19	17.5	2.12
4	10	17–26	21.2	2.79	11	15–24	18.6	3.13
3	5	20–25	21.4	2.19	3	18–25	20.6	3.78
2	5	16–22	19.6	2.61	1	21	21.0	–
<2	–	–	–	–	1	20	20.0	–

t*, time p.i. up to density of 150 HU; t, mean value of t*; SD, standard deviation

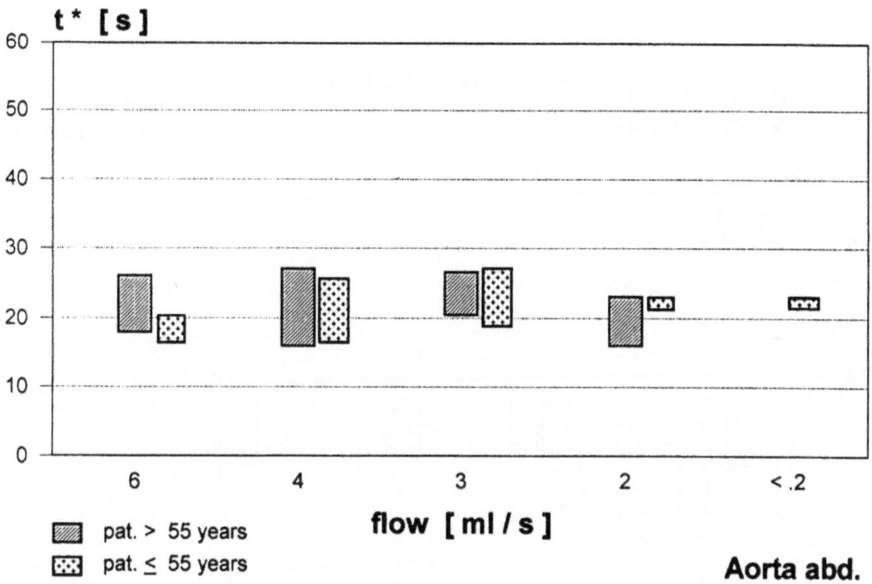

Fig. 1. Abdominal aorta: dependence on t*, flow rate and age of patients

Results

Aorta Abdominalis

Only in 42 of the total of 101 patients a peak could be found; the peak is reached after 17.5 to 27 s after injection start with the older patients and 15 to 25 s with the group of younger patients (Table 1, Fig. 1). The mean difference of 2 s was not significant. For most patients the maximum of contrast medium density occurred before the start of data acquisition. The time density curves declined more slowly with lower flow rate in the ranges of 3 to 6 ml/s. A flow rate up to 3 ml/s did not

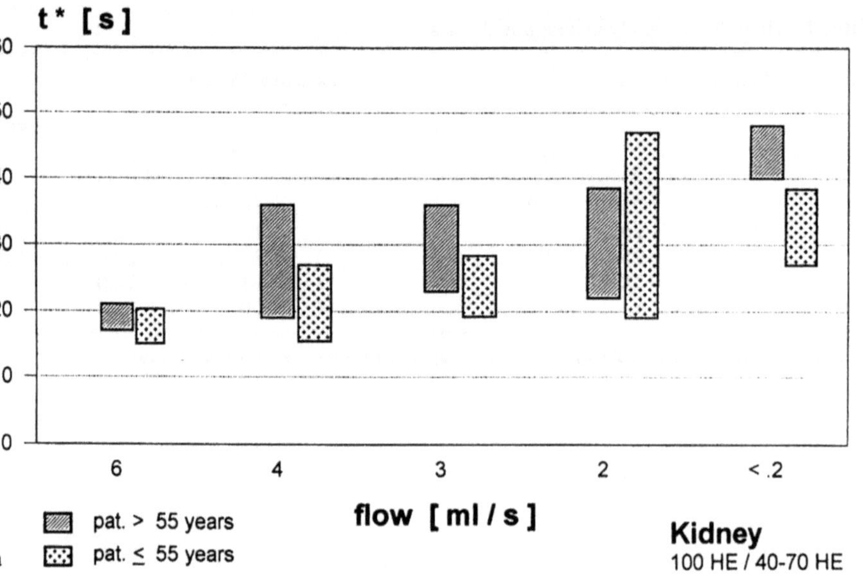

a

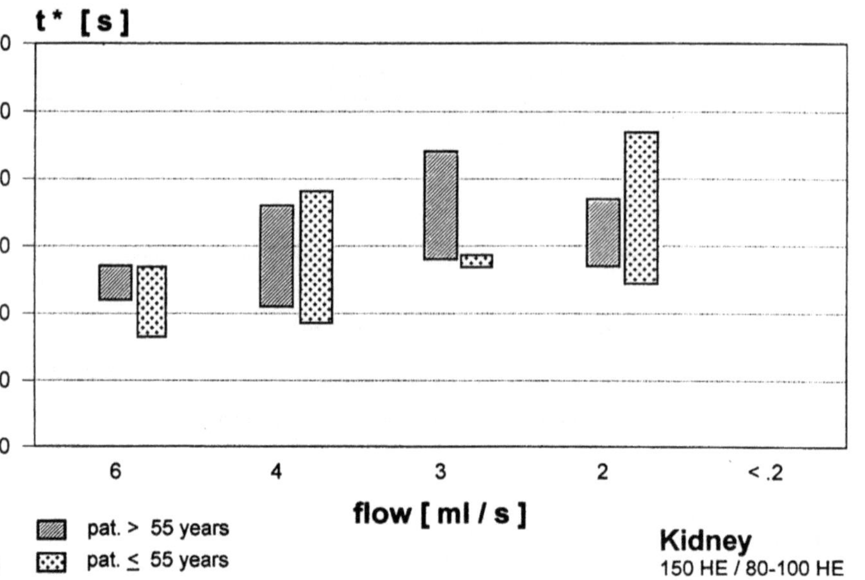

b

Fig. 2 a–c. Kidneys: dependence on t*, flow rate and age of patients (equal conditions see Tables 2, 3 (**a, b**). **c** Dependence onflow rate and enhancement of cortex (-------) and medulla (——)

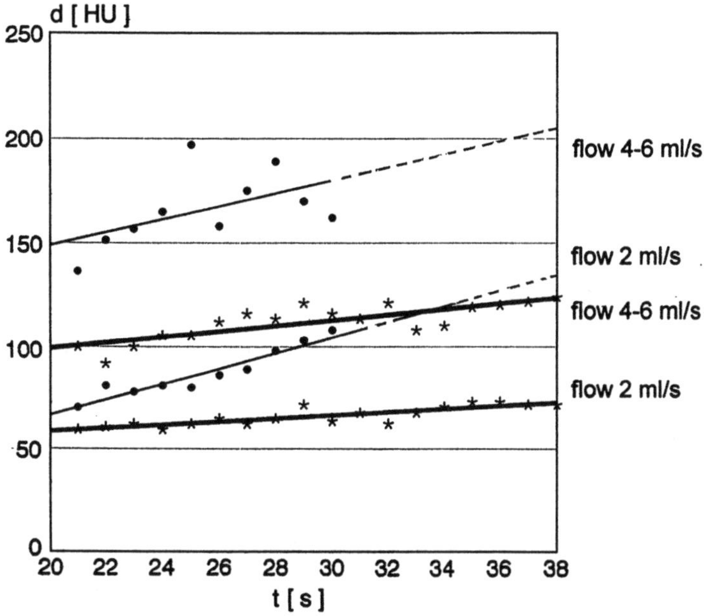

Fig. 2c

change the curve shape. A density of more than 150 HU in the aorta abdominalis was reached only with a flow rate of more than 2 ml/s.

With a start delay above 25 s the density of neighbouring organs increased so that the density difference between aorta and the adjacent structures decreased.

Kidneys

With comparable contrast medium volume a predefined threshold of density was reached earlier with a higher flow rate in the renal cortex and medulla (Tables 2, 3; Fig. 2). The differences decreased with increasing flow rate and decreasing threshold value. The average time for reaching this threshold was longer by 5 s for the group of older patients. The density peaks dependend on flow rate; renal cortex and medulla showed differences in their density curves (Fig. 2c): the enhancement of the renal cortex was more marked with a flow rate of 4–6 ml/s than with a flow of 2 ml/s; the enhancement of the renal medulla was independent on flow rate, there was only a different level of time density curve.

Spleen

An enhancement above a threshold of 100 HU in combination with a marked inhomogenity (delta HU 40–70) occurred in 45 of 55 cases of older patients and in 37 of 42 cases of younger patients if at least 60 ml of contrast medium was applied with a flow of 2 ml/s or more (Tables 4, 5; Fig. 3). Only in the age group up to

Table 2. Time-density study in kidneys

Flow (ml/s)	Patient >55 years				Patient ≤55 years			
	n	t* (s)	t̄ (s)	SD	*n*	t* (s)	t̄ (s)	SD
6	5	17–21	18.8	1.48	2	14–20	16.75	2.5
4	25	19–35	24.4	3.85	16	14–27	19.20	3.7
3	16	23–35	27.7	4.88	5	19–29	25.20	7
2	9	22–38	27.8	5.36	12	19–50	27.30	13.1
<2	2	40–48	44.0	5.6	4	27–40	33.50	9.2

t*, 100 HU of cortex and 40–70 HU of medulla. For other abbreviations see Table 1

Table 3. Time density study in kidneys

Flow (ml/s)	Patient >55 years				Patient ≤55 years			
	n	t* (s)	t̄ (s)	SD	*n*	t* (s)	t̄ (s)	SD
6	5	22–26	23.8	1.48	4	14–26	21.0	4.58
4	18	21–36	28.6	3.85	11	17–40	25.7	7.52
3	13	28–43	35.4	4.88	1	28	–	–
2	4	27–38	34.0	5.36	6	25–50	37.8	10.13
<2	–	–	–	–	–	–	–	–

t*, time p.i. up to density 150 HU of cortex and 80–100 HU of medulla. For other abbreviations see Table 1

55 years this state was reached earlier with increasing flow rate. The (root mean square) deviation of the single values of t* in the older group was nearly twice as high as in the group of younger patients and the deviation increased by a factor of 5 with a flow decreasing from 8 ml/s to 2 ml/s.

The 15 patients that did nto reach the state described above showed no differences with different injection parameters. The state described above was more often reached with 100–150 ml contrast medium given with a flow of 3–4 ml/s than with 50–80 ml contrast medium applied with any different flow above 2 ml/s.

Liver

The mean increase of liver density combined with a visual overcontrasting of arterial or portal vessels was up to a thereshold of 80 HU in 67 cases, 90 HU in 36 cases and 100 HU in only 26 cases of 101 patients (Tables 5, 6). A mean density of 90 HU and more was only reached with flow rates of 3 ml/s and more. In many patients the mean density of the liver was at the start of the spiral CT above the aforementioned threshold. The deviation of single values was extremely high.

Table 4. Time-density study in spleen

Flow (ml/s)	Patient >55 years				Patient ≤55 years			
	n	t* (s)	$\bar{t}$ (s)	SD	*n*	t* (s)	$\bar{t}$ (s)	SD
6	4	19–22	19.6	1.81	4	15–18	16.05	2.12
4	24	18–40	24.0	3.09	15	15–35	21.7	6.39
3	10	24–37	26.0	3.24	4	21–30	25.3	4.51
2	5	16–35	25.0	7.07	5	30–53	38.1	11.28
<2	1	40	40	–	1	32	32	–

t*, time p.i. up to mean density of 100 HU and marked inhomogeneity (delta HU 40–60). For other abbreviations see Table 1

Table 5. Time-density study in the liver

Flow (ml/s)	Patient >55 years				Patient ≤55 years			
	n	t* (s)	$\bar{t}$ (s)	SD	*n*	t* (s)	$\bar{t}$ (s)	SD
6	2	24	24	0	4	14–24	20.5	4.43
4	10	22–47	33	8.23	10	18–36	26.0	5.78
3	7	23–37	29	5.13	3	21–32	27.0	5.56
2	3	18–31	23	7	5	19–52	30.0	13.18
<2	1	51	51	–	3	33–42	37.6	4.51

t*, time p.i. up to mean density of 80 HU. For other abbreviations see Table 1

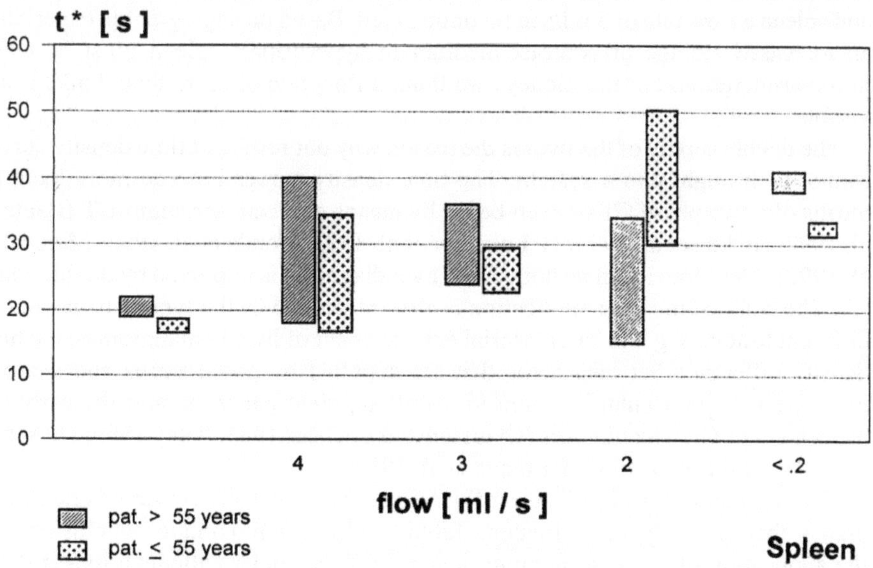

Fig. 3. Spleen: dependence on t*, flow rate and age of patients

Table 6. Time-density study in the liver

Flow (ml/s)	Patient >55 years				Patient ≤55 years			
	n	t* (s)	$\bar{t}$ (s)	SD	*n*	t* (s)	$\bar{t}$ (s)	SD
6	–	–	–	–	3	25–36	33.3	5.72
4	3	29–43	36.3	7.02	8	25–49	37.2	9.28
3	5	33–45	37.4	4.77	–	–	–	–
2	–	–	–	–	2	46–49	47.5	2.12
<2	–	–	–	–	–	–	–	–

t*, time p.i. up to mean density of 100 HU. For other abbreviations see Table 1

Discussion

In spiral CT the functional information derived from contrast medium flow is distributed over the examined volume. By using a protracted bolus injection a functional state shall be maintained during data acquisition over the examined region for a special pathologic process. These requirements lead to a compromise between start delay, a flow rate, necessary volume, and acquisition time. Our retrospective study shows a broad spectrum of individual differences. For the Aorta abdominalis, kidneys, and spleen a classification according to injection parameters is possible. This classification including the pancreas was already found and used for diagnosis by other authors (Bautz et al. 1992; Galanski et al. 1992; Honda et al. 1992; Lenz et al. 1993; Marchal et al. 1991, 1992; Zwicker et al. 1993). Whereas for the aorta abdominalis a flow rate of 2 ml/s is considered to be sufficient for the pancreas and spleen a flow rate of 3 ml/s in recommended. Based on angiographic experience an increased storage of contrast medium in hypertrophic spleen must be taken into consideration. For the kidneys we think a flow rate of more than 2 ml/s is advisable.

The double supply of the liver is the reason why our results of time density curves cannot be brought into a system. The time density curves become more lucid by means of a two phase CT or even better by means of a catheter angio-CT (Bautz et al. 1992; Heiken et al. 1993; Helmberger et al. 1993; Honda et al. 1992; Marchal et al. 1992). Therefore it can be hoped that liver diagnosis is improved by double spiral CT. The contrast medium application is also influenced by the typical behaviour of different lesions, e.g. the early arterial enhancement of liver hemangiomas, the high density difference between areas that are supplied by portal venes and necrotic metastases, hypovascular tumours in a well supplied pancreas, and the early enhancement of Grawitz tumours (Claussen and Lochner 1983; Foley 1989; Heiken et al. 1993; Krahe et al. 1985; Partanen et al. 1984).

The circulatory time is a factor influencing the time density curves of vessels and organs that can only be estimated. Table 7 allows approximate conclusions for the application of contrast medium in spiral CT. For older patients a longer delay (average 5 s) and a higher flow rate are reasonable.

Table 7. Recommended modalities of contrast medium administration

	Delay (s)	Volume (ml)	Flow (ml/s)
Aorta abdominalis	18–25	50–70	2
Kidney (parenchyma)	25–30	100 (60–120)	2–3
Spleen	25–30	80–120	3
Liver (global)	25–70	100–200	3–5

References

Bautz W, Helmberger H, Strotzer M, Lenz M, Gerhardt P (1992) Spiral CT in the Preoperative Evaluation of Vessels of the Upper Abdomen. In: Felix R, Langer M (eds.) Advances in CT II. Springer, Berlin p. 117–123

Claussen C, Lochner B (1983) Dynamische Computertomographie. Springer, Berlin Heidelberg New York

Foley WD (1989) Dynamic hepatic CT. Radiology 170:617–622

Galanski M, Prokop M, Chavan A, Schaefer CM, Nschelsky JE (1992) Spiral volumetric CT as a new screening tool for renal artery stenosis. Radiology 185:181

Heiken JP, Brink JA, Vannier MW (1993) Spiral (Helical) CT. Radiology 189:647–656

Helmberger H, Bautz W, Vogel U, Lenz M (1993) CT-Arterioportographie in Spiraltechnik zum Nachweis von Lebermetastasen. Fortschr. Roentgenstr. 158:410–415

Honda H, Matsuura Y, Onitsuka H, Murakami J, Kaneko K, Murayama S, Kanematsu T, Masuda K (1992) Differential Diagnosis of Hepatic Tumors (Hepatoma, Hemangioma and Metastasis) with CT: Value of Two-Phase Incremental Imaging. AJR 159:735–740

Kalender WA, Vock P, Polcin A, Soucek M (1990) Spiral-CT: Eine neue Technik für Volumenaufnahmen. I. Grundlagen und Methodik. Röntgenpraxis 43:323–330

Kloeppel R, Wittek W (1985) Beitrag zur Injektionstechnik des Kontrastmittelbolus für die Serien-CT. Radiol. diagn. 26:375–380

Krahe B, Harder T, Lackner K (1985) Seriencomputertomographie – Wertigkeit densitometrischer Messungen in der Diagnostik benigner und maligner Läsionen von Leber, Pankreas und Niere. Fortschr. Roentgenstr. 143:28–35

Lenz M, Wunderlich AP, Helmberger H, Gross M (1993) Spiral-CT bei Aortenaneurysmen. Fortschr. Roentgenstr. 158:393–404

Marchal G, Rigauts H, Baert AL (1991) Improved contrast enhancement of the pancreas by spiral scanning. Europ. J. Radiol. 11:221–224

Marchal G, Baert AL (1992) Dynamic CT of the liver. Radiologe 32:211–216

Partanen K, Soimakallio S, Kivimäki T, Syrjänen K, Kormano M (1984) Dynamic topography of the Contrast Enhancement of the Spleen. Europ. J. Radiol. 4:101–106

Zwicker C, Langer M, Langer R, Keske U (1993) Bolusapplikation in der Spiral-CT des Oberbauches. Akt. Radiol. 3:172–176

Maintained Image Quality and Dose Reduction with Spiral CT of the Thorax and Upper Abdomen

K. Cederlund

Introduction

Preoperative computed tomographic (CT) staging of lung cancer includes examination of the lung parenchyma, mediastinal structures, chest wall, liver and adrenals. With spiral CT the whole volume of interest can be covered with one spiral and one i.v. contrast injection. This reduces examination time and contrast medium dose. A third advantage with the spiral CT technique presented here, is reduction of radiation dose.

In this paper we discuss these different parameters and their influence on the diagnostic value of spiral CT in the staging of lungcancer.

Material and Methods

In 500 consecutive patients undergoing CT of the thorax since our Somatom Plus S was installed in September 1993, different scanning techniques have been used to reduce examination time, contrast medium and radiation dose with maintained sufficient image quality. The options offered by our Somatom Plus is a 32-s spiral scan with a maximum tube current of 210 mA, and table feed values of 1–20 mm/s.

Most patients were examined for lung cancer with the following method. With one spiral the distance from the lung apices to the caudal part of the liver was scanned. Depending on the individual distance, table feed was calculated. Slice thickness choosen was 10 mm and mA 210. The contrast medium given was 40 ml of Omnipaque (350 mg I/ml) and directly thereafter 50 ml Omnipaque (140 mg I/ml). Both were given with an automatic injector with 3.0 ml/s and the spiral started 35 s after the start of the contrast injection. All examinations were performed in maximum inspiration.

A minor group of patients were examined with two different techniques at the same session: A, single scanning with continous 10 mm slices; B, spiral scanning with 10 mm slice thickness and table feed 20 mm/s.

In this paper we present our experience in five selected patients using these techniques. To reduce differencies between technique A and B both were performed without contrast medium in these cases. All other parameters were similar in A and B. In order to demonstrate different subtle image quality parameters patients with normal parenchyma (Fig. 1), emphysema, bronchiectasis (Fig. 2), multiple meta-

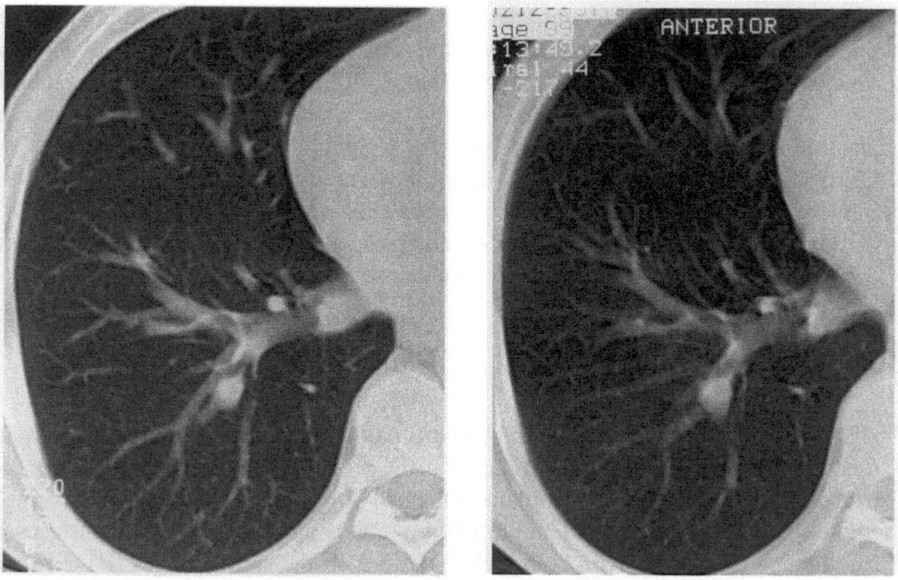

a b

Fig. 1a, b. Normal parenchyma. **a** Single slice 10 mm (technique A). **b** Spiral scan 10 mm (technique B). Tubular structures slightly less demarcated

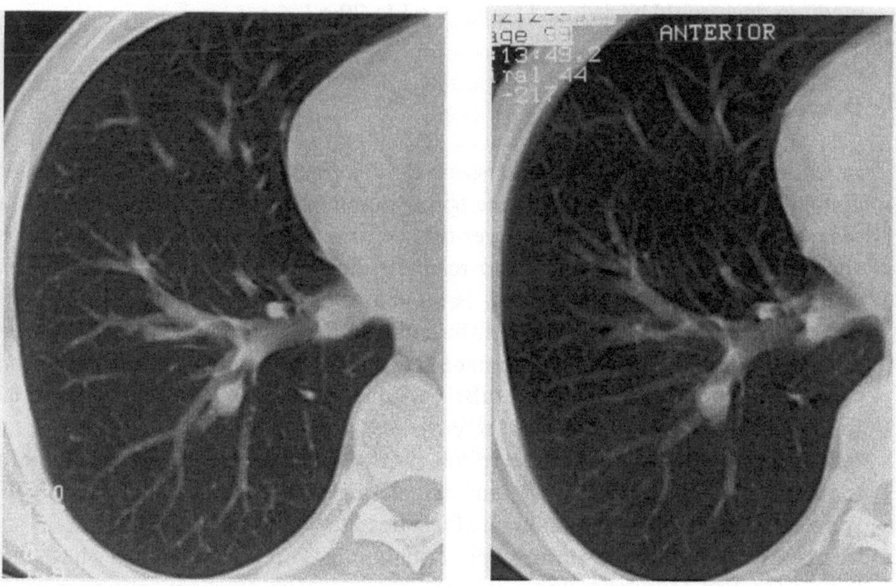

a b

Fig. 2a, b. Patient with bronchiectases. **a** Single slice 10 mm (technique A). Thickened bronchial walls sharply demarcated (*arrow*). **b** Spiral scan 10 mm (technique B). Bronchial walls slightly less demarcated (*open arrow*) stases (Figs. 3, 4) and tuberculosis respectively were selected. All images were reconstructed with a high spatial algorithm (AB 7541) printed on a 3M 969 HQ laser imager with lung window setting (W-2000, C-400). To compare spatial resolution with technique A and B the lung parenchyma images were reviewed at the same anatomical level with special regard to peripheral vessels (their number and sharpness) and to bronchial walls (their thickness and sharpness). All images were reviewed independently by three experienced chest radiologists.

The radiation dose and noise for A and B respectively was measured with a body phantom of cylindrical plexiglass with a diameter of 32 cm.

Results

The difference between technique A and B could be seen on the images as slightly decreased sharpness of small structures as the bronchial walls, especially when they run obliquely to the horizontal plane. This had no impact on the diagnostic value in the selected cases. In the patient with multiple very small (2–5 mm) metastases, all of them could be seen with both techniques but on the spiral images (B) they were less sharply demarcated.

The noise was measured in the phantom study (standard deviation in region of interest with an area of 3 cm) and did not increase with spiral-CT (B) despite reduction of the total mAs with 50%. The radiation dose centrally in the patient was calculated to be 6.2 mGy with technique A and 3.6 mGy with technique B. Examination time was reduced by approximately 50% with spiral technique. The contrast-medium dose could be reduced from 30 g I to 20 g I.

Discussion

In CT staging of lung cancer it is essential to examine the thorax and the upper abdomen. If this can be done with one spiral examination time, contrast medium and radiation dose are reduced. To cover this volume the table feed has to exceed the slice thickness which is known to result in decreased image quality [1–3]. To evaluate if sufficient image quality is maintained with this spiral CT technique in the staging of lung cancer the two different techniques in this study were choosen to demonstrate the largest range of image resolution. In technique B the table feed is twice the nominal slice thickness (also called pitch 2.0) but in routine praxis a table feed of 13–15 mm/s is sufficient to cover the volume of interest. Increasing table feed compared to slice thickness (pitch greater than 1.0) changes the shape of the section sensitivity profile (SSP) and effects the image quality. The examinations were usually free from breathing artifacts despite a breathholding time of 25–30 s in maximum inspiration during spiral scanning. Three experienced chest radiologists reached concensus that sufficient image quality for diagnostic purpose was maintained with spiral CT (B).

One of the great advantages with spiral CT staging of lung cancer is that the contrast-medium dose could be reduced from 30 g I to 20 g I with maintained contrast

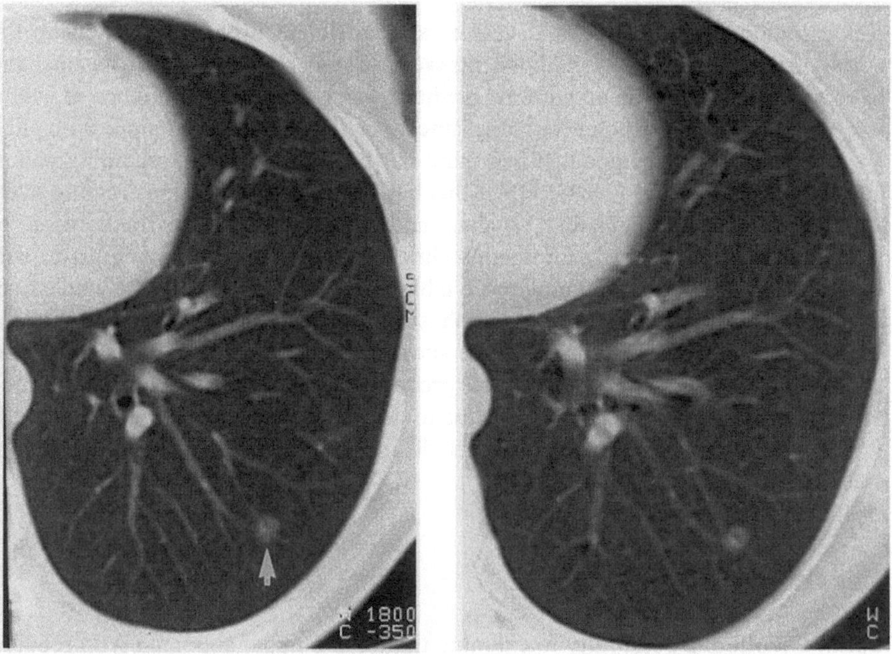

a b

Fig. 3a, b. Patient with metastases. **a** Single slice 10 mm (technique A). Metastases sharply demarcated (*arrow*). **b** Spiral scan 10 mm (technique B). Metastases also clearly seen

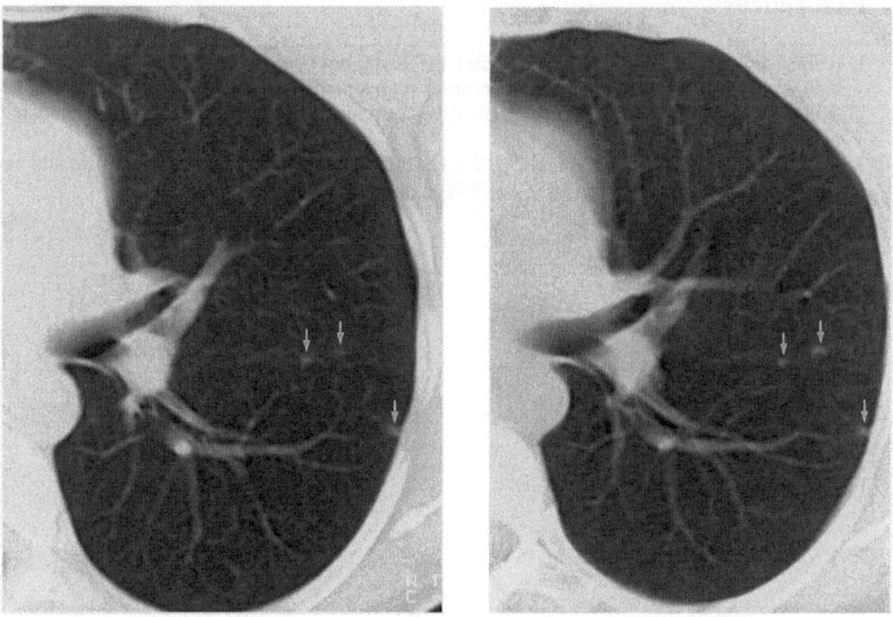

a b

Fig. 4a, b. Same patient as in Fig. 3. Three minimal metastases demonstrated with both techniques (*arrows*) concentration in the mediastinal vessels and sufficient liver enhancement in the portal phase. In the five selected patients we have not compared the mediastinal and liver image quality since no contrast medium was given. Our experience of evaluating the mediastinal structures in lung cancer staging using the technique with pitch greater than 1.0 is very good. When there has been any problem regarding pathology or possible partial volume effect this has been solved by reconstructing overlapping images from existing rawdata and without causing extra contrast or radiation dose and saving examination time. The liver images have been of sufficient quality with the commonly used table feed of 13 – 15 mm/s. The whole liver can be examined in the same contrast phase and we have choosen the portal phase which appears about 45–50 s after the start of the contrast injection. During this "delay time" the thorax is scanned. It is probably not advisable to increase the pitch more when doing a primary liver CT due to decreased image quality caused by different contrast conditions in the abdomen. This is important if liver resection is considered.

Conclusion

Spiral CT offers a possibility to examine thorax and upper abdomen with reduced examination time, contrast medium and radiation dose with maintained image quality.

References

1. Kalender WA, Seissler W, Klotz E, Vock P (1990) Spiral volumetric CT with single-breathhold technique, continous transport, and continous scanner rotation. Radiology 176 : 181 – 183
2. Kalender WA, Polacin A (1991) Physical performance characteristics of spiral CT scanning. Med Phys 18 : 910–915
3. Polacin A, Kalender WA, Marchal G (1992) Evaluation of section sensitivity profiles and image noise in spiral CT Radiology 185 : 29–352

Radiation Exposure in CT Using a Somatom Plus S

U. Golin, D. Borchardt, L. Heuser

Introduction

Computed tomography (CT) examinations play a central rôle in diagnostic radiology. The radiation dose delivered by CT differs greatly from that of projection radiography (Rothenberg and Pentlow 1992). Radiation dose in computed tomography depends on several parameters such as voltage, current, scan time, scan field, rotation angle, filtration, slice thickness and spacing. The final dose distribution in the patient is determined by size, shape and tissue of the patient himself.

In our study we used thermoluminescent dosimetry in an anthropomorphic phantom which provides the organ tissues and will be described below.

Purpose

The purpose of this study was the determination of the organ dosages for standard and helical CT examinations using a SOMATOM PLUS S.

Material and Methods

For the determination of radiation we used thermoluminescent dosimeters (TLD) (lithium-fluoride rods) which were calibrated prior to use. The evaluation of the TLDs was carried out with a 2000A/B-system (Harshaw). The TLDs were placed in special inserts in a humanoid phantom (Fig. 1). This phantom correspons to a complete body consisting of 35 slices. It is composed of skeleton, lung, and soft tissue equivalents. In order to measure the dose at the female breast and the male gonads TLDs were put into the tubes of "butterflies" (infusion sets). These were fixed at the corresponding place on the phantom. The phantom was placed on the patient's table. Special attention was paid to lay the phantom into the centre of the gantry. We performed standard examinations with a SOMATOM PLUS S for the head including the sinonasal cavity, the chest, and the abdomen with auto sequences. Spiral CT was carried out for the chest, the sinonasal cavity (SNC), and a combination of auto sequence and spiral CT simulating the evaluation of a renal lesion. In the latter case we performed 10-mm contiguous slices from the diaphragms to the end of the kidneys and added a 5 mm spiral CT of the kidneys. The CT of the SNC should simulate the search of midfacial fractures from the hard palate to the frontal sinuses. The lumbar

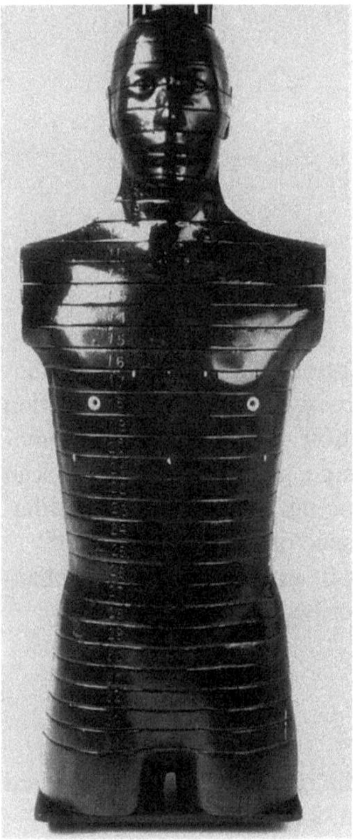

Fig. 1. Humanoid phantom

spinal CT examined the last three segments. The protocol of each examintion is to be seen at the table below (Table 1). Each examination was performed ten times, because our initial experiences had shown that single examinations produced data with great variation. This ten-fold exposure was carried out at least twice. The results were averaged. In our standard examinations we do not perform overlapping slices.

Results

For CT examinations of the head simulating the search for an intracranial lesion the mean radiation dose for the orbit was 4.8 mSv. Attention was paid that in choosing an appropriate gantry angulation the radiation beam avoided the orbit and the eye lens respectively. The CT of the SNC which included the orbit totally resulted in an orbit dose of 16.3/16.7 mSv (2-mm slices autosequence/2 mm spiral CT). The mean skull dose was 34.1 mSv. The details can be found in Table 2.

The 10-mm autosequence CT of the chest led to a mean dose of 22.1 mSv for the lung, 19.0 mSv for the skin, and 22.6 mSv for the female breast. In a 10-mm spiral CT of the chest the dosages were 20.8 mSv for the lung, 18.6 mSv for the skin, and 21.5 for the female breast. These data lay within the variation of the accurracy of the TLDs. A 5-mm spiral CT of the hilar region produced a mean radiation dose of

Table 1. Examination protocols

Examination protocol
CCT

Programme: Base orb

Posterior fossa	**Cerebrum**
Algorithm: standard	
Slice thickness: 3 mm	5 mm
mA: 500	500 mA
Scan time: 2 s	2 s
Table feed: 6 mm	8 mm
Number of scans: 5	11
Voltage: 120 kV	
Gantry tilt: –9°	

Examination protocol
Sinonasal cavitiy

Programme: Inner ear	Base orb
Autosequence	**Spiral**
Algorithm: high	High
Slice thickness: 2 mm	2 mm
mA: 170	165 mA
Scan time: 2 s	39 × 1 s
Table feed: 2 mm	Table speed: 2 mm/s
Number of scans: 38	
Voltage: 120 kV	
Gantry tilt: 0°	

Examination Protocol
Chest

Programme: Lung

Autosequence	**Spiral**
Algorithm: standard	Standard
Slice thickness: 10 mm	10 mm
mA: 145	145 mA
Scan time: 1 s	26 × 1 s
Table feed: 10 mm	Table speed: 10 mm/s
Number of scans: 27	
Voltage: 137 kV	
Gantry tilt: 0°	

Examination protocol
Abdomen

Programme: abdomen

Autosequence	**Spiral**
Algorithm: standard	Standard
Slice thickness: 10 mm	5 mm
mA: 210	210 mA
Scan time: 1 s	29 × 1 s
Table feed: 10 mm	Table speed: 5 mm/s
Number of scans: 27	
Voltage: 120 kV	
Gantry tilt: 0°	

Examination protocol
Spine

Programme: spine

Autosequence
Algorithm: standard
Slice thickness: 3 mm
mA: 440
Scan time: 2 s
Table feed 3 mm
Total number of scans: 26
Voltage: 137 kV
Gantry tilt: according to the angulation of the intervertebral disc space of the last three segments

Table 2. Head examinations (organ doses in mSv)

Examination	Cranial CT	Sinonasal cavity 2-mm spiral CT	Sinonasal cavity CT 2-mm slices
Orbit	4.8	16.7	16.3
Parotid gland	28.8	17.6	17.9
Submandibular gland	2.1	1.3	1.5
Thyroid	1.4	0.8	0.8
Cervical spinal cord	4.9	2.3	2.1
Cerebellum	28.4	15.6	15.2
Cerebrum	33.8	3.3	3.5
Skull	34.1	–	–

Table 3. Chest examinations (organ doses in mSv)

Examination	Chest CT autosequence (10 mm)	Spiral CT chest (10 mm)	Spiral CT hilar region (5 mm)
Thyroid	3.5	3.9	1.1
Cervical spinal cord	1.4	1.3	0.8
Thoracic spinal cord	17.2	17.5	13.8
Thoracic vertebra	17.5	17.6	12.5
Sternum	21.8	22.8	17.0
Lung	22.1	20.8	14.4
			6.2
Colon transversum	2.9	2.7	0.6
Kidney	1.8	1.9	0.5
Liver	4.3	3.5	0.9
Breast	22.6	21.5	15.3
Skin	19.0	18.6	–

Table 4. Abdominal and spinal examinations (organ doses in mSv)

Examination	Abdominal CT	Renal spiral CT	Upper abdominal CT with renal spiral CT	Lumbar spinal CT
Lumbar spinal cord	15.9	13.7	21.5	31.1
Lumbar vertebra	17.1	14.8	22.8	29.8
Lung	15.3	18.5	21.6	–
Kidney	23.9	18.0	39.3	11.3
Liver	24.1	21.6	41.5	4.4
Colon transversum	28.5	20.0	40.4	5.5
Rectum	18.8	0.7	1.2	3.7
Uterus	**15.3**	0.5	1.2	3.8
Ovary	19.4	0.7	1.2	10.7
Testis	6.4	0.6	0.8	1.9
Urinary vessel	14.9	6.5	1.2	4.2
Skin	26.6	24	45.4	9.7

14.4 mSv in the midparts of the lung and 6.2 mSv in the lower parts of the lung. The mean breast dose was 15.3 mSv. For further details we refer to Table 3.

In an abdominal CT with contiguous 10-mm slices from the diaphragm to the symphysis the mean dose for the lower parts of the lung was 15.3 mSv, for the liver 24.1 mSv, for the colon transversum/rectum 28.5/18.8 mSv, for the bladder 14.9 mSv, for the uterus 15.3 mSv, and for the female/male gonads 19.4/6.4 mSv. For the evaluation of a renal lesion the liver received a mean dose of 41.5 mSv, the kidneys 39.3 mSv, the colon transversum 40.4 mSv, and the skin 45.4 mSv. The single performance of a renal 5-mm spiral CT showed that for the directly exposed region the data of a single renal spiral CT and the abdominal CT can be added. The regions which are not directly in the radiation beam receive dosages which cannot be added because of the different scattered radiation.

Lumbar spinal CT with contiguous 3-mm slices produced a mean kidney dose of 11.3 mSv, a mean ovary dose of 10.7 mSv and mean uterus dose of 3.8 mSv. The details of the organ doses of abdominal CT examination including lumbar spine CT can be found in Table 4.

The spiral CT produces the same dosage as the standard CT with contiguous slices provided comparable parameters are used.

Discussion

There are a few studies dealing with the orbit or eye lens dose for computed tomography of the head. The dosages range between 2.3 mSv for females and 3.0 mSv for males respectively (Panzer and Zankl 1993) and 5.58 mSv (Yeoman et al. 1992). In all these studies a direct exposure of the orbit was avoided. With our orbit dose of 4.8 mSv we lie within to normal range. Yeoman et al. (1992) found that there is a great difference of dose if the beam angulation passes through the eye (43.44 mSv). The severity of posterior fossa artifacts was not significantly different. Another study (Torizuka et al. 1992) showed that the change of the baseline from the orbitomeatal line to a line parallel to the hard palate decreased the radiation dose to the lens from 12.7 cGy to 0.274 cGy without loss of information.

In our investigation a contiguous 2-mm slice CT or a 2-mm spiral CT for the evaluation of midfacial fractures produced an orbit dose of 16.7/16.3 mSv. The spiral CT with the possibility of reconstruction offers a dose reduction because a second coronal CT is not necessary.

In our cranial CT as well as in the chest CT the dose for the thyroid is slightly higher than the doses in the literature (Panzer and Zankl 1988; Nishizawa et al. 1991), whereas the lung dose is approximately the same [22.1 mSv in our study as compared to 19.6 mSv (Nishizawa et al. 1991) and 21.6 mSv (Panzer and Zankl 1988)]. Nishizawa et al. (1991) reported a quite low dose of 15.9 mSv for the female breast. In our study we found 22.6 mSv for contiguous slices and 21.5 mSv for spiral CT; this is comparable to the dose of 23.4 mSv of Panzer and Zankl (1988).

In a 10-mm contiguous abdominal CT the liver received a dose of 24.1 mSv comparable to the 27.77 mSv of Nishizawa et al. (1991). Usual standard CT examinations of the upper abdomen involve a prior native CT series and a series with the administration of contrast media. Therefore the organ dose may rise considerably as to be seen in our example of the simulation of the evaluation of a renal lesion.

We found a relatively high ovary dose during a pelvis CT (19.4 mSv) as compared to other studies [15.14 mSv in Nishizawa et al. (1991) and 16.9 mSv in Panzer and Zankl (1988)]. This also applies to the male gonads. In our series we found a dose of 6.4 mSv, whereas other studies report doses below 1.4 mSv (Panzer and Zankl 1988; Nishizawa et al. 1991).

Following the recommendation of the German Society of Radiology and the German Society of Medical Physics an exact determination of the embryo dose should be undertaken if the uterus dose exceeds 20 mSv (see Panzer and Zankl 1988). A field study in Germany showed that in 50% of all cases of pregnant women undergoing a pelvic CT the embryo dose was higher than 20 mSv (Panzer et al. 1988). In our study the uterus dose of 15.3 mSv is below this threshold.

For a standard CT of the lumbar spine examining the last three segments we found an uterus dose of 3.8 mSv. It should be noted that the mean ovary dose was relatively high (10.7 mSv). We did not find any comparable data in the literature dealing with the dose measurement for a spinal CT.

Conclusion

Our study shows that the mean organ doses with our SOMATOM PLUS S compare with the literature. The uterus dose of 15.3 mSv for an pelvic CT is clearly below the mean average.

It is important to note that when comparable parameters are used (such as the same volume and the same milliampere second value) spiral CT produces the same doses as standard CT with single contiguous slices, as to be seen in our examples of the chest CT and the sinonasal cavity CT.

In order to minimize the radiation dose the ALARA (as low as reasonably achievable) principle of X-ray examinations should also be observed for CT examinations.

References

1. Nishizawa K, Maruyama T, Takayama M, Okada M, Hachiya J-I, Furuya Y (1991) Determinations of organ doses and effective dose equivalents from computed tomographic examination. Br J Radiol 64 : 20 – 28
2. Panzer W, Scheurer C, Drexler G, Regulla D (1988) Feldstudie zur Ermittlung von Dosiswerten bei der Computertomographie. 149 : 534 – 538
3. Panzer W, Zankl M (1993) Die Strahlenexposition des Patienten bei computertomographischen Untersuchungen. Röntgenpraxis 46 : 15 – 18
4. Rothenberg LN, Pentlow KS (1992) Radiation dose in CT. Radio Graphics 12 : 1225 – 1243
5. Torizuka T, Hayakawa K, Satoh Y, Tanaka F, Saitoh H, Okuno Y, Ogura A, Nakayama Y, Konishi J (1992) High-resolution CT of the temporal bone: a modified baseline. Radiology 184 : 109 – 111
6. Yeoman LJ, Howarth L, Britten A, Cotterill A, Adam EJ (1992) Gantry angulation in brain CT: dosage implications, effect on posterior fossa artifacts, and current international practice. Radiology 184 : 113 – 116

Optimization of the Irradiation of the Splenic Region by CT Angiography

W. WITTMOSER, J. DUNST, L. KEILHOLZ, K. MAATSCH, P. WEBER

Introduction

The irradiation of the splenic region in patients with Hodgkin's disease or non-Hodgkin's lymphomas is complicated by the great variability in shape and location of the spleen and the lymphatic vessels (especially the nodi lymphatici pancreatici superiores) beside the splenic artery. On the other side the tolerance dose of the kidneys ($TD_{5/5} = 23$ Gy for the total organ, EMAMI et al. 1991) is quite low in comparison to the intented dose of 30–40 Gy in the reference point. As a matter of fact irradiation fields must be collimated individually to avoid unnecessary irradiation of the left kidney. Therefore we have looked for a suitable imaging system that permits exact treatment planning.

Materials and Methods

Patients planned to be irradiated in the splenic region are examined as a matter of routine with spiral computed tomography SIEMENS SOMATOM PLUS-S with ANGIO-CT software to visualize the interesting structures. We choose a slice thickness of 2 or 3 mm and a table feed of 4 or 5 mm with a current of 180 mA or 210 mA at maximal spiral length. The procedure is made at medium depth of inspiration. To improve the image quality, stopping of respiration is necessary, though it is quite educative to see the respiratory shift of the organs. Our favourite contrast medium is SCHERING OMNIPAQUE 300, that is less aggressive than the 350 type. We recommend a contrast medium flow of 4 ml/s and a total volume of 120 ml with a delay time of 15–17 s and the injection of normal saline afterwards. For to achieve optimal image quality, a remote controlled injector is necessary – we use an ULRICH XD 5500. It may also be useful (see later) to inject 20 or 30 ml contrast medium prior to the examination procedure for the imaging of the renal pelvis.

The received tomograms must be firstly edited erasing some of the bony elements (for instance the ribs) to avoid a disturbing superposion with the structures to be imaged. In contrast to diagnostic purposes we leave the spine and parts of the ribs on the right hand side to obtain landmarks (Fig. 1a–b). Then the angiograms are evaluated with the maximum-intensity-projection-algorithm (MIP).

Analogous to this proceeding, the first simulation is carried out injecting contrast medium to image the pelvis of the kidneys. Then the radiographs are made in the typical geometry in anterior-posterior and posterior-anterior direction (Fig. 2a).

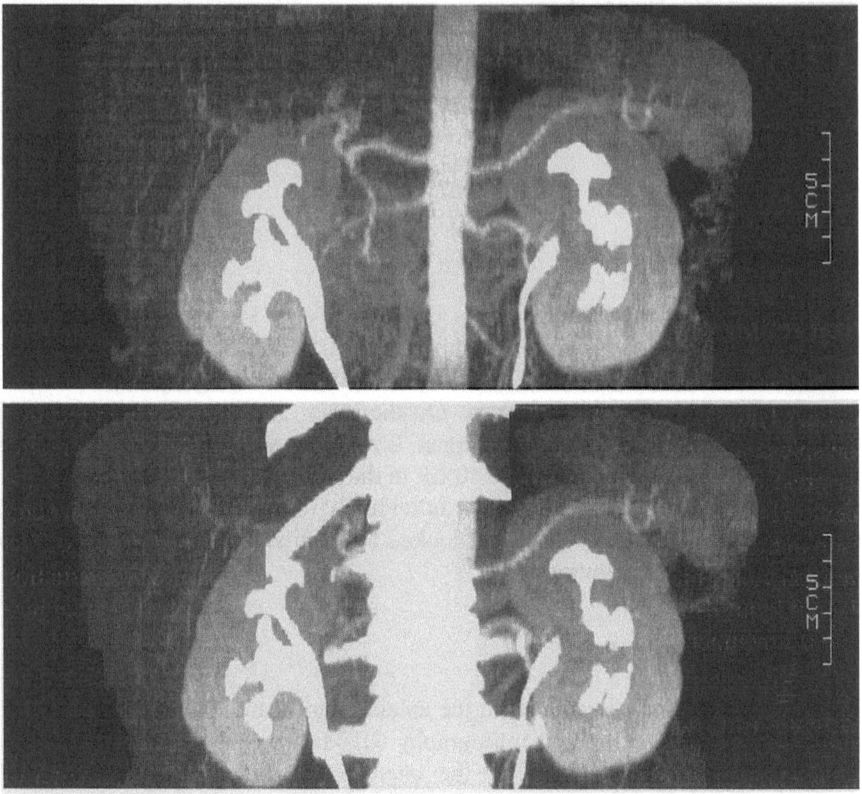

a

b

Fig. 1a–b. Computed tomography angiograms editted in different ways. **a** Erasing all bones to concentrate on the vascular system. **b** Leaving parts of the ribs and the spine for treatment planning purposes

After that the CT reconstructions (Fig. 2c) are compared with the images from the localization at the analog system SIEMENS SUBTRASKOP to mark the main structures (usually: spleen, splenic artery, left kidney) on the localization films as a pattern for constructing individual shielding blocks.

As the last step, the moulden blocks are fitted in and the contour is marked on the patient's skin during the second localization.

Theoretical Remarks

Two points should be discussed when CT angiography is applied for treatment planning purposes: Images achieved from the Angio-CT software (and other programs like 3D) are parallel projections, comparable with the observer's-eye-view from endless distance in treatment planning systems. To construct individual blocks exactly, the beam divergence must be regarded using the beam's-eye-view. On the other side, the interesting structures are located in a thin slice of about 10 cm or less

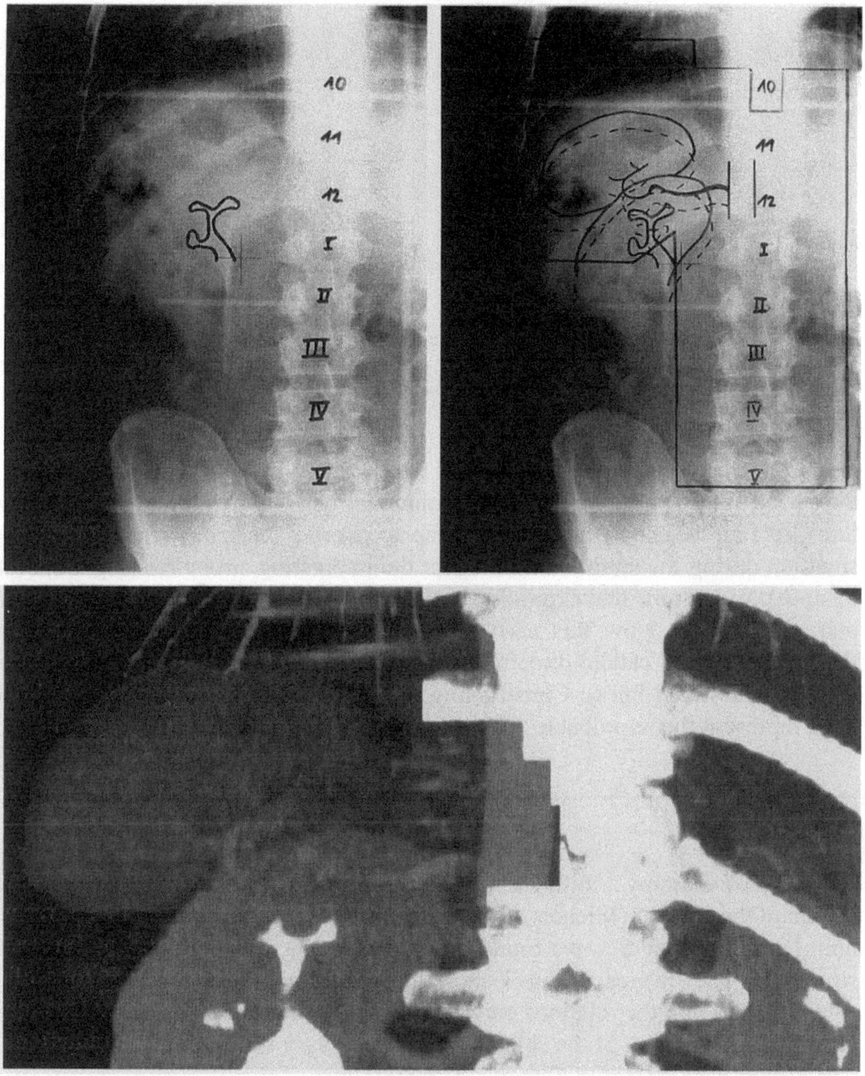

a b c

Fig. 2a–c. A 34-year-old man with Hodgkin's disease stage IIIA. **a** Posterior-anterior radiograph from first simulation with partially marked pelvis of the left kidney. **b** Same radiograph after transferring the interesting structures from the computed tomographic angiogram in **c** and marking the contour of the block. *Unbroken* (*broken*) lines using the kidney pelvis (spine) as reference structure

in comparison to a focus skin distance (irradiation geometry) of about 120 cm. That is the reason why the deviation due to this geometrical problem is minimal and amounts less than 1 cm.

Greater differences between the images from the simulation and the angiograms are explained with different respiratory behaviors: During localization or irradiation, the patient respirates plainly and continually in contrast to the spiral CT exa-

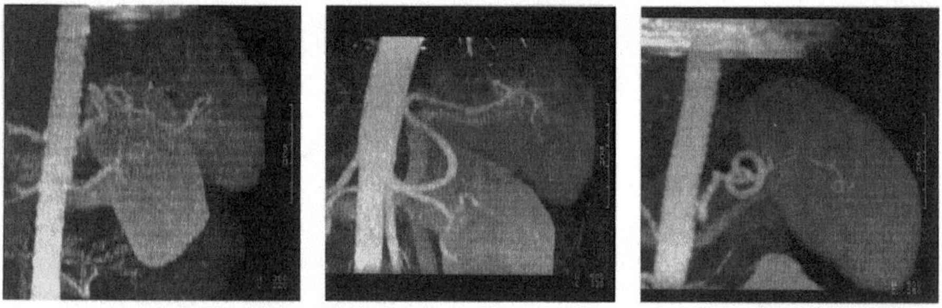

a b c

Fig. 3. Variations of the splenic artery and the location of spleen and left kidney. The possibility of shielding the upper part of the left kidney is quite different as demonstrated in three typical cases. Notice the varied tortuosity of the splenic artery

mination, where a deeper inspiration is necessary to be able to stop respiration for the period of the spiral. We solve this problem by using two different reference structures: At first we match the two radiographs covering the spine – that represents the situation during the spiral – and transfer the interesting structures (Fig. 2b, broken contour). We assume that expiration induces in first approximation an organ shift in cranial direction. Now this shift is simulated by moving the radiograph from the localization in caudal direction to match the marked pelvis of the left kidney (Fig. 2b, unbroken lines). Constructing the block contour we suppose the broken lines represent the unprobable "worst case" of inspiration during irradiation.

Results

"All texts of anatomy... follow a fairly uniform pattern in illustrating the vascularization of the spleen" (Michels 1955). Michels criticized this fact, and we agree with him. During our studies, we found great topographical varieties of the interesting structures. The images in Fig. 3 show three different, representative runs of the splenic artery and the relations between the spleen and the left kidney. This makes clear that the imaging of the splenic area is necessary for optimized irradiation.

Conclusion

CT angiography provides images with a high quality, the invasivity is minimal and the examination time short – normally less than 25 min to receive the reconstructions. Another advantages to be mentioned is the high information of a three-dimensional data set – the examination can also be used for other diagnostic or planning purposes – and the easy access to CT for radiotherapists.

Integration of the MIP algorithm in modern three-dimensional treatment planning systems would be surely useful for to allow visualization of vessels and highly perfused structures during radiotherapy planning procedures. In the future the problem of respiratory deviations will be possibly solved by ultra fast CTs.

References

Abrams HL (1971) Splenic Arteriography. In: Abrams HL (Ed) Angiography. Little, Brown and Company, Boston, p 1003–1027
Emami B, Lyman J et al. (1991) Tolerance of Normal Tissue to Therapeutic Irradiation. Int. J. Radiation Oncology Biol. Phys. 21 : 109–122
Kalender W, Polacin A et al. (1992) Current Status and New Perspectives in Spiral CT. In: Felix R, Langer M (Eds) Advances in CT II. Springer Berlin Heidelberg New York, p 87–94
Kalender W (1993) Quo vadis CT? CT im Jahr Zweitausend. electromedica 61 : 30–39
von Lanz T, Wachsmuth W (1993) Praktische Anatomie Teil 6: Bd.2. Bauch. Springer, Berlin Heidelberg New York
Michels NA (1955) Blood Supply and Anatomy of the Upper Abdominal Organs. Lippincott, Philadelphia Montreal, p 201–235
Napel S, Marks MP et al. (1992) CT Angiography with Spiral CT and Maximum Intensity Projection. Radiology 185 : 607–610
Perez CA, Brady LW (1987) Principles and Practice of Radiation Oncology. Lippincott, Philadelphia
Rubin GD, Napel S et al. (1992) Spiral CT creates 3-D neuro, body angiograms. Diagnostic Imaging Aug. 1992 : 66–75
Rubin GD, Dake MD et al. (1993) Three-dimensional Spiral CT Angiography of the Abdomen: Initial Clinical Experience. Radiology 186 : 147–152
Siemens Medical Systems, Inc. (1993) The Clinical Benefits of: CT Angiography. CT Marketing Devision Iselin, New Jersey

Spiral CT in Treatment Planning of Intraoperative Radiotherapy

A. Nilles, C. Ehritt-Braun, G. Bruggmoser, N. Hodapp, H. Frommhold, M. Langer

Introduction

Gastric carcinoma is a malignancy with an unfavorable prognosis due to a high rate of regional failure after standard therapy of surgical resection. External beam radiation is given only in palliative intent. High doses to control neoplastic disease cannot be achieved in the upper abdomen without significant normal tissue toxicity.

Intraoperative radiotherapy (IORT) offers a reasonable alternative to treat gastric cancer in delivering high doses of radiation to the regional lymph node area without damaging the surrounding tissue including the radiosensitive organs, for instance bile duct, bowel, spinal cord, kidneys, adrenal glands and smaller vessels. Abe – the first in using electrons in patients with advanced gastric carcinoma – observed a significant increase in survival rate and decrease in local recurrent tumor growth in patients with advanced tumor stage treated with additional IORT compared to similar stages treated by surgery alone [1–3]. Quality assurance is important in such a treatment as effect and success have to be verified quantitatively. Thus the best imaging techniques available are mandatory for a satisfactory documentation of the treated volume.

Before surgery tumor site and size and the patient's anatomy have to be known to plan the IORT procedure including shape and size of the cone to be used and the estimated penetration depth of the radiation. In using spiral computed tomography (SCT) and 3-D reconstruction of the coeliac trunc with its major vessels these questions can be answered easily and sufficiently [7].

Material and Method

From February 1991 to February 1994, 36 patients with gastric cancer received intraoperative electron beam radiotherapy (IORT) after gastrectomy or distal resection and extended lymphadenectomy. The IORT field included: tumor bed, coeliac trunc, common hepatic artery and the regional lymphatic drainage area of compartment II. To plan the IORT procedure spiral CT of the abdomen with 3-D reconstruction of the visceral vessels in frontal and sagittal view was performed (Table 1). The appropriate target volume including cone size and electron energy could be planned with regard to the spinal cord, pancreas, bile-duct, kidneys and adrenal glands (Figs. 1, 2). Special shaped cones could be constructed in a preplanning phase before surgery, lead shielding could be provided if necessary.

Table 1. Scan parameters for spiral computed tomography

I.	Slice	5 mm
	Table feed	5 mm
	Increment	5 mm
	Time	2 × 1 s/slice
	Voltage	120 kV
	Power	165 mAs
II.	Flow rate	3 ml/s
	Volume	80 ml
	Start delay	20 s

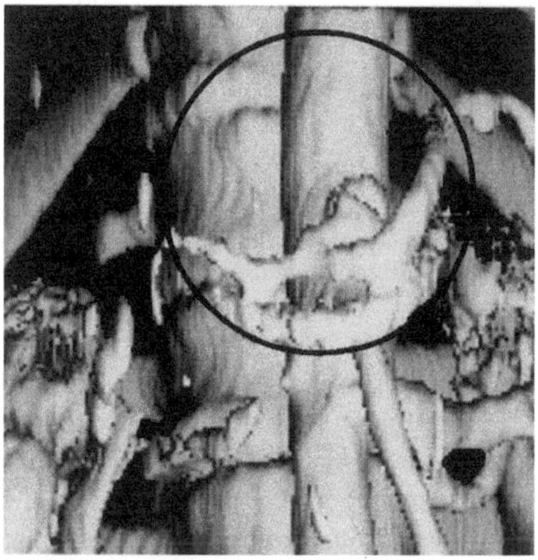

Fig. 1. Intraoperative radiotherapy preplanning of the target volume (*circle*) in the frontal view of a 3-D reconstruction from spiral computed tomography

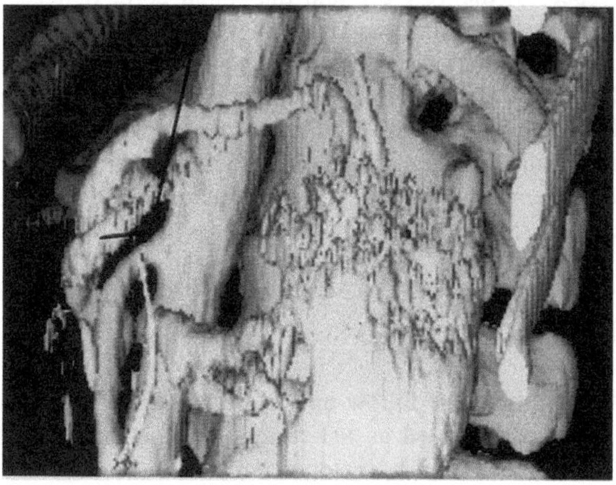

Fig. 2. Intraoperative radiotherapy preplanning of cone position in the sagittal view of a 3-D reconstruction from spiral computed tomography

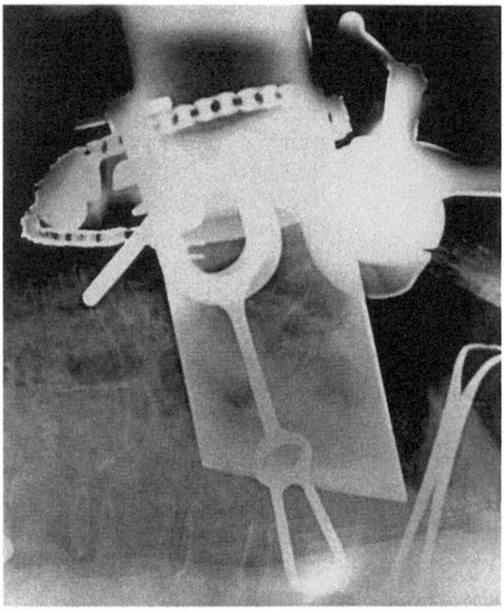

Fig. 3. Visualisation of the positioned cone by lateral X-ray photograph during surgery before intraoperative radiotherapy

Surgery generally took place in the IORT operation theater with the installed electron linear accelerator (Siemens Mevatron KE) providing electron energies ranging from 6–21 MeV. After tumor resection, extended lymphadenectomy of compartment I and II and exclusion of lymph node metastasis in compartment III [6] – suspicious lymph nodes were histologically evaluated during surgery – the actual situation was compared with the pre-planning. Radiotherapist, surgeon and physicist together chose the appropriate cone and electron energy. The positioned cone was visualized by a lateral X-ray radiography to control its actual position with respect to the vertebra and the spinal cord, if necessary corrections were made (Fig. 3). The cone was fixed with two separate holders to prevent its dislocation during the docking maneuver (Fig. 4). After the patient's transfer to the linear accelerator the alignement of the treatment head with the cone was done via a touchless laser docking system [5]. During the IORT procedure, a video camera focused on the irradiated area displayed the actual situation, documented by a video printer. After removing the cone, the field margins were marked with titanium clips for later control.

Results

During the close follow-up we observed no complications related to IORT. From 36 patients treated as listed above 22 patients are alive without tumor disease. 14 have died, eight developed peritoneal spread, four metastatic disease, one died perioperatively, and only one showed local recurrent disease within the clip-marked IORT target volume as displayed by spiral CT examination at the site of left macro-

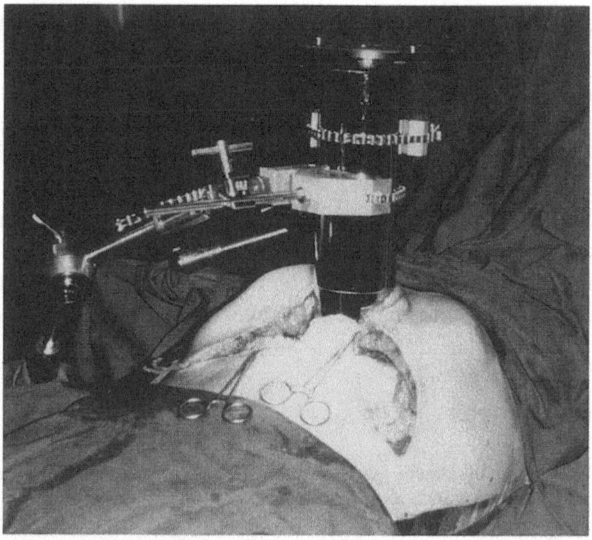

Fig. 4. Cone ready for irradiation fixed with two separate holders

scopic disease (R_2 resection). This case revealed 25 Gy not to be a sufficient dose for R_2 resection with remaining macroscopic disease. In these cases higher doses or other treatment schedules have to be considered.

Discussion

Spiral CT offers undeniable advantages: its fast performance and reduced amount of contrast media qualifies this method for the elder patients as well. The continuous examination and independence of breath excursions provide excellent diagnostic statements. The possibility of 3-D reconstruction of visceral vessels reveals an excellent means to plan IORT: cone size and -shape can be predicted and special irregular shaped cones can be constructed before surgery; the target volume can be determined and discussed with the surgeons in advance; the electron energy and consecutively penetration depth can be evaluated before treatment.

The presentation of the resulting dose distribution together with the 3-D-reconstructed organs is of less importance. The reason therefore is, that density inhomogenities play a rather minor role and that only in a few cases field matching is necessary. Nevertheless the abilities of the "beams-eye-view" module of a modern 3-D treatment planning system should be used [4]. Helpful hints when choosing the angle for beam incidence or planning the individual beam shape can be gained with the help of this tool. Although the preoperative CT cannot reveal the actual situation during surgery it represents a good approximation and its use may reduce the preirradiation setup time considerably. The verification of the cone position is facilitated by comparing the intraoperative radiographs with digitally reconstructed radiographs (DRR) from corresponding directions, calculated from the 3-D-CT-matrix with the help of the therapy planing system.

Conclusion

Spiral CT offers two decisive possibilities within one examination: perfect and quick diagnostic evaluation and contrast medium reduction and by means of 3-D reconstruction a good method to plan IORT. Planning tools of modern 3-D therapy planning systems as "beam's -eye-view" or DRR can be very helpful.

References

1. Abe M, Takahashi M, Yabumoto E, Onoyama Y, Torizuka K, Tobe T, Mori K (1975) Techniques, Indications and Results of Intraoperative Radiotherapy of advanced cancers. Radiology 116:693–702
2. Abe M, Takahashi M, Yabumoto E, Adachi H, Yoshii M, Mori K (1980) Clinical Experiences with Intraoperative Radiotherapy of Locally Advanced Cancers. Cancer 45:40–48
3. Abe M, Shibamoto Y, Takahashi M, Manabe T, Tobe T, Inamoto T (1987) Intraoperative Radiotherapy in Carcinoma of the Stomach and Pancreas. World J. Surg. 11:459–464
4. Goitein M, Abrams M, Rowell D, Pollari H, Wiles J (1983) Multi-Dimensional Treatment Planning: II:Beam's Eye-View Back Projection, and Projection Through CT Sections. Int. J. Radiat. Oncol. Biol. Phys. 9:789–797
5. Hogstrom KR, Boyer AL, Shiu AS, Ochran TG, Kirsner SM, Krispel F, Rich T (1990) Design of Metallic Electron Beam Cones for an Intraoperative Therapy Linear Accelerator. Int. J. Radiat. Oncol. Biol. Phys. 18:1223–1232
6. Japanese Research Society for Gastric Cancer (1981) The General Rules for the Gastric Cancer Study in Surgery and Pathology. Jpn. J. Surg. 11:127–139
7. Rubin GD, Dake MD, Napel SA, McDonnell CH, Jeffrey RB (1993) Three-dimensional Spiral-CT Angiography of the Abdomen: Initial Clinical Experience. Radiology 186:147–152

Spiral CT: In Vitro Measurement of Stenoses

G. WITTENBERG, R. SCHINDLER, A. TRUSEN, G. SCHULTZ, M. JENETT, M. KELLNER, A. TSCHAMMLER, D. HAHN

Introduction

Since the introduction of continuous volume scanning within short time using spiral computed tomography (SCT), it is possible to get three-dimensional (3-D) reconstructions of the vessels without superimposed structures in all required projections [1, 6]. First clinical applications of the less invasive SCT-angiography demonstrate a good morphological correlation with arterial vessel visualization [2–5]. Also first in-vitro measurement of eccentric stenoses using SCT show a high correlation ($r = 0.89 - 0.99$) between real and measured degrees of stenosis [7]. In this study we evaluate the influence of different SCT parameters, like slice thickness, table speed and reconstruction interval on the measured degrees of stenosis.

Materials and Methods

Phantoms

The phantoms were made out of wax with a density about –100 HU. As the inner lumen of the phantoms 4, 6 and 8 mm were choosen similiar to the great branches of the abdominal aorta. Concentric stenoses with a lumen narrowing of 30%, 50%, 70% and 90% were simulated. The length of the stenoses was 3 mm.

The phantoms were filled with diluted contrast agent with a density of 220 HU comparible to the density of the abdominal aorta after i. v. administration of contrast medium. During the examination the models were placed into a covered water basin aligned in x-, y- or z-direction.

Spiral CT

All examinations were done on a Somatom Plus Scanner with a 24-s SCT option. The slice thickness was 1 mm, 2 mm and 5 mm. The table speed was varied between 1 mm/s and 5 mm/s. Using a slice thickness of 2 mm the table speed was increased up to a pitch of 2. For image reconstruction the standard algorithm and a reconstruction interval of 1 mm or 2 mm was used. For the examinations 120 kV and 125 mA were used.

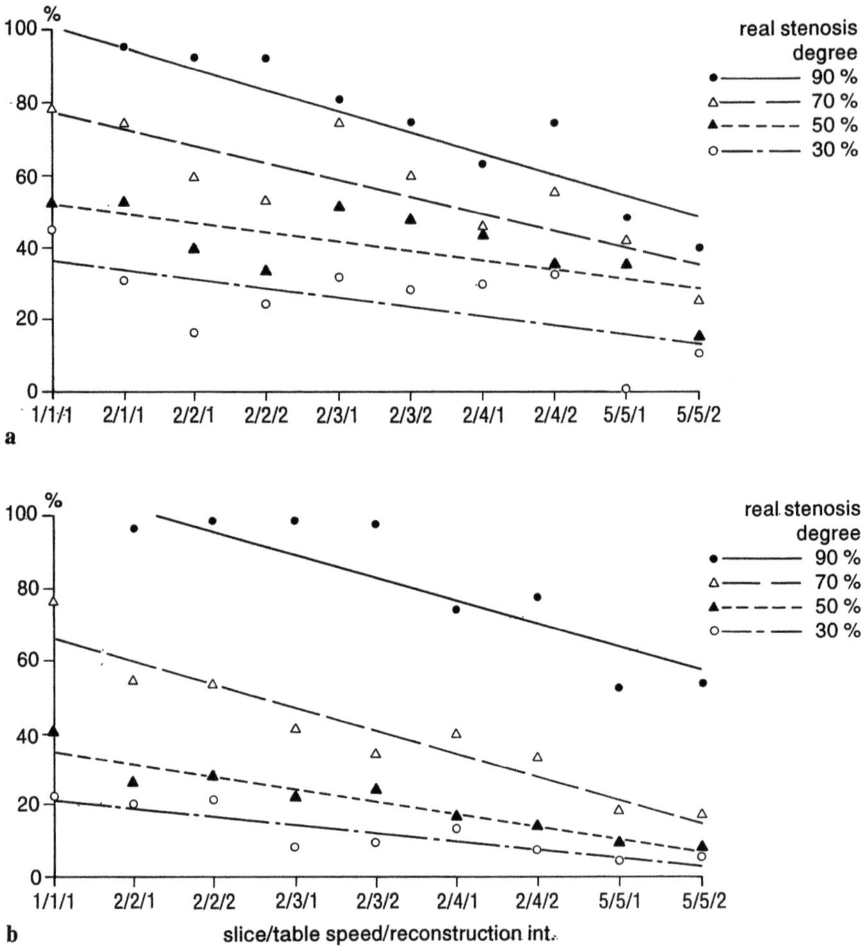

Fig. 1a, b. The 4-mm models aligned in z-direction: results obtained for measurement technique **a** and visual assessment **b** of stenosis degrees with increasing spiral computed tomography parameters

An other purpose of the study was to find a reconstruction algorithm with the best correlation between real and measured stenoses degrees by changing the SCT parameters. For image reconstruction soft detail, soft, standard and high algorithm was evaluated.

We also evaluated the tube current in order to improve the stenoses detection. The tube current was changed between 85 mA, 125 mA, 165 mA and 210 mA. Slice thickness and table speed was also increased for the measurements. Image reconstruction was performed by using the standard algorithm.

Table 1. Results of determination of stenosis degrees by means of measurement techniques in 6-mm models aligned in x-direction

Slice/table speed/reconstruction interval	Linear correlation coefficient	Regression straight line equation
1/1/1	$r = 0.9987$	$y = 0.9435\,x + 10.6$
2/1/1	$r = 0.9947$	$y = 0.7910\,x + 21.7$
2/1/2	$r = 0.9760$	$y = 0.5640\,x + 26.7$
2/2/1	$r = 0.9623$	$y = 0.9302\,x + 17.2$
2/2/2	$r = 0.9919$	$y = 0.9534\,x + 13.5$
2/3/1	$r = 0.9940$	$y = 0.8217\,x + 26.4$
2/3/2	$r = 0.9802$	$y = 1.0927\,x + 6.5$
2/4/1	$r = 0.9708$	$y = 0.8431\,x + 27.6$
2/4/2	$r = 0.9975$	$y = 0.8113\,x + 29.0$
5/5/1	$r = 0.9838$	$y = 0.8777\,x + 25.3$
5/5/2	$r = 0.9747$	$y = 0.8168\,x + 30.9$

Evaluation of the Data

Determination of the stenoses degrees was carried out by:

1. Electronic lumen width measurement and/or interpolation with the help of single split-images and computation of the degrees of stenosis.
2. Visual assessment of the degree of stenosis with three-dimensional reconstructions (512 matrix, treshold 100 HU) by five radiologists. For the statistical analysis the mean degree of stenosis was calculated.

For statistical analysis linear correlation coefficients and regression straight line equations were used.

To show the influence of the SCT parameters concerning the detection of the stenoses degrees in a similiar way compensating straight lines were drawn through the obtained results for different values of slice thickness, table speed and reconstruction interval.

Results

Slice Thickness, Table Speed, Reconstruction Interval

By aligning the phantoms in z-direction the stenoses degrees were undercalculated/underestimated with increasing slice thickness, table speed and reconstruction interval. The greatest effects were seen in the smallest models, the 4-mm phantoms. Using a slice thickness of 5 mm (pitch = 1) the 90% stenosis of the 4-mm phantom was estimated to a stenosis degree of 50%. In Fig. 1 the results for the 4-mm phantoms for both determination techniques are shown.

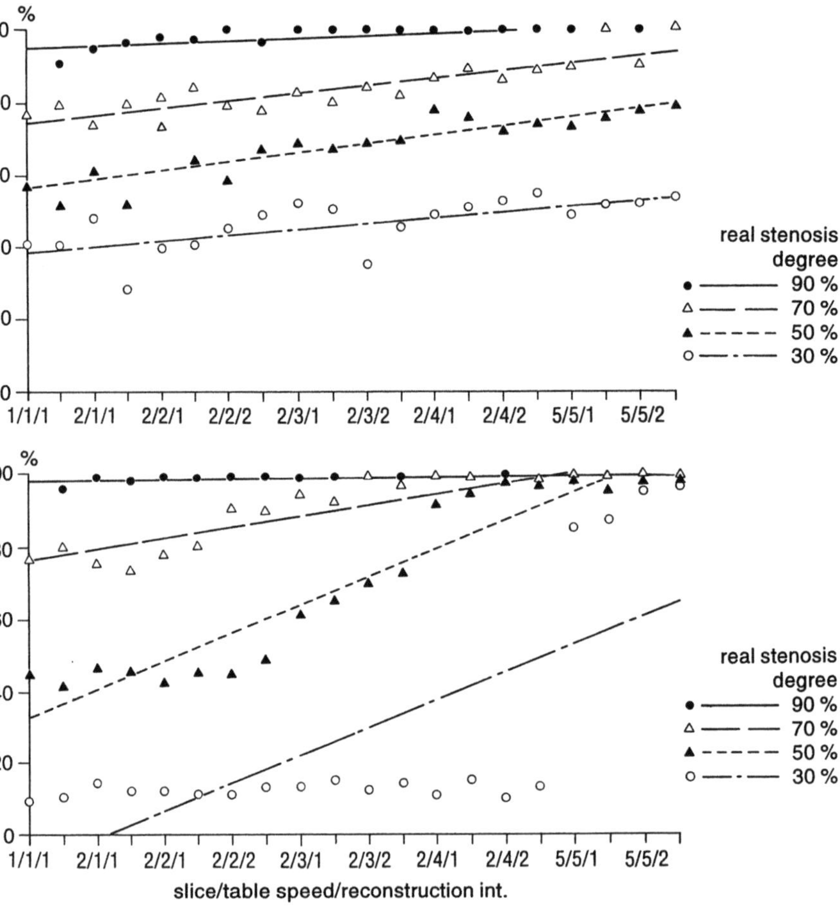

a b

Fig. 2a, b. The 6-mm models aligned in x- and y-direction: results obtained for measurement technique **a** and visual assessment **b** of stenoses degrees with increasing spiral computed tomography parameters

By aligning the models in x- or y- direction the stenoses degrees were overcalculated/overestimated with increasing SCT parameters. The visual assessment of the 30% stenosis of the 4-mm model resulted in a degree of stenosis of 100% by using 5 mm as slice thickness (pitch = 1). In Fig. 2 the results of the 6-mm phantoms are demonstrated for this alignment.

The linear correlation coefficients varied between $r = 0.8$ and $r = 0.99$, but the regression straight line equation deteriorate with increasing of slice thickness, table speed and reconstruction interval. For example the results of the 6-mm phantoms aligned in x-direction are shown in Table 1.

Reconstruction Algorithm

Performing image reconstruction using standard algorithm resulted in the smallest increase/decrease – depending on the model alignment – of the compensating line.

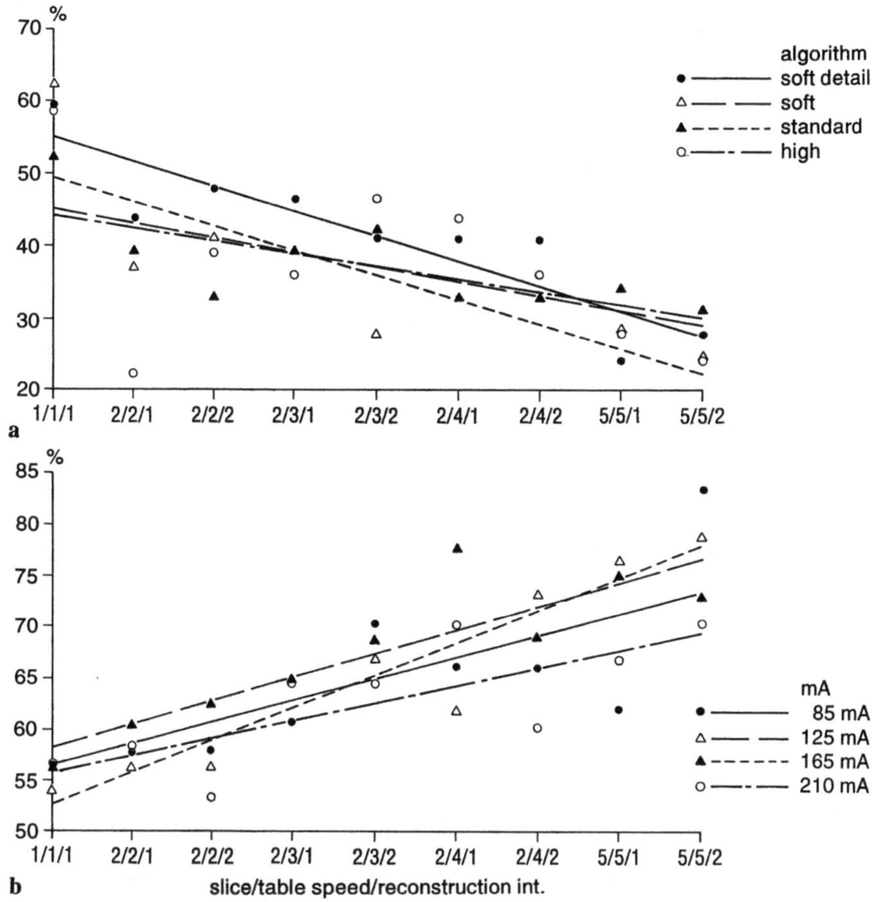

Fig. 3a, b. Results of determination of stenosis degree using different algorithms for image reconstruction **a** or different tube currents for data acquisition **b**.
a Algorithm: a model aligned in z-direction (stenosis degre: 50%) was examined with increasing spiral computed tomography (CT) parameters. The smallest decrease of the compensating straight line is seen using standard algorithm for image reconstruction.
b Tube current: a model aligned in x-direction (stenosis degree: 50%) was measured with increasing spiral CT parameters. The smallest increase of the compensating straight line is seen using a tube current of 210$24mA

This means that the deviation of stenosis degree was the smallest of the evaluated algorithms by using different SCT parameters (Fig. 3a).

Tube Current

The best results of stenosis degree determination were obtained using 210 mA (Fig. 3b). Also the 3-D image reconstructions were improved using higher tube currents (Fig. 4).

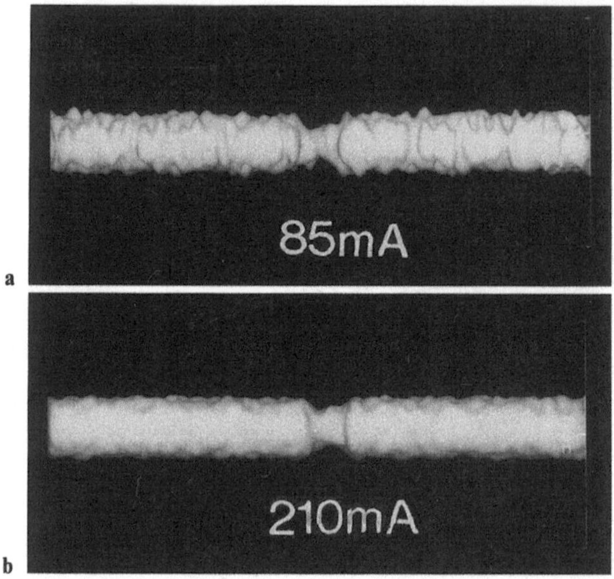

Fig. 4. Tube current: image noise is reduced using 210 mA for tube current and therefore image quality is improved

Discussion

Angiography is still the method of choice for the evaluation of vascular alterations. Up to now clinical applications of the less invasive SCT angiography demonstrate a good morphological correlation to angiography [2–5]. In addition to the free vessel view SCT visualizes the surrounding anatomy. The obtained high correlation ($r = 0.8-0.99$) between real and measured degree of stenosis agree with the results of the former study where the linear correlation coefficients varied between $r = 0.89$ and $r = 0.99$ [7]. However it should be mentioned that both studies were performed under optimized conditions. Scanning patients there are a lot of possibilities for producing artefacts, e.g. arterial pulsation or breathing. An other possibility of stenosis degree deviation is to choose a great slice thickness and table speed. Both options result in an increased or decreased stenosis degree depending on the vascular direction. Therefore it is important to remark the results of our study and do spiral CT angiography only by using:

1. A small slice thickness, a small table speed and a small reconstruction interval.
2. Standard algorithm for image reconstruction.
3. For data acquisition 120 kV and 210 mA.

By attention to these rules it is possible to use SCT angiography, e.g. as a screening method in arterial hypertension to exclude a renovascular cause.

References

1. Kalender WA, Vock P, Polacin A, Soucek M (1990) Spiral-CT: Eine neue Technik für Volumenaufnahmen. I. Grundlagen und Methodik. Röntgenpraxis 43 : 323 – 330
2. Napel S, Marks M, Rubin GD, Dake MD, McDonnell CH, Song SM, Enzmann DR, Jeffrey RB (1992) CT angiography with Spiral CT and maximum intensity projection. Radiology 185 : 607 – 610
3. Rubin GD, Dake MD, Napel SA, McDonnell CH, Jeffrey RB (1993) Three-dimensional Spiral CT angiography of the abdomen: Initial clinical experience. Radiology 186 : 147 – 152
4. Rubin GD, Dake MD, Napel S, Jeffrey RB, McDonnell CH, Sommer FG, Wexler L, Williams DM (1994) Spiral CT of renal artery stenosis: Comparison of three-dimensional rendering techniques. Radiology 190 : 181 – 189
5. Schwartz RB, Jones KM, Chernoff DM, Mukherji SK, Khorsani R, Tice HM, Kikinis R, Hooton SM, Stieg PE, Polak JF (1992) Common carotid artery bifurcation: Evaluation with Spiral CT. Radiology 185 : 513 – 519
6. Soucek M, Vock P, Daepp M, Kalender W (1990) Spiral-CT: Eine neue Technik für Volumenaufnahmen. II. Klinische Anwendungsmöglichkeiten. Röntgenpraxis 43 : 365 – 375
7. Wittenberg G, Jenett M, Tschammler A, Krahe Th (1993) In-vitro measurement of stenoses with Spiral CT. In: Lemke H-U, Inamura K, Jaffe CC, Felix R (Hrsg) Computer Assisted Radiology. Springer-Verlag, Berlin Heidelberg New York, S 501 – 506

Skeleton

Chairmen: W.A. Kalender, V. Metz

Generation of Surgical Models by Spiral CT and Stereolithography

W. A. KALENDER, A. POLACIN, H. HEINRITZ, H. HIRSCHFELDER, U. HIRSCHFELDER, M. SMET

Introduction

The use of anatomical models for surgical planning and simulation based on computed tomography (CT) scanning has been proposed early (Alberti 1979). First trials were started in the 1980s (Vannier et al. 1983, Mankovich 1985); they were based on conventional slice-by-slice CT as means for creating the 3D data and on cutting or milling machines to generate the models. The quality of models created by this approach was limited in most cases. The advent of spiral CT scanning which allows to produce 3D data sets with less effort, but with inherently higher 3D spatial resolution and the introduction of layer manufacturing techniques (LMT) which allow to produce anatomical models of arbitrary complexity with very high resolution offered a new basis for these efforts. Here we report on our approach to routinely provide high quality models and on preliminary clinical experience. This effort is partly funded by the European Union as BRITE project PHIDIAS (laser photopolymerisation models based on medical imaging: a development improving the accuracy of surgery). As for other groups (e.g. Brennan et al. 1992, Klein et al. 1992, Kreiborg and Dahl 1993, Fleiter et al. 1994), stereolithography presently is the LMT of highest interest to us.

High Resolution 3D Imaging with Spiral CT

Spiral CT scanning is based on slip-ring technology and was first implemented on a SOMATOM PLUS. First clinical results were presented in 1989 (Kalender et al. 1990; Vock et al. 1990); the technique and its clinical applications were the primary focus of previous SOMATOM PLUS User Meetings. While scan times were limited initially and thick slices were used predominantly to cover adequate volumes, spiral CT techniques have been improved in several respects and can now be considered mature.

For high-resolution 3D imaging – and for generation of anatomical models as in our case –, resolution along the body's longitudinal axis, the z-axis, is of decisive importance. While spatial resolution in the scan plane, i.e. the x/y-plane, is better than 1 mm in all scan and reconstruction modes and thereby fully adequate for our applications, z-axis resolution is limited by the slice width of 1 or several millimeters. It is clear and generally accepted that thin slices have to be chosen to limit negative effects of slice thickness on 3D spatial resolution. It is not clear to the same

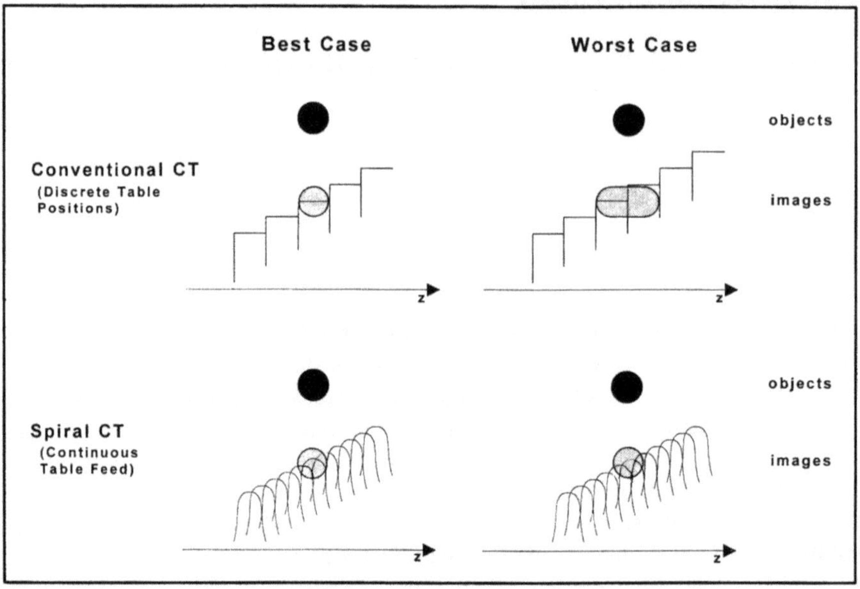

a

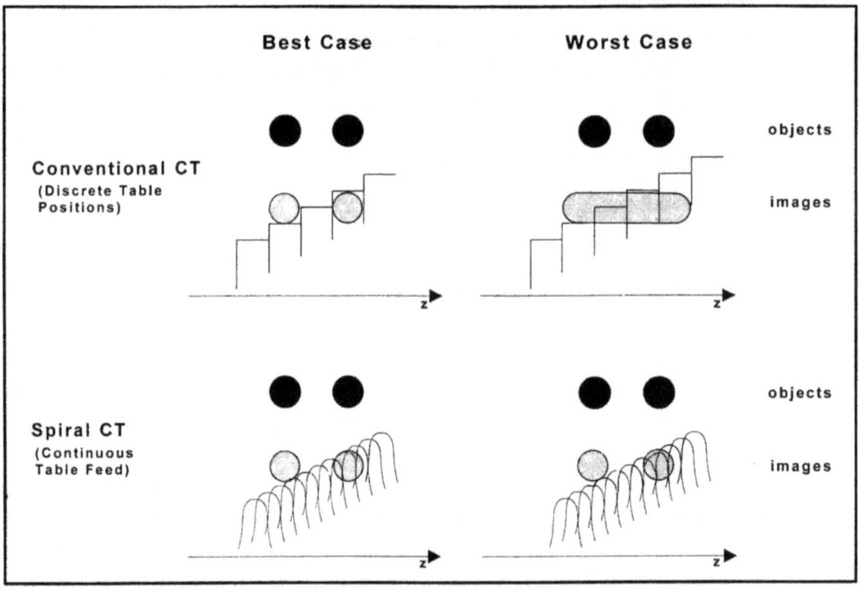

b

Fig. 1a, b. Comparison of contrast and spatial resolution for conventional and for spiral computed tomography (CT). **a,b** Schematic presentation of the dependence of resolution on sampling along the z-axis, i.e. the number of images available. Performance in conventional CT varies with the random relationship of scan pattern and lesion location while spiral CT can always offer optimal performance. **c,d** Phantom experiments verified that contrast and spatial separation of spheres are significantly better in spiral CT (from Kalender et al. 1994)

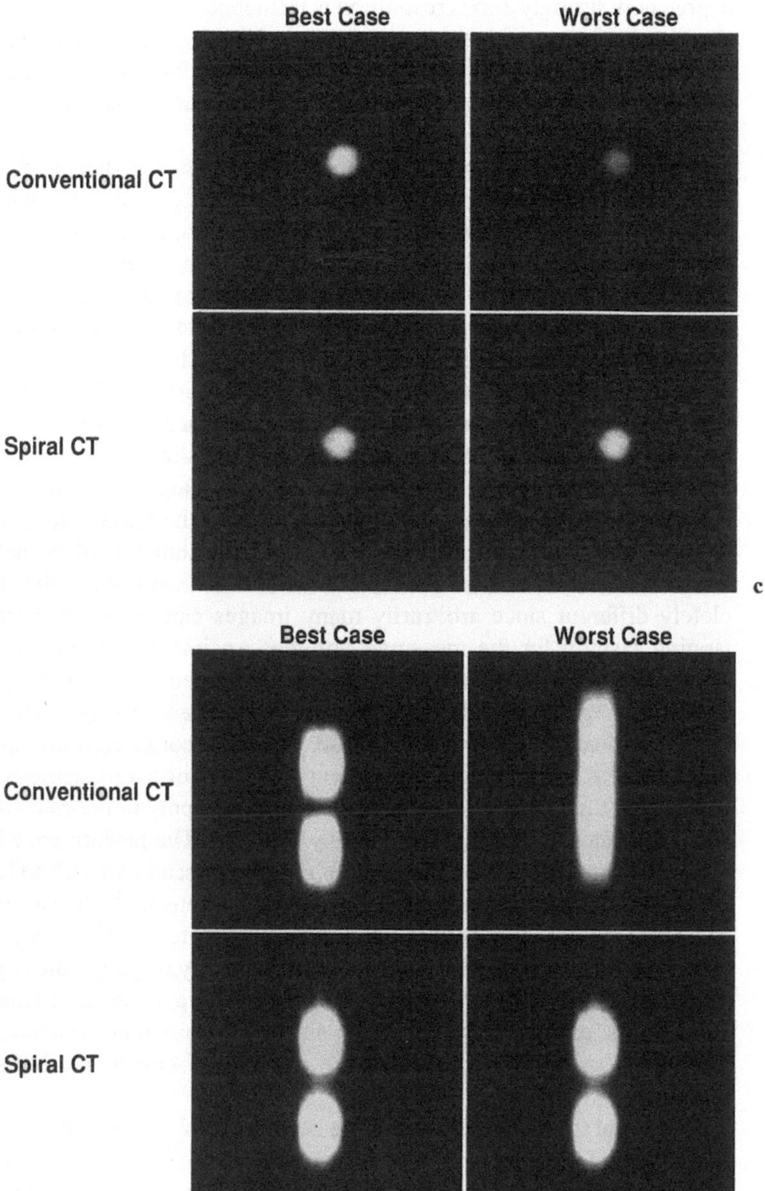
Best Case
Worst Case
Conventional CT
Spiral CT
c
Best Case
Worst Case
Conventional CT
Spiral CT
d

Fig. 1c, d

degree how strongly z-axis resolution is influenced by spiral CT data acquisition and slice interpolation with the concommitant broadening of slice sensitivity profiles (SSP) (Kalender and Polacin 1991; Polacin et al. 1993). It is often assumed that the SSP degradation in Spiral CT will necessarily cause a degradation in z-axis resolution.

We have evaluated this problem in detail by basic considerations, simulations and phantom experiments to show that opposing effects dominate (Kalender et al. 1994). While SSPs in spiral CT are slightly broadened as compared to conventional CT, the sampling rate due to the continuous scanning is much higher since images can be calculated at any point in the scan volume. To explain the respective differences and the priniciple advantages resulting from this fact, let us consider the search for focal lesions. These naturally occur at random sites which are not known at the beginning of the diagnostic procedure. How well they will be imaged three-dimensionally with conventional CT depends on how well the chosen scan pattern fits the random positions of the lesions. In the best possible case, the slices are chosen such that center of slice and center of lesion coincide: in this case, maximum contrast will be reached. With the same probability the center of the lesion can also coincide with the border of two adjacent slices: in this case, the contrast will be halved for lesions with a diameter of half the slice thickness or less. In spiral CT, the situation is completely different since arbitrarily many images can be reconstructed in an overlapping fashion for the measured volume. An image with maximal contrast can always be made available. It needs not be mentioned that these images are calculated retrospectively from the volume once scanned and that no further scan with the related exposure is necessary. These principle considerations are illustrated in Fig. 1a where – in a thought experiment – a sphere of 5 mm diameter is imaged with 5 mm slice thickness. Analogous considerations apply to the case of two lesions of equal diameter to be imaged separately (Fig. 1b). The performance in conventional CT will always depend on the random relation of scan pattern and lesion positions. In spiral CT, maximal performance can always be ensured when a sufficient number of images are reconstructed. Thus, from a priniciple point of view, spiral CT offers significant advantages with respect to image quality inspite of the slight degradation of SSPs. These differences in performance have been confirmed in detail by simulations, experiments (Fig. 1c, d) and specimen studies (Kalender et al. 1994). Therefore, spiral CT constitutes the method of choice for high-resolution 3D imaging.

Our spiral CT examinations for the generation of anatomical models were carried out with the following parameters: slice thickness of 2 mm or less, table feed of 1 to 4 mm/s; double spiral technique of 2×40 s in most cases (Spiral DXP option); reconstruction with SLIM interpolation algorithm and STANDARD convolution kernel.

Generation of Surgical Models with Stereolithography

Stereolithography (SL) represents a so-called layer manufacturing technique, a process where arbitrarily complex three-dimensional models supplied in the form of

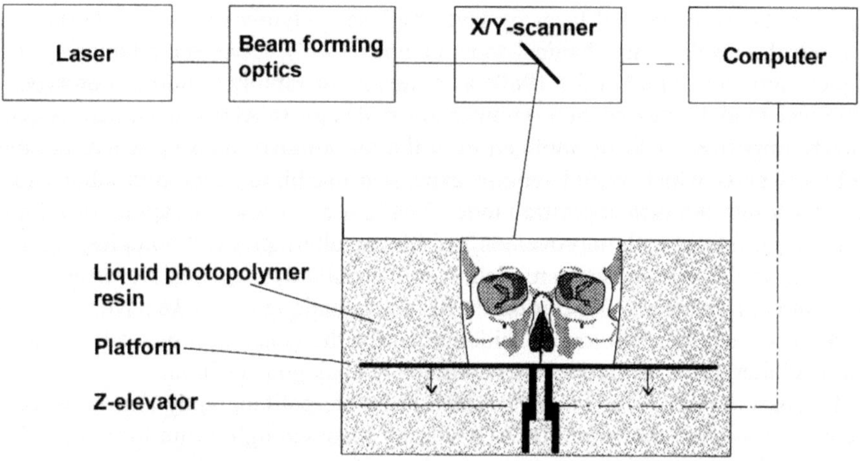

a

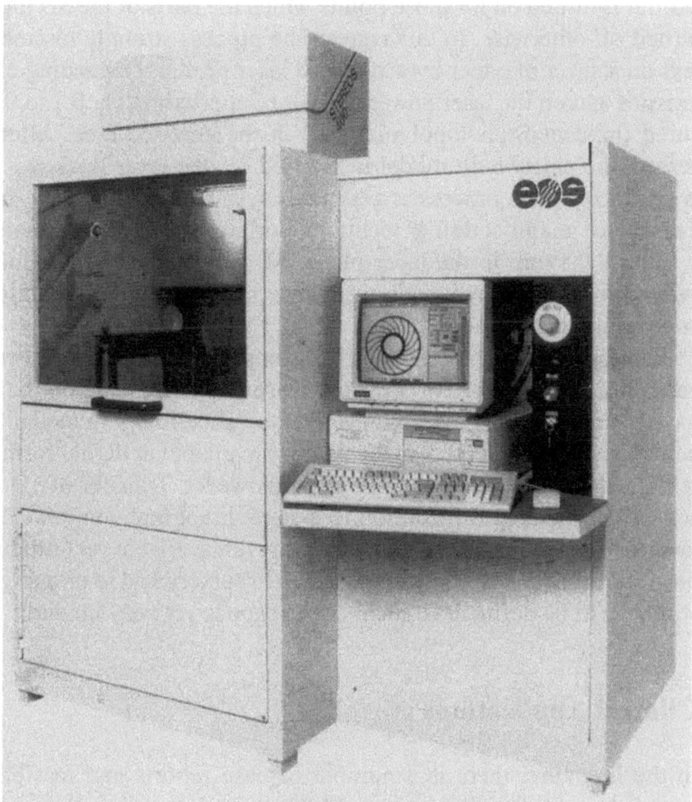

b

Fig. 2a, b. Stereolithography. **a** Illustration of the principle of building models layer by layer. **b** Photograph of a stereolithography unit (photo courtesy of EOS GmbH, Munich, Germany) digital data are generated layer by layer by laser polymerisation of a liquid resin without the need for mechanical tools (Jacobs 1992). Layer manufacturing techniques were developed in the 1980s as a means for rapidly building prototypes of technical models created by computer-aided design (CAD) procedures. A particularly important field of application is the automotive industry where complex technical parts which would require excessive machining time and labor can be created within hours as a plastic model. LMTs are at present a rapidly developing technological field with improvements of SL and alternative technologies, e.g. laser sintering and fused deposition modeling, still constantly evolving. Nevertheless, we will limit our present considerations to SL, the technique which we have used in our work. The basic concept and considerations for the generation of medical models apply to alternative techniques in a completely analogous fashion.

The basic principle of model generation by stereolithography and a respective technical setup are shown in Fig. 2. A sharply focussed light beam from a UV laser is steered by an x/y mirror system over the surface of a liquid photopolymer resin bath; it is turned on for those points which are parts of the 3D model to be built and turned off otherwise. In this respect the process strongly resembles the printing of text on a sheet of paper by a standard laser printer. Depending on the resin characteristics and on the laser power, a layer of approximately 0.1 to 0.4 mm thickness is cured (hardened, photopolymerized) in the exposed area. After one layer is processed, the partly built model is lowered by one layer thickness and the next layer is produced. This process is repeated layer by layer until the model is complete. This layer manufacturing technique offers an intrinsic resolution of typically 0.1 mm × 0.1 mm in the layer plane. SL can therefore reproduce the information offered from CT or magnetic resonance imaging (MRI) with high fidelity without any significant degradation.

The use of SL or other LMTs for generating medical models might be considered straightforward for two obvious reasons: (1) the data on the anatomical model have been acquired "layer by layer" if the slice-imaging modalities CT or MR are being used as the source; (2) the data are available in digital form. A lot of work has remained and still remains to be done, however. Transfer of 3D model data from a scanner or medical workstation to a stereolithography unit is still difficult as conventions or standards for data formats are not available yet (although initiatives have been started). Quality control measures to specify and to ensure geometric accuracy still have to be defined. Clinical experience is yet very limited.

Clinical Applications

In the literature, there is a number of case reports and feasibility studies on the use of stereolithography or other LMTs in medicine (e.g. Brennan et al. 1992; Klein et al. 1992, Kreiborg and Dahl 1993, Fleiter et al. 1994). There are no extended

Fig. 3a, b. Patient with fibrous dysplasia of the frontal sinus system involving the right orbit. **a** Multiplanar reformation and 3D display. **b** Anatomical model which illustrates very well to which extent the orbital roof is infiltrated.

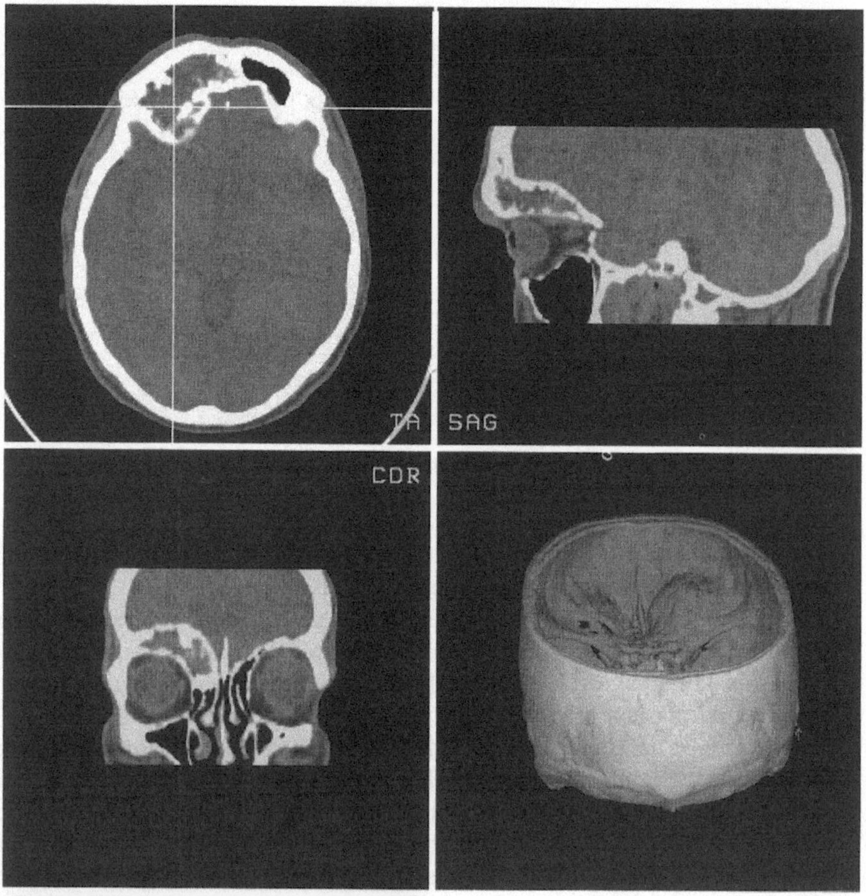

a

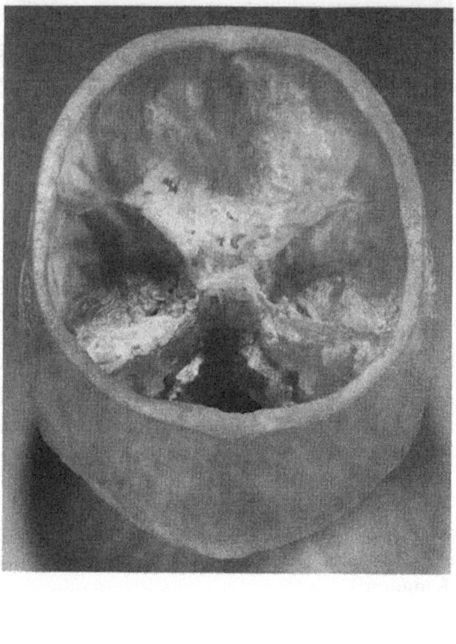

b

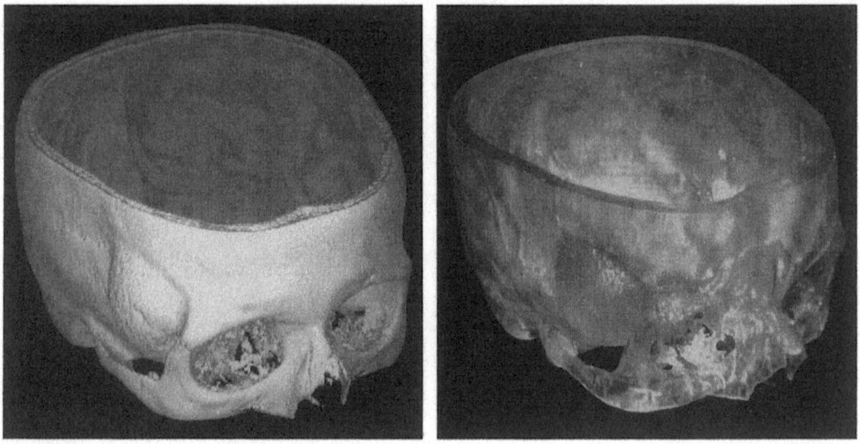
a b

Fig. 4a, b. Patient with a temporal bone osteoma. a 3D display. b Anatomical model

clinical studies or validations available yet, however. While the potential is apparent and often discussed, practical experience is still limited.

Applications have been suggested for many surgical procedures involving complex skeletal anatomy, e.g. for skull plasties, craniosynostosis, trauma in the maxillofacial region, orthodontic and paradontic cases, spinal trauma, pelvic fractures and dysplasias, congenital and acquired malformations of the foot or hand. Some examples are shown in Figs. 3, 4. A review of these applications and particular demands on the technical parameters has recently been given (Smet 1994). It can be expected that the time needed in complicated surgical cases can be significantly reduced with planning and simulation based on anatomical models and that the quality may be higher due to the possibility of preparatory steps. Some very important demands from clinicians and surgeons are of practical nature: they are asking for routine availability of models within hours and at low cost. Applications will be limited in number until this aim will be reached. Work now in progress has the potential to bring about significant improvements soon.

Outlook

Rapid prototyping techniques are of very high interest in general. They are considered a key technology by the European Union, and they receive a high priority with respect to funding of research and development projects in industry. It can be expected that technical progress will result which also will have positive implications on medical applications. Project PHIDIAS[1] aims to contribute to the solution of a number of open problems listed above. Standardization of data transfer is one

[1] Partners in project PHIDIAS are the Interdisciplinary Research Unit for Radiological Imaging at the University of Leuven (Belgium), Siemens Medical Systems (Germany), Materialise N.V. (Belgium), and Zeneca Specialties (United Kingdom)

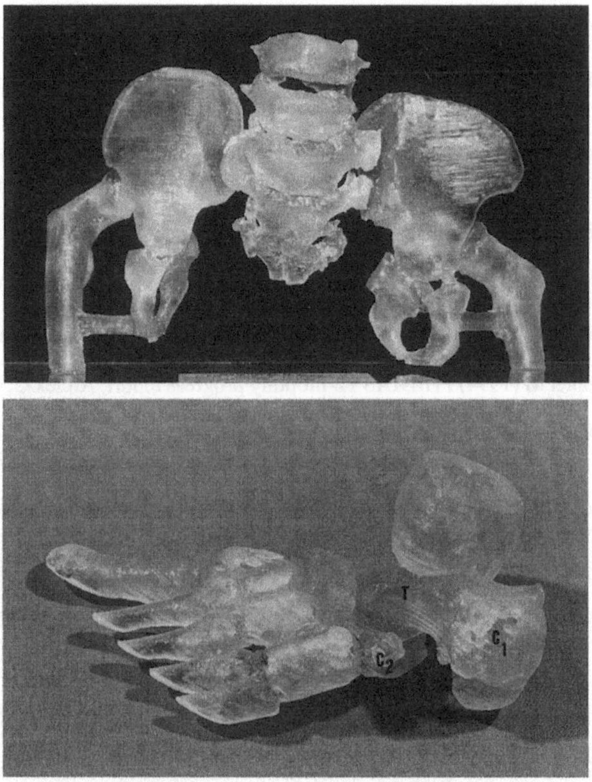

Fig. 5a, b. Anatomical models of the hip (a.) and the calcaneus (b.). **a** Bladder extrophy in a 4 y. female leading to an open pelvis. **b** Wrongly fused calcaneus after fracturing into two pieces (C_1, C_2) in a 11 y. female

objective which should help to make models available routinely with less effort. Production within 24 h is the goal. Cost reduction is a further practical aim. To add colour to the models, to process multiple objects, to provide fusion of CT and MRI results are some of the equally challenging goals which may at the same time expand the range of potential applications of rapid prototyping in medicine.

References

Alberti C (1980) Three-dimensional CT and structure models. Br J Radiol 53 : 261 – 262

Brennan P, Stucki H, Ghezal A, Stucki P, Fuchs W (1992) Three-dimensional printing from Somatom Plus CT data. In: Felix R, Langer M (Eds.) Advances in CT II. Berlin, Springer, pp. 207 – 210

Fleiter T et al. (1994) Preoperative planning and follow-up with spiral CT and stereolithographic models in craniofacial surgery. In: Pokieser H, Lechner G (Eds.) Advances in CT III. Berlin, Springer, pp. 149

Jacobs P (1992) Rapid Prototyping & Manufacturing. Fundamentals of Stereolithography. Dearborn: Society of Manufacturing Engineers

Kalender WA, Seissler W, Klotz E, Vock P (1990) Spiral volumetric CT with single-breath-hold technique, continuous transport, and continuous scanner rotation. Radiology 176 : 181 – 183

Kalender W, Polacin A (1991) Physical performance characteristics of spiral CT scanning. Med Phys 18:910–915
Kalender W, Polacin A, Suess C (1994) A comparison of conventional and spiral CT with regard to contrast and spatial resolution: An experimental study on the detection of spherical lesions. J Comp Assist Tomogr 18:167–176
Klein HM, Schneider W, Nawrath J, Gernot T, Voy ED, Krasny R (1992) Stereolithographische Modellfertigung auf der Basis dreidimensional rekonstruierter CT-Schnittbildfolgen. Fortschr Röntgenstr 156:5
Kreiborg S, Dahl E (1993) Cranial base and face in mandibulofacial dysostosis. American J Medical Genetics 47:753–760
Mankovich N (1985) The use of computerized tomographic (CT) scans for display and prostheses construction. SPIE Proc 535
Polacin A, Kalender WA, Marchal G (1992) Evaluation of section sensitivity profiles and image noise in spiral CT. Radiology 185:29–35
Smet M (1994) PHIDIAS 12-monthly progress report, Annex C: Quality requirements for medical models. Leuven
Vannier MW, March JL, Gado MH, et al. (1983) Clinical applications of three dimensional surface reconstruction from CT scans: Experience with 250 patient studies. Electromedica 51: 122–131
Vock P, Soucek M, Daepp M, Kalender WA (1990) Lung: spiral volumetric CT with single-breath-hold technique. Radiology 176:864–867

Preoperative Planning and Follow-Up with Spiral CT and Stereolithographic Models in Craniofacial Surgery

T. Fleiter, R. Hoffmann, R. Niemeier, C.D. Claussen

Introduction

Severe fractures, tumor resection and craniofacial malformations require detailed preoperative planning and post-surgery follow up. With spiral computed tomography (SCT) it became possible to acquire high-resolution, motion artifact reduced images of this region in less time compared to conventional single-slice CT. Additional 3D reconstructions are preferred by the surgeons to get more preoperative information about the anatomical structures, position of fragments and tumor extension. Although several progresses were made according to image quality and 3D imaging, there has always been a missing link between the preoperative planning and the surgical procedure itself. The aim of the study was to evaluate the use of spiral CT and solid 3D-stereolithographic models to overcome this disadvantage and the use of spiral CT in follow-up examinations.

Material and Methods

According to the complex bone structures of the craniofacial region and the limited 3D information within conventional multiaxial radiographs, which are commonly used by the surgeons for detailed procedure plannings, most of the 28 examined cases were done on patients with severe fractures or dysplasia of this region. All patients were scanned with spiral CTs, using 1- or 2-mm slice thickness and table feed. The increment between two images was always equal to the original slice thickness. Two or three contiguous 40 s spiral CTs were needed to scan the whole region of interest. All raw-data were stored to provide post-examination recalculations. Radiation dose-reduced spiral CTs were used in all follow-up studies. The therefore slightly increased noise-level of the images was diminished with medium edge-enhancement reconstruction algorithms.

The images were 3D reformatted with the 3D software package of the Somatom Plus S to control the scanning procedure and to provide an 3D overview. All areas of certain interest were reconstructed by primary zooming of the stored raw data. Images were reformatted with standard frontal, lateral, dorsal and caudal views and additional oblique 3D projections.

Complex cases were selected for the generation of stereolithographic models. Extraction of bone structures and the transskription into a stereolithographic file was done with a seperate imaging system and a particular software (Mimics/Materialise). The stereolithographic models were exposed with a standard stereolithographic machine (3D-Systems).

Results

Although there are still detectable differences between high-resolution conventional CT and spiral CT, all 3D reconstructions of spiral CT images were superior compared to the conventional 3D-images, which is mainly caused by the reduction of patient movements during the examination and the slight smoothing effect of the spiral CT. Most important was the reduction of examination time: Patients with severe craniofacial fractures could be primary examined without relaxation and general anesthesia as well as children with craniofacial malformations. No additional scans were needed for diagnostic or therapeutic reasons. The overall image quality of follow-up studies was improved by the use of titanium implant materials, which lead to reduced artifacts.

In all cases the 3D representation of the scanned region was preferred by the surgeons for preoperative planning, although primary diagnosis still remains on the interpretation of axial images. The primary spiral CT was sufficient for both requirements. The 3D solid models were used for precise preoperative resection planning and implant fitting with conventional surgical tools. In all cases preformed implants and supporting devices were of sufficient shape and led to a reduction of needed operation which was, however, not exactly measurable (Figs. 1–10).

Discussion

The advantages of 3D visualisations have been proven in several studies [1–4]. But in most cases it is still used only as a kind of presentation tool. As 3D image quality depends on several scan and reconstruction parameters [5] spiral CT is a basic assumption for primary scanning, 3D representation and solid 3D model generation with stereolithography. Although these models add real new therapeutic aspects to 3D procedures, it is in most cases still used as an – unfortunately very expensive – presentation tool [6].

Improvements of the scanning procedure like double-spiral technique, advanced interactive image manipulation and automized seperation of interesting structures will be the next steps towards precise preoperative resection planning and implant construction. The shape of these implants can be calculated within the 3D reconstruction and transferred via stereolithography into direct casting of biocompatible and implantable materials [7]. Several applications of this technique are going to become available and have to be proved in further studies.

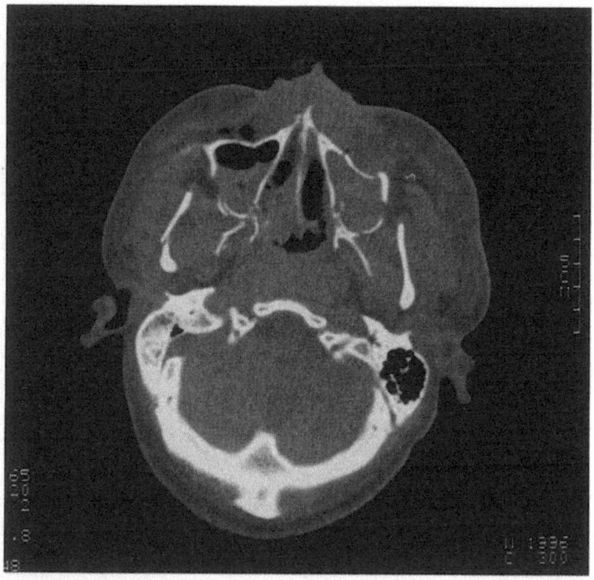

Fig. 1. Spiral CT of a patient with severe frontal impression after car accident. Several fractures of maxilla and fractured mandibula are detectable

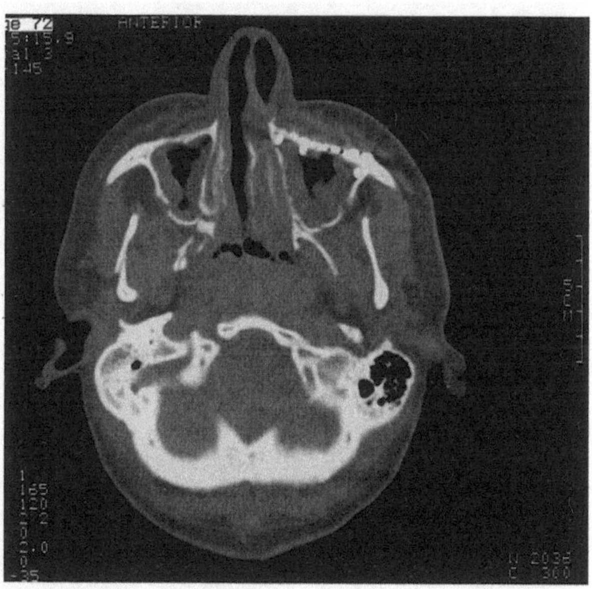

Fig. 2. Same patient as in Fig. 1 after reconstruction with titanium miniplates. Note the slight artifacts caused by the implants

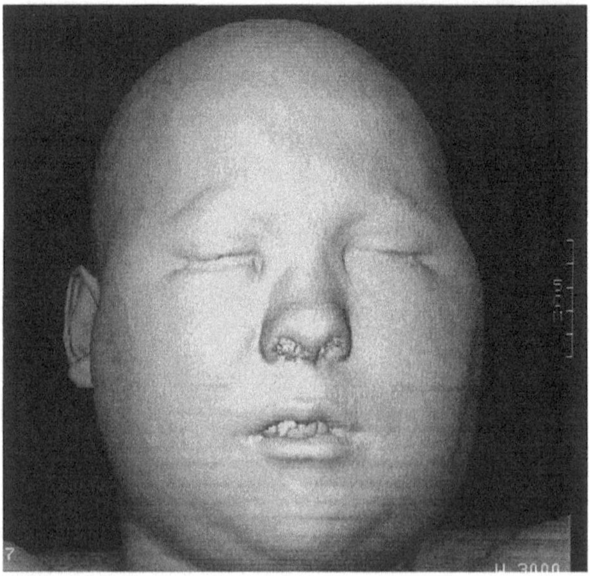

Fig. 3. Surface reconstruction of a patient, primary scanned with spiral CT after accident

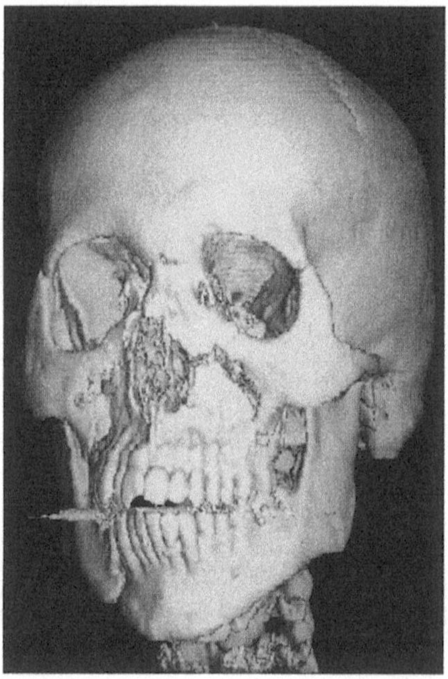

Fig. 4

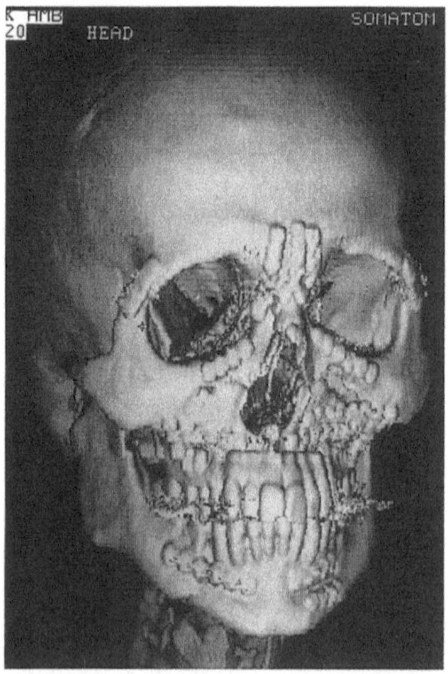

Fig. 5

Fig. 4. Same patient as in Fig. 3, demonstrating slip off fractures of right maxilla and mandibula

Fig. 5. Same patient as in Fig. 3 after reconstructive surgery. Artifacts are only caused by patient movement between two contiguous spiral CT and teeth inlays, whereas there are only slight artifacts caused by the miniplates

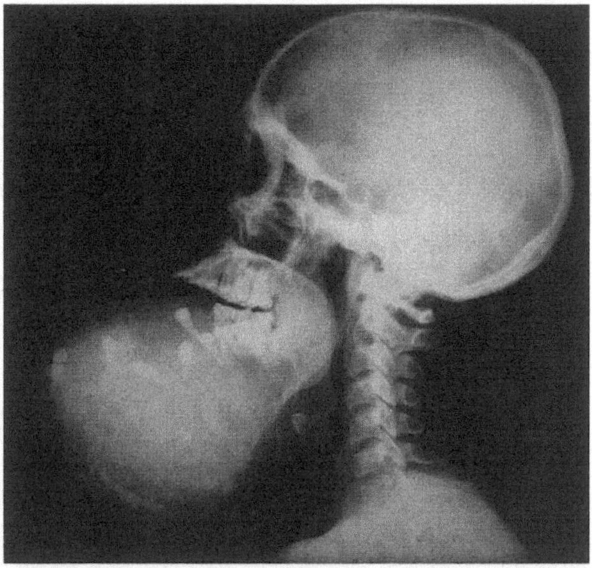

Fig. 6. Lateral view of a patient with extreme, slow growing osteosarcoma of the mandibula. All teeth in the frontal part of the tumor remained vital

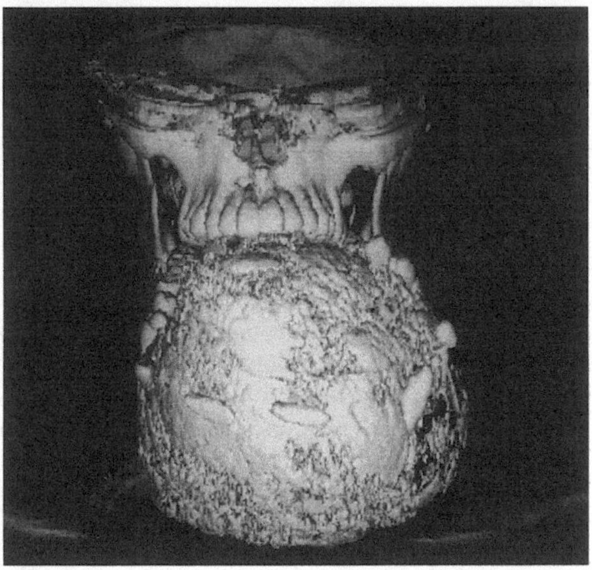

Fig. 7. First attempt to scan the patient with conventional single slice CT. The scanning had to be stopped dued to massive motionartefacts

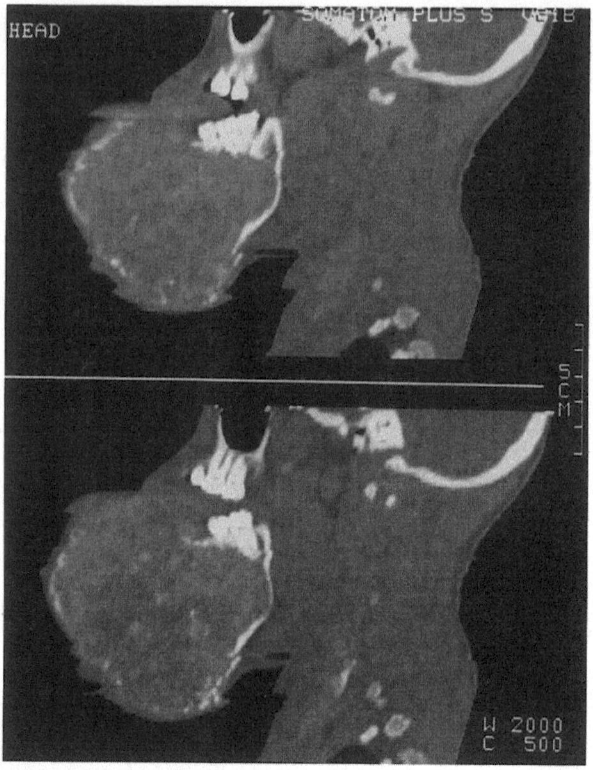

Fig. 8. Sagittal reconstruction of Fig. 7 demonstrating the motion artifacts which were not detectable in the original axial scans

Summary

Preoperative planning and computer assisted surgery techniques are going to be used in several medical specialities. Recent progresses have been made according to precision and accuracy of the scanning by the use of spiral CT. It became possible to acquire high-resolution, motionartifact-reduced images of the complex craniofacial bone structures with contiguous spiral CTs. But up to now there is still a missing link between the preoperative diagnosis and planning with axial and 3D-reformatted spiral CTs and the surgical procedure.

The integrated use of spiral CT and stereolithographic models provides a new alternative to overcome this disadvantage.

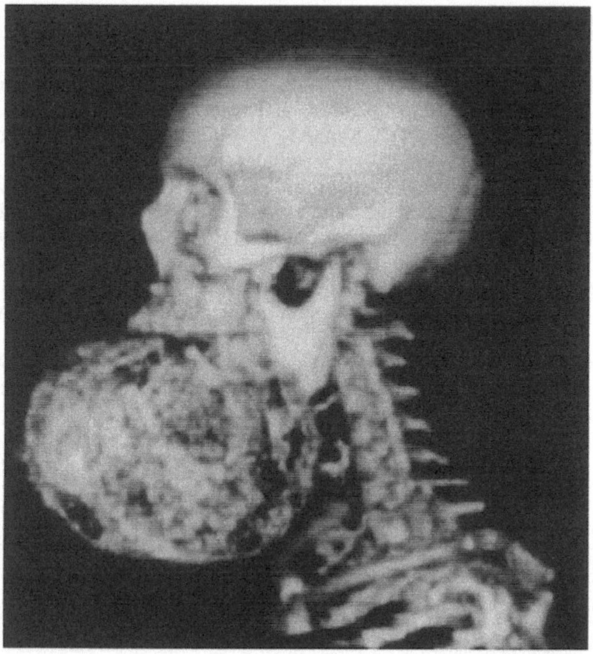

Fig. 9. 3D-reformatted contiguous spiral CT of the same patient as Figs. 7 and 8 with plain decreased artifacts

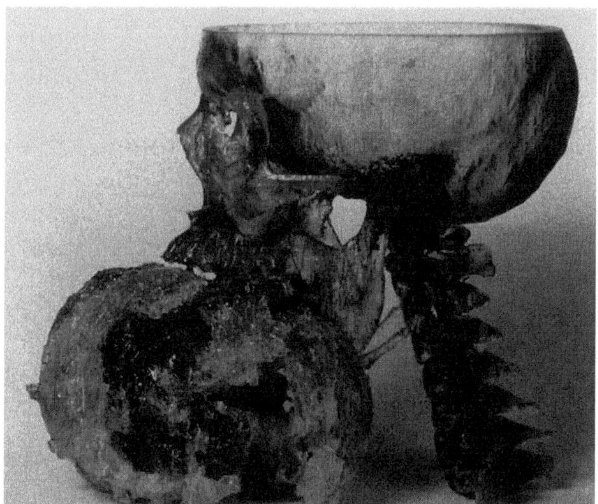

Fig. 10. Corresponding stereolithographic model which was used for preoperative resection planning and mandibula implant fitting

References

1. Vannier MW, Marsch, JL, Warren JO (1984) Three Dimensional CT reconstruction images for craniofacial surgical planning and evaluation. Radiology 150 : 179 – 184
2. Burk DL,.Mears DC, Kennedy WH, Cooperstein LA, Herbert DL (1985) Threedimensional computed tomography of acetabular fractures. Radiology 155 : 183 – 186
3. Wojcik WG, Edeiken-monroe BS, Harris JH (1987) Three-dimensional computed tomography in acute cervical spine trauma: a preliminary report. Skeletal Radiology 16 : 261 – 269
4. Soyer P, Roche A, Gad M et al. (1991) Preoperative segmental localisation of hepatic metastases: Utility of three-dimensional CT during arterial portography. Radiology 180 : 653 – 658
5. Ney DR, Fishman EK, Magid D et al. (1991) Three-dimensional volumetric display of CT-Data: Effect of scan parameters upon image quality. Journal of Computer Assisted Tomography 15 : 875 – 885
6. Klein HM, Schneider W, Alzen G, Voy ED, Günther RW (1992) Pediatric craniofacial surgery: comparison of milling and stereolithography for model manufactoring. Pediatr. Radiol. 22 : 458 – 460
7. Jonck LM, Grobbelaar CJ (1990) Ionos Bone Cement (Glas-Ionomer): An Experimental and Clinical Evaluation in Joint Replacement. Clinical Materials 6 : 323 – 359

Scanning Protocol for Advanced 3D Reconstruction of Joints Using the Double Spiral CT Technique

H. HIRSCHFELDER, P. WEBER, U. HIRSCHFELDER

Introduction

The benefit of 3D reconstructions based on transaxial computed tomographic (CT) images is still a subject of much discussion among radiologists. This question has been answered for orthopedic surgeons and orthodontists: They require 3D display. In orthopedic examinations of limb joints or bodering on the spinal column and orthodontic evaluation of the facial skull, the question of the shape and position of the joint pairs is of primary importance. In contrast, the question of structure is often only of secondary importance for the clinician. One typical example of this is a dysplasia of the hip, where the congruence and position of the joint pairs are of decisive diagnostic and therapeutic relevance. An evaluation of the bony structure by CT must be clarified only in borderline cases involving poor bone stock if there is any doubt as to whether planned therapeutic measures can be performed for this very reason.

Within the framework of CT examinations 3D surface reconstruction in combination with multiplanar reconstruction is a suitable method of answering these orthopedic and orthodontic indications. The required information on bone structures thus remain intact. In our clinic, CT examinations of joints therefore routinely include a 3D reconstruction. More than half of all CT examinations involving limb joint are requested mainly for the demand of a 3D display.

For about 3 years, we are having the possibility of utilizing the spiral CT technique [4], which we employ almost exclusively to generate 3D data files. In the rapid course of development of the spiral CT technique, it has in the meantime proved possible to develop optimized CT scan parameters for rapid post-scan processing of three-dimensional displays.

Profile Measurements

During the last user conference in Berlin 2 years ago, the use of the spiral CT technique for 3D reconstructions was judged critically by some participants [1] and quite positively by others [3]. Since the "step-by-step" CT technique still represents the "golden standard", the first question posed was whether, in comparison to this method, spiral CT also provides a similarly favorable basis for producing 3D reconstructions.

Profile evaluations of phantom studies were performed for this purpose: A gap containing a material equivalent to 50 HU and varying in thickness (from 1 to 5 mm)

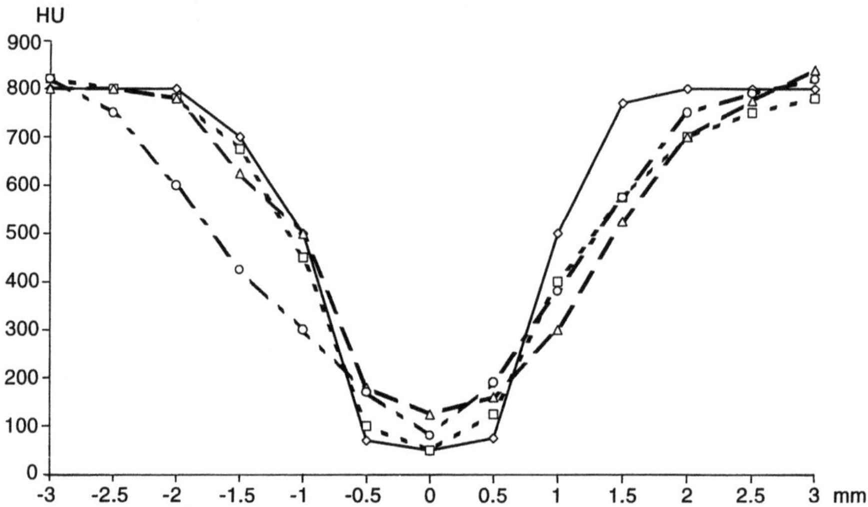

Fig. 1. Sensitivity profiles of phantom measurement under different scan conditions (120 kV, 165 mA, gap 2-mm, 1-mm increment). ●, 1-mm conventional scanning, 1-mm increment; □, 1-mm spiral scanning, 1-mm table feed/s; △, 1-mm spiral scanning, 2-mm table feed/s; ○, 2-mm conventional scanning, 1-mm increment

was attached to a phantom with a diameter of 2 cm and a density of 800 HU and scanned in water. Since the critical point in spiral CT technique is the Z axis, this gap was located parallel to the scan plane. After examing various different scan parameters, a reconstruction along the Z axis and a profile evaluation via the precision of display of the gap and in the form of a sensitivity profile are performed (Fig. 1).

Basic Spiral CT Technique

Findings in the evaluation of profiles show that spiral scans performed with a 1-mm slice thickness, and using the "slim" profile according to the rebinning method [5] yield a nearly equally good display of the profile studies for phantom gaps of 2 mm and more as the conventional scanning technique does with a slice thickness of 1 mm and otherwise identical scanning conditions (Fig. 1). Even for phantom integrated gaps of 1 mm and less, the values obtained were acceptable. Although a verifiable difference could be found in the profiles, this proved difficult to detect through the evaluation of clinical images.

An increase of the scan's slice thickness resulted in the expected reduction of the inclination in the profile pattern both with the conventional technique and with the spiral CT. That means that, for a true-to-life 3D reconstruction, the slices used should be as thin as possible, i.e. a slice thickness of 1 mm should be selected.

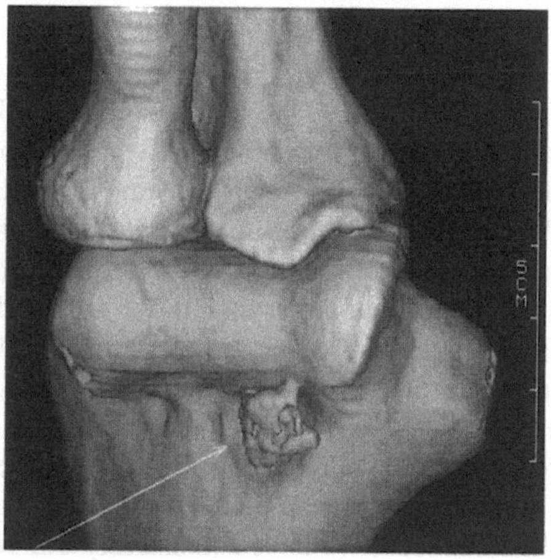

Fig. 2. A 3D reconstruction of the elbow and 1-mm DXP double spiral technique. The loose bony structure (*arrow*) was not detected on conventional radiogram or MRI

DXP Double Spiral Technique

The current generation of SOMATOM PLUS scanners feature a maximum scan length of 40 s with a minimal dose of 125 or 165 mA, which corresponds to a scanning volume of 40 mm with a 1-mm slice thickness. This is often insufficient to display larger joints together with the mated joints and, thus, to reach a clinically relevant diagnosis. In order to compensate for this disadvantage, we now regularly utilize the "DXP double spiral technique" in the "long" version, which has been available to us since August 1993. This gives us the possibility of connecting two spiral CT data files back-to-back, thus doubling the volume of the scan (Fig. 2). The joining of multiple spiral CT scans had already been employed at an earlier date. However, a disturbing "step effect" which occurred at the overlapping positions could not be avoided in clinical practice. This was due to the fact that the interspiral delay of up to 3 min proved much too long [1]. Depending on the prevailing scanning conditions, the current DXP technique can reduce this delay to max. 25 s. As a result, an examination employing the DXP spiral technique does not take longer than 105 s for the patient.

The diagnostic value of the primary images as a basis for a 3D reconstruction is of course no different here than for the basic spiral CT technique, since the parameters remain unchanged except for the fact that the area examined here is twice as long owing to the double spiral. The volume of a scan thus acquired is sufficient to satisfy the demand for clinically useful application of 3D reconstructions of limb joints.

Doubled Table Feed (Pitch 2)

For the past 2 years we have also been gathering experience in the use of accelerated table feeds [2, 5]: When a given slice thickness is used for spiral CT, a table feed of up to twice the speed is selected instead of one with the same speed. Studies conducted by us using the above mentioned phantom have shown that, under consistent utilization of rebinning [5], the profiles obtained from the evaluation of the profile studies are even better than those obtained by conventional CT with twice the slice thickness and an increment of 1 mm (Fig. 1). As long as extremely fine disturbances in the surface profile are not important for the clinical indication and evaluation, e.g. as in the case with fracture lines, this technique can readily be used for 3D reconstruction (Fig. 3). Various different effects are thus attained: In cases where a small scan volume is planned the patient's dose rate can be cut in half by doubling the table feed. We have consistently utilized this benefit in connection with examinations of children and adolescents. On the other hand the scan volume can also be doubled. As a result, a scan volume of almost 160 mm can be attained with the optimum slice thickness of 1 mm by utilizing the DXP long double spiral technique and double table feed. This volume seems to be sufficient for most orthopedic and orthodontic indications.

Scan Protocols

Therefore, for an optimal 3D reconstruction with the framework of orthopedic and orthodontic indications, we have been routinely using the spiral technique with 120 kV and 125 or 165 mA for our current examinations. Image reconstruction is performed for the primary slices in the standard kernel with the "slim" profile and an increment of 1 mm. We select the single spiral, double spiral or double table feed depending on the size of the joint in question and the clinical indication involved:

- 1-mm spiral CT with 1-mm table feed for the evaluation of fine structures in small joints (wrist, ankle, mandibular joint)
- 1-mm double spiral CT with 1-mm table feed for the evaluation of fine structures in larger joints (knee, elbow, calcaneus; Fig. 3)
- 1-mm spiral CT with double table feed for large joints when shape and position are of primary importance for the clinical indication
- 1-mm double spiral CT with double table feed for examination of the shape and position of entire anatomical regions (pelvis, lumbar or cervical spine, deformation of limbs, facial skull; Fig. 4)
- An even larger scan volume is required only in very rare cases, e.g. for the evaluation of the entire spine column in scoliosis: In these rare cases, we still use a 2-mm slice thickness in connection with the Double Spiral technique and a double table feed. Reconstruction of the primary slices is performed with a 2-mm increment due to the limited capacity which the suitable slices have for a subsequent 3D reconstruction.

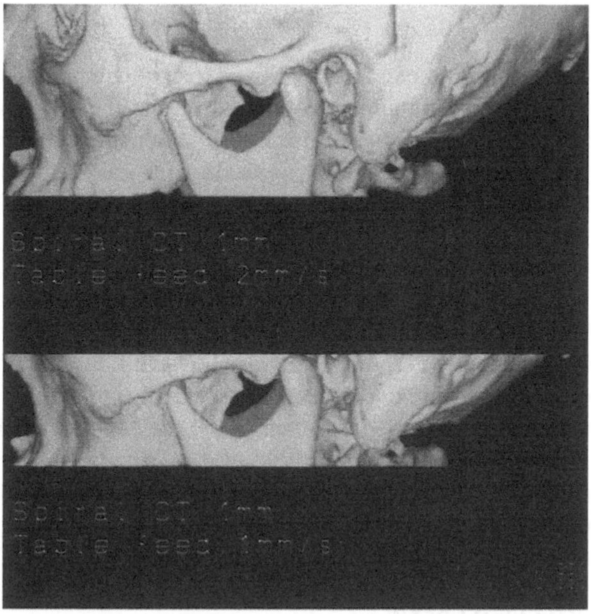

Fig. 3. A 3D reconstruction of the jaw. Above 1-mm spiral scanning, 2-mm table feed/s; below 1-mm spiral scanning, 1-mm table feed/s

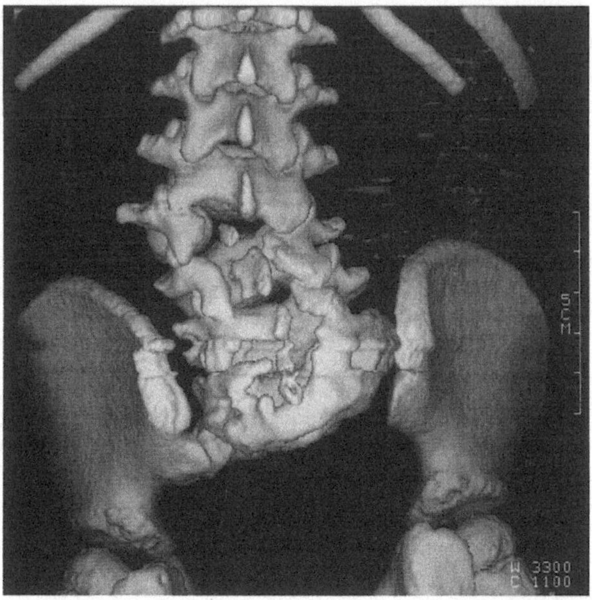

Fig. 4. A 3D reconstruction of the lumbar spine in a caudal regression syndrome; 1-mm DXP double spiral technique with pitch 2

Discussion

This scan parameter can be utilized to examine peripheral joints or for studies of the entire visceral cranium. Problems are caused by the low dose rate when generating primary slices of the hip for obese patients and by the poor signal-to-noise ratio when displaying shoulder joints. In such cases, the dose rate must be increased, resulting in a reduced scan volume in spiral CT. In case the region thus scanned proves too small for clinical evaluation, a conventional step-by-step scanning technique must eventually be resorted to in such cases.

If, in addition to a shape-and-position analysis via 3D display in the standard kernel, a structural analysis of the matching joint generated from the primary slices is also required, spiral CT will enable the desired clinical diagnosis without increased exposure to radiation by repeatedly generating the primary images from the mandatorily recorded raw-data file in the edge-enhancing kernel.

On the other hand, the value of a 3D display of joints is often overestimated by surgeons: Not only the display of the 3D surface is important, but also the display of the joint in the three dimensions using a multiplanar reconstruction for complete radiological acquisition of an intraarticular process. This can easily be done by using the current 3D reconstruction software in the "Reformatting" technique on the SOMATOM PLUS.

The question of whether a three-dimensional display and the display of a joint in three dimensions are useful must be decided by the orthopedic surgeon and/or orthodontist in charge. Full utilization of the possibilities now offered by the SOMATOM PLUS makes it possible to process the existing data from a spiral CT scan parallel to the display of the primary slices without any problems in relation to time or computing power. As a result, the radiologist can easily "cater to the service demands" of the operating orthopedic surgeon or orthodontist following this image processing.

References

1. Fleiter T, Rieber A, Wakat P, Brambs HJ, Claussen CD (1992) Optimized Scan Modes and Reconstruction Techniques for Three-Dimensional Display of Bone Structures. In: Felix R, Langer M (eds.) Advances in CT II. Springer, Berlin Heidelberg New York, pp 155–161
2. Hirschfelder H, Hirschfelder U, Polacin A, Kalender WA (1992) 3D Imaging of Joints with Spiral CT: Choice of Parameters and Comparison with Conventional CT. (abst) Radiology 185, p. 117
3. Hupke R, Ezrielev J, Fisler R (1992) Three-Dimensional Imaging in CT. In: Felix R, Langer M (eds.) Advances in CT II. Springer, Berlin Heidelberg New York, pp 147–154
4. Kalender WA, Seissler W, Klotz E, Vock P (1990) Spiral Volumetric CT with Single-Breath-Hold Technique, Continous Transport and Continous Scanner Rotation. Radiology 176, pp 181–183
5. Polacin A, Kalender WA, Marchal G (1992) Evaluation of Section Sensitivity Profiles and Image Noise in Spiral CT. Radiology 185, pp 29–35

Dental CT: A New Diagnostic Tool in Dental Radiology Based on Double Spiral CT

U. Hirschfelder, H. Hirschfelder, J. Regn

Introduction

In the beginning of 1990, dental computed tomography (CT) software program was developed which offers the possibility of reconstructing panoramic and transaxial images of the maxilla and the mandible from CT data files [1, 5, 6] for analyzing dento-skeletal relationships in mulitplanar anatomical overviews. Up to 7 successive panoramic images running parallel to the jaw and various reformattings of varying distance and length arranged perpendicular to the centric panoramic line provide new possibilities of gaining insights into the morphology of the maxillo-mandibular system. Until now, this software was primarily utilized for diagnosis and planning of dental implantations [1]. Initial clinical experience has, however, shown that the narrowly restricted range of indications involved in implantology can be extended to include other fields of dentistry [4], whereby a large scan volume is required. The spiral CT scanning technique [2, 3, 7, 8], and especially its newest development, the double spiral CT scanning technique (DXP), seem to offer interesting perspectives in this regard.

These must be explored while evaluating such questions as: which examination parameters are desirable or acceptable in view of the quality of the dental image, which dental indications this scanning method is relevant to, and what advantages of dental CT can be recognized based on the data file from DXP examination. Implantological aspects are not taken into account here.

Patients

All previous experience with dental CT is based on findings resulting from CT studies of 55 predominantly adolescent patients mainly aged between 7 and 18 years performed at the Department of Orthodontics at the University of Erlangen-Nuremberg, Germany.

Clinical Indication

The indication for CT examination and clinical testing of the dental CT software program among this group of patients primarily resulted from the need to exactly clarify the topographically false position of displaced tooth germs and structural anomalies of the jawbone.

Table 1. Scan parameters (DXP) and image reconstruction

Scan time	1 s
Slice thickness	1 mm
Dose	120–165 mA
Table feed/speed	1 mm/2 mm
Image reconstruction	Slim
Increment	1 mm
Zoom	Approx. 3.5
Algorithm	Utrahigh
Window/center	3500/800

Method of Examination

Twenty patients were examined with the dynamic screening mode and 35 patients with the spiral CT scanning technique. Double spiral CT was used in 20 cases. Both single and double table feeds were utilized, depending on the volume being examined. The CT examination was performed in a superextended cranial position and a straight gantry setting, with the patient's head being positioned and fixed according to the medio-sagittal plane of the facial skull and the occlusal plane. All patient examinations were performed under identical conditions (Table 1).

In order to determine the differences between simple and double table feed (DXP 1/1 and 1/2) with regard to image qualitiy and the size of the reconstruction volume, a macerated skull was scanned from the tip of the chin toward the cranium under the above conditions. For comparison, the jaw region was scanned in a further study employing 2 mm slice thickness and single table feed (XP 2/2).

In a further processing of CT data files via dental CT software, the reconstruction of 6 more panoramic lines was presented after carfully defining the central panoramic line. The maximum lenth of the paraxial images was defined as 30 mm with a distance between a distance between secondary slices of 1 mm.

Results

Image Quality and Survey

Previous experiences with dental CT have pointed out that two factors are decisive whith regard to a wide range of indications:

- A good general survey displaying the entire upper and lower jaw.
- High image quality showing a maximum of morphological details.

The findings shown in Tables 2 and 3 indicate, that, depending on table feed, CT examinations employing the DXP technique with a slice thickness of 1 mm and single table feed offers sufficiently large reconstruction volumes for dental CT. To a large extent, this scan parameters fulfill the requirement for optimal surveyability

Table 2. Examination and reconstruction volume with qualitative Evaluation of the DXP-CT scanning technique for dental CT

	Scanning range/ reconstruction range	Region	General survey in dental CT	Quality of dental scans
1/1 DXP	8 cm	Subregion: maxilla or mandible	–	+++
1/2 DXP	16 cm	Maxilla and mandible	+++	++
2/2 XP	8 cm	Subregion: maxilla or mandible	–	–

+++, outstanding; ++, good; –, restricted

Table 3. Reconstruction of the dental CT from spiral CT data files: evaluation for locally defined and comprehensive dental problems

	Local problem	Clinical application of dental CT	Comprehensive problem	Clinical application of dental CT
1/1 DXP	+++	*Maxilla or mandible* Displaced teeth Structural anomalies	–	–
1/2 DXP	++	Displaced teeth within the maxilla and the mandible Structural anomalies	+++	*Maxilla and mandible* Multiple teeth displacements Multiple structural anomalies
2/2 XP	(+)	Dental disorders	–	–

+++, DXP scanning technique well suited; ++, DXP scanning technique suitable; (+), DXP scanning technique not well suited; –, DXP scanning technique unsuitable

of the teeth and the jaws accompanied by high image quality. Comparing the different scan parameters it is evident, that the spacial resolution of the DXP 1/1 scan technique with 1 mm slice thickness and single table feed insures the best results with regard to contour definition and the display of spongiosa over a scanning range of 8 cm (Fig. 1a).

Depending on the facial and jaw anatomy, with DXP 1/1 technique only subregions of the stomatognathic system can be scanned. The general survey in the dental CT panoramic and paraxial images must therefore be generally assessed as "restricted". In comparison, the blurred, unclear image detail of dental CT based on spiral CT using 2-mm slice thickness and a single table feed must be classified as inadequate despite the 1-mm increment. Since a loss of diagnostically valuable information is to be expected, scanning with a 2-mm slice thickness is unsuitable for dental CT (Fig. 1b).

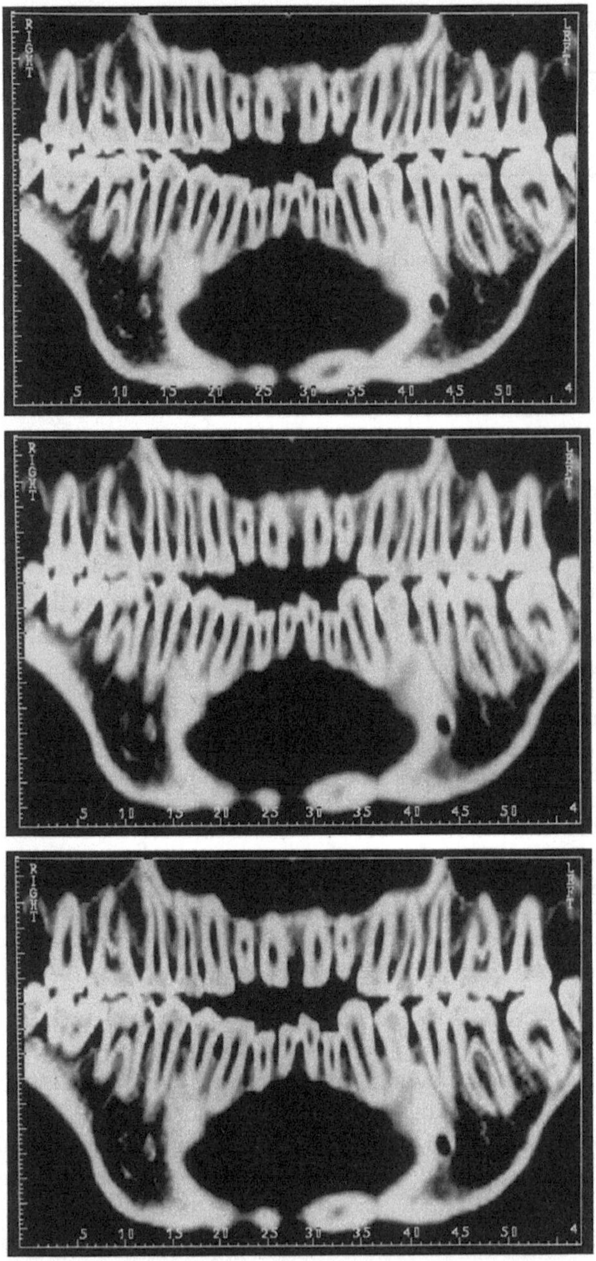

a

b

c

Fig. 1a–c. Spiral CT: comparison of three combinations of slice thickness and table feed. **a** DXP 1 mm/1 mm: high image quality; **b** XP 2 mm/2 mm: inadequate image quality; **c** DXP 1 mm/2 mm: good image quality

In view of the required survey and image quality requirements, the DXP 1/2 technique can be regarded as very interesting. With a reconstruction volume of 16 cm the total stomatognathic system including the maxillary sinus, the tooth and root relationships to the buccal and lingual cortical bone and the mandibular canal can be analysed with astonishing clarity. With regard to the image quality, there is slightly increased blurring effect to be seen resulting from double table feed. However, this does not seriously impair the diagnostic possibilities (Fig. 1c). From this perspective, recommendations for the most favorable scanning parameters can be derived for locally defined and comprehensive dental problems (Table 3).

Clinical Applications

Clinical experience in the application of this scanning technique has pointed out, that dental CT can be used as an efficient diagnostic tool (a) for three dimensional determination of the position of displaced tooth germs, and (b) for evaluating the bony jaw density and diagnosing structural abnormalities.

For this diagnostic aim spiral CT has proven to be an excellent scanning method especially for children and adolescents, due to its extremely short examination time, good image quality and prescripted low radiation dose.

Example 1. An 11-year-old female patient had developmental disturbances of the dentition: congenitally missing of the upper second premolars, displacement of the upper canines and of the upper first bicuspid on the right hand side.

Dental CT in the analysis of the seven panoramic displays located between the palatinal and labial side and the corresponding paraxial reformattings exhibit clearly the palatinal malposition and the mesial inclination of the upper canines, whereby the right canine is dislocated in a more dorsal position than the left one. Around the crowns of these displaced teeth a cystic enlargement of the dental sac is clearly verifiable. The upper first bicuspid on the right hand side shows also a defective palatinal position with a 55° mesio-distal inclination and an 81° palatinal inclination towards the occlusal plane (Fig. 2a, b).

By using dental CT it was consequently possible to determine the topography of these defective tooth position exactly and to utilize this specific morphologic information for selective and coordinated treatment planning of surgical and orthodontic procedures.

Example 2. An 8-year-old boy had a total cleft lip palate on the right hand side and dental disturbances. The panoramic views of the dental CTs point out a 53° mesial inclination of the canine and at the same degree a distal inclination of the lateral incisor on the right hand side toward the region of the cleft palate. The bony defect measures an average width of 6.8 mm at the height of the displaced canine and 13 mm at the height of the nasal apertures (Fig. 3).

Example 3. A seven-year-old female patient had multiple dentitional disorders in the upper and lower jaw. Dental CT, panoramic and paraxial images, of this patient provide detailed information on serious disturbances of the stomatognatic system:

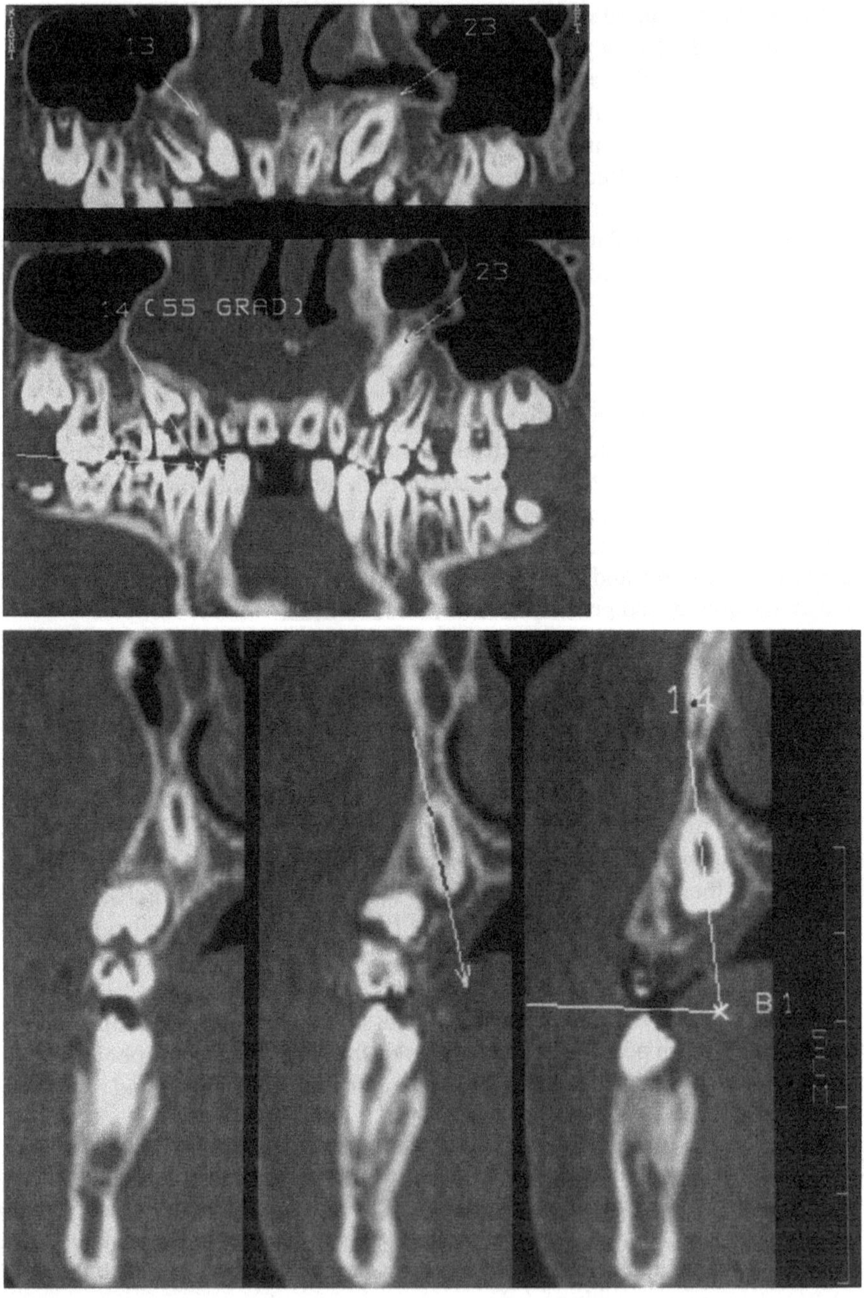

a

b

Fig. 2a,b. DXP 1 mm/1 mm: displacement of the upper canines and the first bicuspid (described in text)

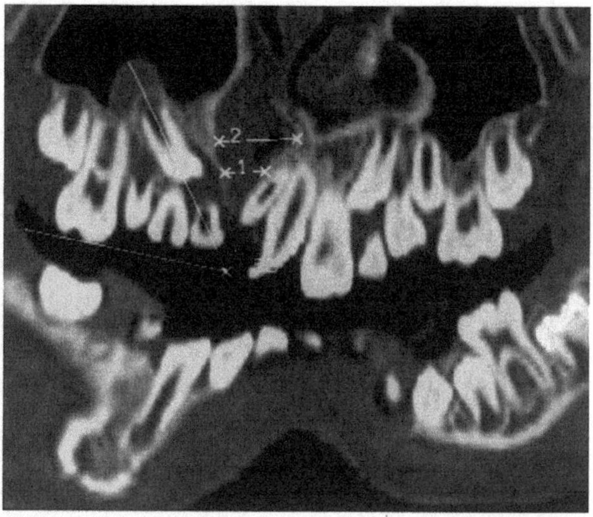

Fig. 3. DXP 1 mm/2 mm: cleft lip palate and dental malpositions (described in text)

nearly horizontal displaced and rotated upper central incisors with extensive cysts around their crowns (Fig. 4a). This malposition is caused by displaced upper canines pressing on the cranial root surface of these teeth (Fig. 4c). Furthermore, there are atypically disto-inclined first molars with distal cystic formations to be recognized and transverse distal first bicuspid on the left hand side, which is also surrounded by an extensive cyst (Fig. 4b). The lower canines are displaced, too, lying beneath the roots of the lower incisors (Fig. 4a). The knowledge of these abnormalities offers an outstanding basis for therapeutic considerations.

Discussion

The clinical application of dental CT indicates that this software program is superior for three dimensional analysis of malformations of the dentition and abnormalities of the jawbone structure. This represents a considerable gain of valuable diagnostic information required for an efficient, problem-related therapeutic concept. One prerequesit for this is the need of a sufficiently large scan volume with a slice thickness of 1 mm. This is insured by double spiral CT in a very short examination time and reduced radiation dose. These factors are especially important when examining children and adolescents, since the anatomically exact determination of atypically located tooth germs, which are relatively often seen in these age-group, is required with regard to surgical and orthodontic therapy planning.

In contrast to conventional radiological methods of examination, a main advantage exhibited by dental CT is based on the distortion- and overlap-free reconstructions, which allow dental and structural abnormalities metrically to objectify.

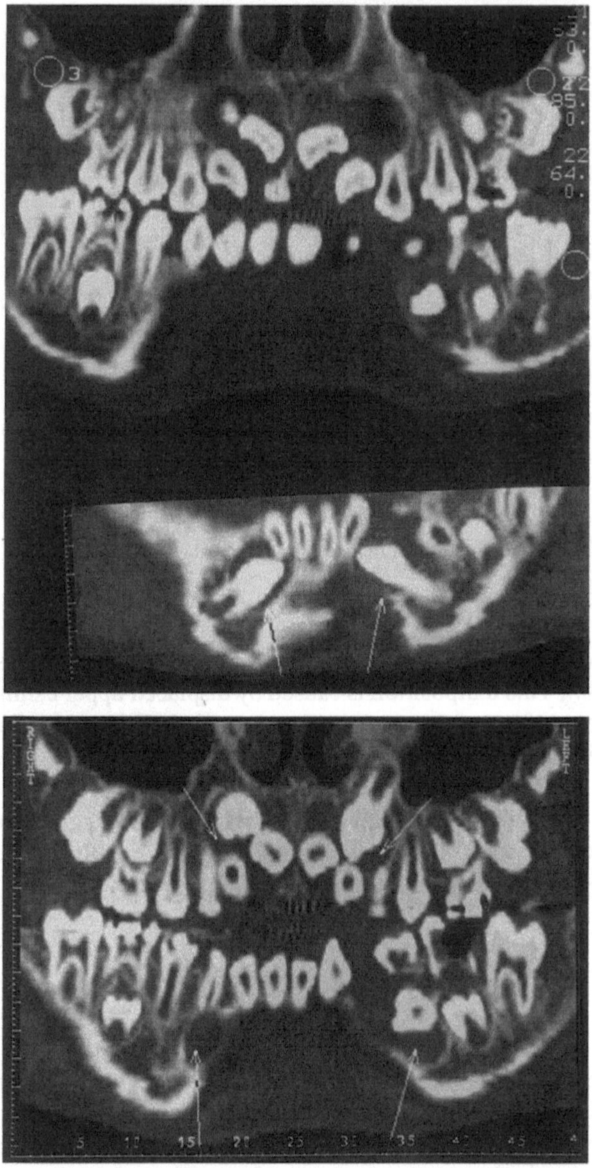

a

b

Fig. 4a–c. DXP 1 mm/2 mm: multiple dentitional disorders (described in text)

The decisive advantage of DXP scanning technique is also to be seen in the possibility of calculating the reconstructions of the primary slices additionally in the standard mode in order to generate 3D surface reconstructions of the skull on this basis. Optimal possibilities are thus provided for diagnosing dento-facial malformations with only a single X-ray.

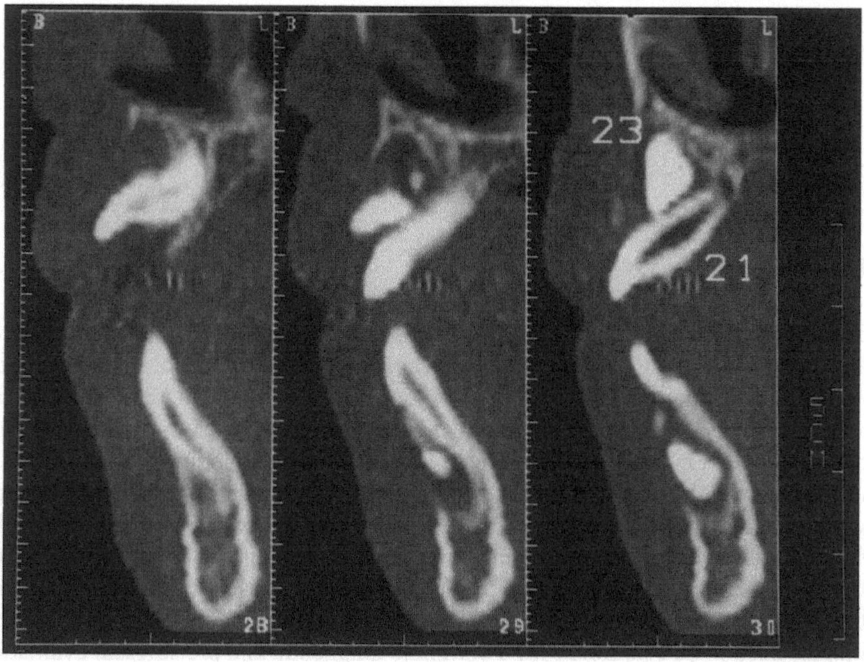

Fig. 4c

References

1. Casselman JW, Deryckere F, Hermans R, Declerq C, Neyt L, Pattyn G, Meeus L, Vandevoorde P, Steyaert L, Devos V (1991) Dental Scan: CT software program used in the anatomical evaluation of the mandible and maxilla in the perspective of endosseous implant surgery. Fortschr Röntgenstr 155:4–10
2. Hirschfelder U (1992) Die Spiral-CT-Aufnahmetechnik – erste Erfahrungen für kieferorthopädische Fragestellungen. Fortschr. Kieferorthop. 53:247–253
3. Hirschfelder U, Hirschfelder H (1993) Einsatz neuer CT-Techniken für kieferorthopädische Fragestellungen. Dtsch Zahnärztl Z 48:128–133
4. Hirschfelder U (1994) Die Panorama-Übersichtsaufnahme: Dental-CT versus Orthopantomographie. Fortschr Kieferorthop 55:14–20
5. Hupke R, Ezrielev J (1992) A new Imaging Aid: Dental CT. In: Felix R, Langer M (Hrsg): Advances in CT II. Springer, Berlin-Heidelberg-New York, p 211–219
6. Imhof K (1992) Dental-CT: Ein neues Programm zur Planung und Überprüfung von Kieferimplantaten. Elektromedica 60:26–29
7. Kalender W, Vock P, Polacain A, Soucek M (1990) Spiral-CT: Eine neue Technik für Volumenaufnahmen. I. Grundlagen und Methodik. Röntgenpraxis 43:323–330
8. Kalender W, Polacin A, Marchal G, Baert AL (1992) Current Status and New Perspectives in Spiral CT. In: Felix R, Langer M (Hrsg): Advances in CT II. Springer, Berlin-Heidelberg-New York, p 85–94

Craniofacial Malformations: 3D Spiral CT Evaluation

M. Dragani, A. Tartaro, C. delli Pizzi, C. Colosimo, L. Bonomo

Introduction

Spiral computed tomography (SCT) differs from standard CT in that it can study anatomic volumes in a few seconds with a single geometric spiral scan. The continous volumetric acquisition of data allows, at the end of the scan, the reconstruction of planar images at each level of the volume acquired, with the most suitable algorithm and field of view (FOV). The speed of image acquisition allowed for both uncooperative and pediatric patients to be examined. In addition, the radiation dose was about half that of the standard CT. Greater post-processing possibilities of the spiral CT allow for considerable improvement of three-dimensional (3D) images in terms of spatial resolution. These features of spiral CT seem particularly useful in the study of pediatric patients with cranio-facial malformations where 2D- and 3D images need to be elaborated for a complete diagnostic and pre surgical evaluation. The aim of this study is to analyse the diagnostic quality and utility of the axial, multiplanar and 3D images obtained with the spiral CT for the study of cranio-facial malformations.

Material and Methods

Twenty-one patients ranging in age from 1 month to 4 years with cranio-facial malformations (16 craniosynostoses, three sphenoid dysplasias, two progressive facial dysplasias) were included in the study. In six patients with craniosynostosis the spiral examination was carried out after the first cranioplastic operation while in three patients the examination was carried out both before and after the first surgical operation. The spiral CT examination was carried out with a Somaton Plus scanner: acquisition time 20–24 s (mAs 165, kw 120); slice thicknes 5 mm; table feed 5 mm/s. The axial slices were reconstructed in overlapping minimum increases of 2 mm on the longitudinal axis. In all cases the algorithm of 360° LI and the "soft" (Kernel 4.5) were used for the reconstruction of axial images. The MPR were carried out on sagittal and coronal planes after the study of brain and orbital-facial structures. For the 3D reconstructions we used "surface rendering" software with an average threshold of 140 HU for the skull and –200 HU for the soft parts. The 3D reconstructions were carried out with standard (frontal, back, bottom, top, right and left lateral views) and oblique rotational views. Illumination and smoothing were also performed on the reconstructed surfaces.

Table 1. Location of craniosynostosis in 16 patients

Sutures	Affected (%)
Lambdoid	37
Sagittal	43
Metopic	20
Coronal	60

Results

In none of the patients studied was anaesthesia or any other pharmacological sedation necessary. On children of less than one year the exam was almost always carried out during spontaneous sleep. On older children, who were first shown round the scanning room, the exam was carried out without problems while they were awake. Never was it necessary to repeat the spiral scan nor carry out further standard technique scans. We founded two cases of trigonocephaly, four of scaphocephaly, six of plagiocephaly, one of oxycephaly and three of brachiocephaly. In three of these cases craniolacunae were also found. The axial spiral images and MPR showed three cases of hydrocephalus together with craniosynostosis, a dermoid, a plessiform neuroma and a lipoma with agenesia of the corpus callosum. The image quality was always satisfactory and there were no artefact movements. The coronal sutures were best evaluated on the frontal view, and 45° – 315° rotational views. The sagittal sutures were best evaluated on "aerial view" looking at the top of the skull. The lambdoid sutures were best seen on 135° to 225° rotational views. The metopic sutures were best evaluated on frontal view. The locations of the suture fusion in the16 patients are provided in Table 1.

Discussion

The advantages of spiral CT in comparison with conventional CT are the rapid acquisition volume, the lower radiation dose, the possibility of having better reconstruction of images and retrospectively, on all the levels of volume acquired, allowing images with different FOV and algorithm (3, 4, 8). This favours the study of pediatric patients by reducing the necessity for sedation especially in craniofacial malformations where CT examination procedure involves the study of the brain and the 3D study of the skull; 3D CT allows for the most accurate diagnosis of craniosynostosis. Besides, the 3D view of the skull permits information to be passed easily from the radiologist to the neurosurgeon, allowing the surgical operation to be planned. The results of our study underline how the spiral CT simplifies considerably the examination procedure of craniofacial malformations, reducing the acquisition time of the exam notably. A single volumetric scan (maximum duration: 24 s) is all that is needed to give the information necessary for brain study and a 3D study of the skull and facial bone. If we consider that the 3D spiral image quality is at least

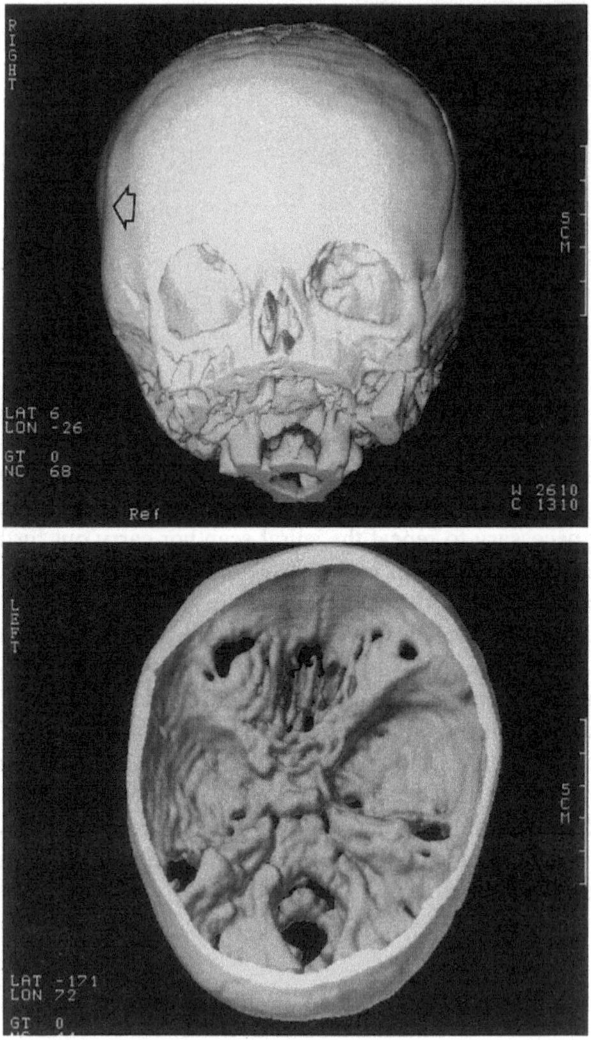

a

b

Fig. 1a, b

on a par with the traditional 3D CT images, considering the substantial reduction in examination time and dose for the patient, the spiral CT technique may indeed be proposed in the 3D study of cranio-facial malformations.

Summary

Spiral CT technique provides rapid acquisitions of large anatomic volumes reducing radiation dose to the patients; in the acquired volume axial slices, conventional mul-

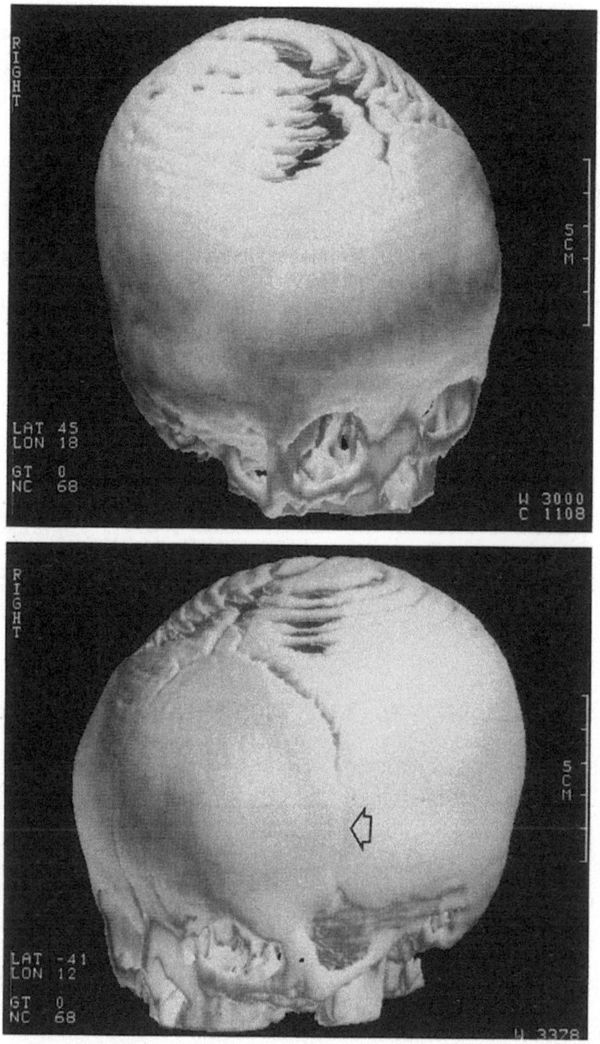

c

d

Fig. 1c, d

tiplaner images and 3D reformations may be reconstructed by means of adequate selection of FOVs and algorithms. These possibilities make spiral CT the method of choice to completely evaluate cranio-facial anomalies in the pediatric population. Our experience includes spiral CT studies of 21 children affected by cranio-facial malformations (16 craniosynostoses, three sphenoid dysplasias, two progressive facial dysplasias). Somatom Plus CT scanner was used; the technical parameters were the following: acquisition time 20–24 s, 165 mAs, 120 kV, slice thickness 5 mm, table feed 5 mm/s. In all patients spiral CT studies were obtained without anaesthesia or sedation and resulted in good quality diagnostic depiction of both craniofacial anomalies and associated intracranial pathology. We conclude that craniofacial malformations in pediatric population represent specific indication for spiral CT study.

References

1. Clauser L et al. (1990) 3D imaging in cranio maxillofacial surgery. The surgeon's point of view. Neuroradiologia 2 (suppl 4) 19
2. Hemmy DC et al. (1983) Three dimensional reconstruction of cranio-facial deformities using computed tomography. Neurosurgery 13 : 534–541
3. Kalendar WA et al. (1990) Spiral volumetric CT with single breath-hold technique, continuos transport, and continuos scanner rotation. Radiology 176 : 181–183

Inclination and Version of the Acetabular Cup: Measurement of Angle in CT after Scaling

R. Sokiranski, R. Niemeier, C.D. Claussen

Introduction

To describe the position of an implanted acetabular cup the version and inclination angles are measured by conventional X-rays (Fig. 1). Our investigations and those of other working groups [1, 2] lead to the following statements:

- The precision of the measurements depends a lot on investigation conditions which are difficult to control.
- The differentiation of retro- or ante version is not possible with only one radiograph.
- There are different mathematical definitions as well for the version- and for the inclination angle and often authors have examined other angles than there defined and referred to in their work.

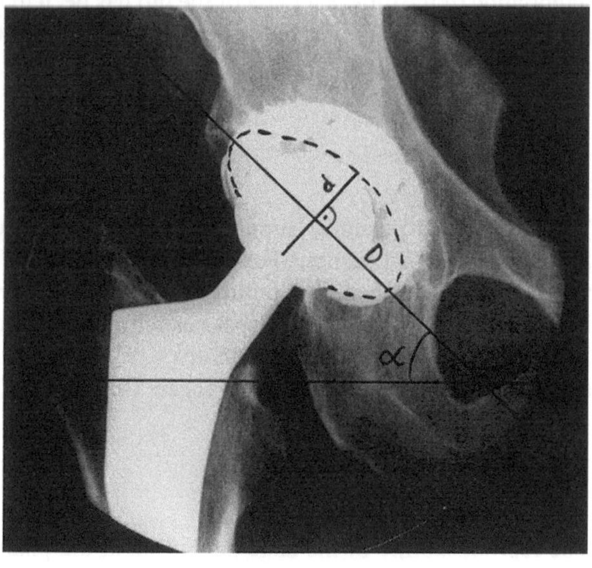

Fig. 1. Measurements of the inclination and version angel on conventional X-ray

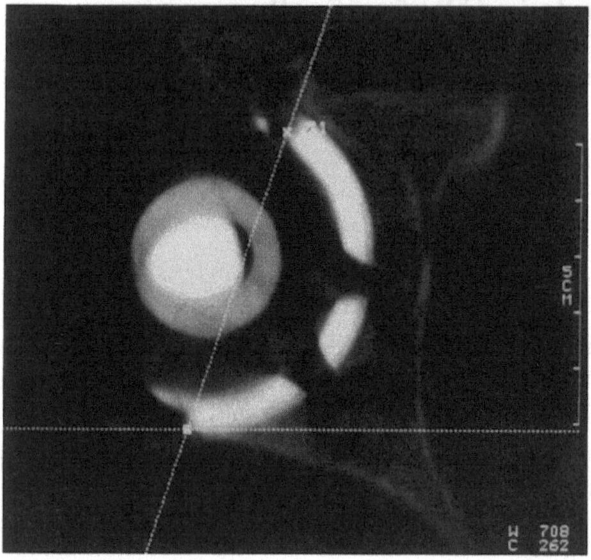

Fig. 2. Example of an implanted acetabulum cup in a patient. Reconstruction after scaling down raw daty by a factor of 10

The use of computer tomography (CT) for these measurements in the past was restricted due to metal artefacts. By a recently developed CT program [3] the differentiation of the different parts of the hip has been made possible by a rescaling of the CT values (Fig. 2). For this a correct recording of three-dimensional cup parameters is now possible.

Methods

We examined a phantom simulating controllable acetabular cup positions in a Somatom Plus S CT scanner. For the different positions we took X-rays in a.p. direction (Fig. 3) and two axial sections in CT (Fig. 4). The X-rays have been digitized before measurement. In the CT sections the circular marking wire is imaged for each section by two points. The coordinates x, y, and z for the measured four points are sufficient for the calculation of all angles (Fig. 5).

Results

The reproducability of the angels adjusted at the phantom was less than $\pm 1°$. The correspondence between the chosen angle and those found by the X-ray method showed a standard deviation of $\pm 0.7°$ for the inclination and ± 0.6 for the version. The angles read from the CT images revealed a substantial deviation in comparison

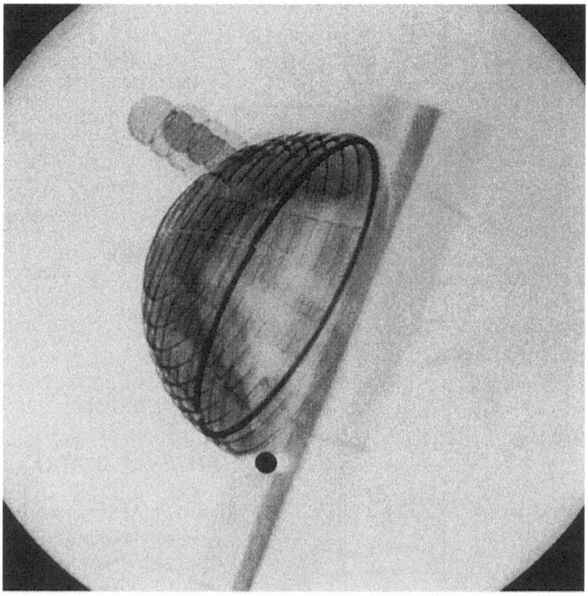

Fig. 3. X-ray of an acetabulum cup in a.p. direction. Version 20° and inclination 45°

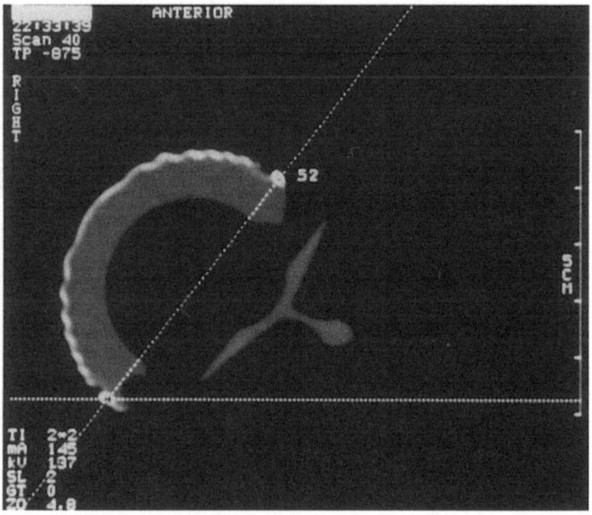

Fig. 4. Axial section in CT. The marking wire is imaged by two points

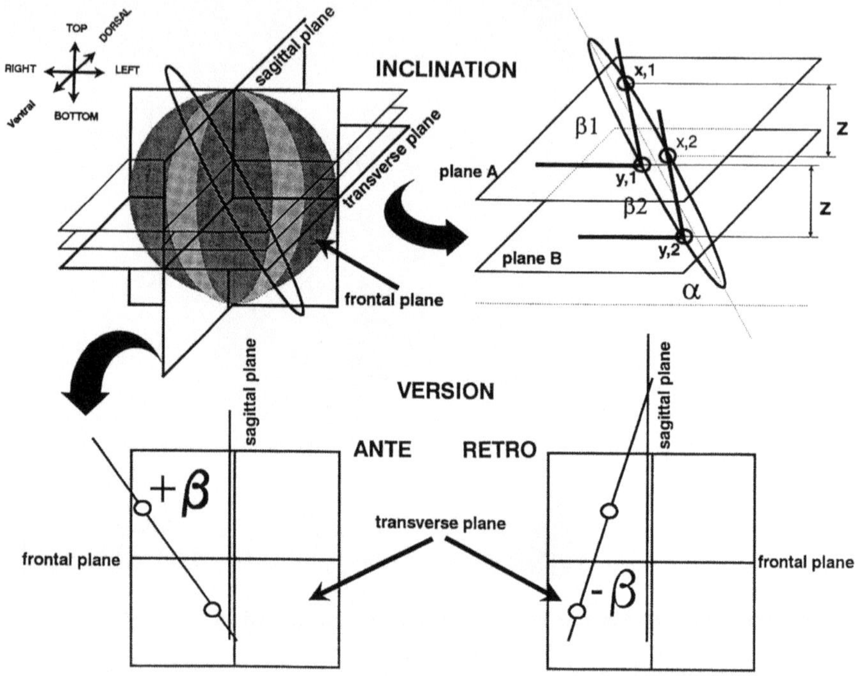

Fig. 5. Two axial sections. In each section are tow points of the marking wire

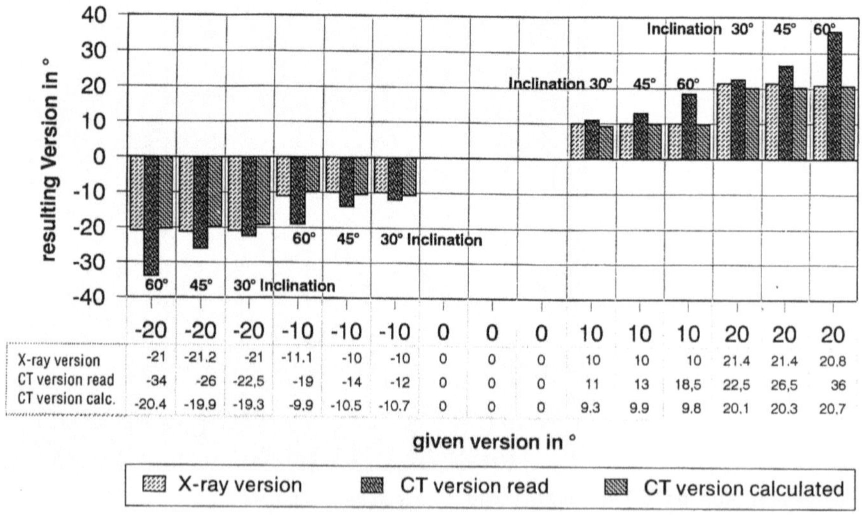

given version in °	-20	-20	-20	-10	-10	-10	0	0	0	10	10	10	20	20	20
X-ray version	-21	-21.2	-21	-11.1	-10	-10	0	0	0	10	10	10	21.4	21.4	20.8
CT version read	-34	-26	-22,5	-19	-14	-12	0	0	0	11	13	18,5	22,5	26,5	36
CT version calc.	-20.4	-19.9	-19.3	-9.9	-10.5	-10.7	0	0	0	9.3	9.9	9.8	20.1	20.3	20.7

Fig. 6. Version dependence of the inclination. Very high deviation between angle read from CT and real angle

$$\sin^2\alpha_2 = \frac{1}{1+\cot^2\alpha_1\,\cos^2\beta_2} \qquad \alpha_2 = \text{CT inclination}$$

$$\cos^2\alpha_1 = \frac{1}{1+\tan^2\alpha_2\,\cos^2\beta_2} \qquad \alpha_1 = \text{con. X-ray inclination}$$

$$\sin^2\beta_1 = \frac{\sin^2\beta_2}{1+\cot^2\alpha_1\,\cos^2\beta_2} \qquad \beta_2 = \text{con. X-ray version}$$

$$\sin^2\beta_2 = \frac{\cos^2\beta_1}{1+\sin^2\beta_1\,\cot^2\alpha_1} \qquad \beta_1 = \text{CT version}$$

Fig. 7. Converting equations for inclination and version in CT and in conventional X-ray

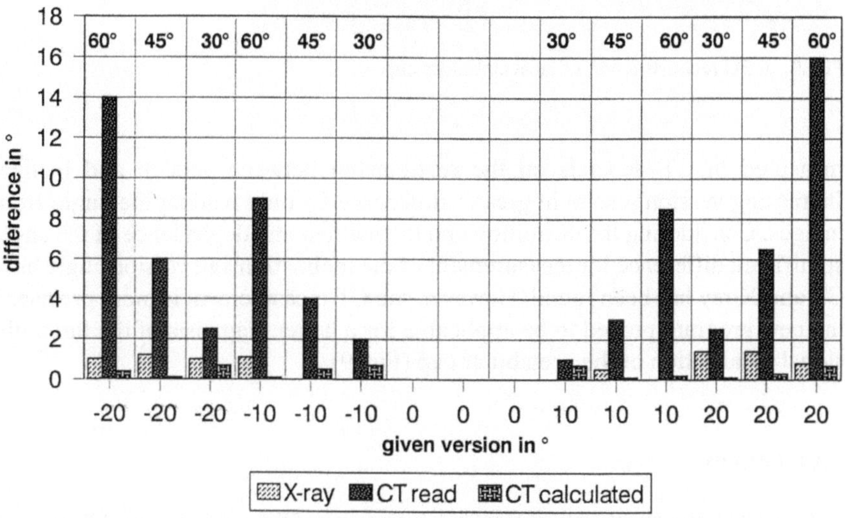

Fig. 8. The differences between the true angle and the angle measured in CT

with the adjusted (real) angle (Fig. 6). The cause of that was the different definition of the individual angle-defining plains. Considering these differences and after corresponding rearrangement of the formula (Fig. 7) the duration was $\pm 0.7°$ for the inclination and $\pm 0.3°$ for the version between the real angle and the angles calculated from the CT coordinates (Fig. 8).

Discussion

By phantom investigations we proved that both methods can be used for the measurement of the angles. The difference between the true angle and the angle we

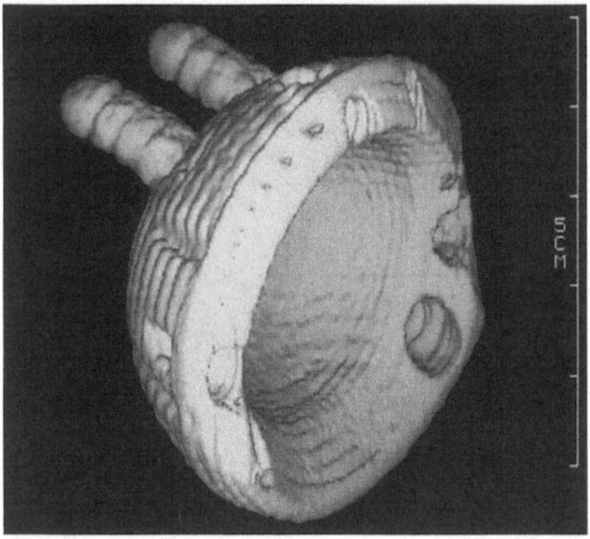

Fig. 9. A 3D reconstruction of an acetabulum cup

measured in CT depends on the relationship between version and inclination. Increasing version results in greater difference by only reading the angle from CT images. Considering the definition and the mathematic dependence of the angle, no significant difference for measurement of the inclination and version angle between CT and X-ray has been found. However, the CT measurement is more precise. Thus the new program proved to be applicable for a better diagnosis of the three-dimensional localisation of the acetabular cup (Fig. 9).

References

1. Ackland M, Bourne W, Uhthoff H (1986) Anteversion of the acetabular cup. J Bone Joint Surgery (Br) 1986;68-B. No. 3 : 409–413
2. Petersson H, Gentz C-F, Lindberg HO, Carlsson A (1982) Radiologic evaluation of the position of the acetabular component of the total hip prothesis. Acta Radiologica Diagnosis 23 Fase. 3A: 259–263
3. Klotz E, Kalender W, Sokiranski R, Felsenberg D (1990) Algorithms for the reduction of CT artefacts caused by metallic implants. SPIE Medical Imaging IV Vol. 1234 : 642–650

Mandibular and Temporomandibular Joint Pathology: Standard Approach with the Somatom Plus 3-D CT Software Program

C.H. Buitrago-Téllez, R. Wächter, F.J. Ferstl, P. Stoll, M. Langer

Introduction

The diagnosis of mandibular and temporomandibular pathology is difficult task because of the morphological changes associated with trauma, deformities, degenerative disorders or neoplasms. Three-dimensional computed tomography (3-D CT) has been introduced as an important aid in the assessment of craniofacial bones including the mandible [5], especially in the setting of skeletal deformities [4, 7], trauma [1] and preoperative evaluation [6, 8]. Because reproducibility is essential for inter- and intraindividual comparison of 3-D CT examinations, the lack of standardization of 3-D image views represent a relevant clinical and radiological question. In the routine different views from any projection may be obtained resulting in different 3-D studies, which depend on the specific clinical cases and physician. Moreover, some 3-D image projections may not be adequate to demonstrate particular findings according to the superimposition of bony structures or artefacts.

For that reason, the current study was conducted to determine the 3-D image views providing the most valuable anatomical and pathological information of osseous parts of the mandible and the temporomandibular joint (TMJ).

Patients and Methods

Twenty-three patients with mandibular or temporomandibular joint disorders were evaluated. The average age was 34 years (range: 18–50 years). There were 16 male and seven female patients. Table 1 shows the covered pathological spectrum. Axial 2-D CT studies were generated for all patients using diverse CT techniques: one group ($n = 13$) with serial, contiguous non-overlapping 2-mm slices, a second group ($n = 9$) with serial 1-mm slices at the TMJ level and one spiral CT (2 mm × 2 mm × 1 mm).

The 3-D reconstructions were generated using the binary-thresholding algorithm (threshold value: 150 HU) described by Herman in 1988 [2].

The following 3-D image views were reformatted in all patients according to specific parameters:

- Lateral rotations (R = rotation) using a tilt (T) of $-10°$: R $\pm 60°$, $\pm 90°$, $\pm 115°$, $\pm 140°$

Table 1. Clinical study population

	Patients (n)
Mandible	*16*
Trauma	5
Tumor/tumor+like lesions	6
Osteomyelitis	2
Atrophy or deformity	3
Temporomandibular joint	*7*
Trauma (Fracture/luxation)	2
Ankylosis	2
Arthrosis	1
Hyperplasia of the condylar process	2

- Frontal rotations (T = tilt) using a rotation (R) of 0°: T −10°, −25°, −95°, −115°
- Cut sections from
  - A dorsal 3-D view (R 180°/T 8°) up to the dorsal margin of the glenoid fossa.
  - An oblique 3-D view (R ±105°/T −7°) parallel to the lingual aspect of the ascending mandibular ramus.
- 2-D reconstructions (coronal, sagittal, axial and oblique) based upon:
  - A lateral 3-D view (R 90°/T 0°)
  - A frontal 3-D view (R 0°/T 0°)
  - A cranial 3-D view (R 0°/T 110°)

Because the reproducibility of patient head position is critical for the definition of standardized views, the 2-D reconstructions based on the lateral 3-D view was imaged first to corroborate the symmetry of the mandible condyles on a coronal reconstruction. When a slight rotation was necessary to obtain a symmetrical display of the condyles, this value in degree (e.g. R ± 3°) was added or subtracted to the standard frontal view of R 0°.

After completing all 3-D views, cut-sections and 2-D reconstructions, the anatomical and pathological depiction of the most relevant mandibular and TMJ bony regions were evaluated by one radiologist and one maxillofacial surgeon using a fivepoint score system (1 = not visible; 2 = poor; 3 = moderate; 4 = satisfactory; 5 = optimal diagnostic image quality). The gold standard were the 2-D axial CT images together with the clinical and surgical informations. A direct comparison of the axial 2-D CT studies and the 3-D reconstructions was not performed as it was already subject of an own previous investigation [1].

Results

TMJ Structures

The 3-D CT views demonstrating the highest scores for the depiction of the glenoid fossa of the TMJ and the mandible condyle were the R ±140°/T −10° view in the lateral rotation, the R 0°/T −115° projection in the frontal rotation, the dorsal cut section based on the R 180°/T 8° 3-D image and the 2-D reconstruction based on the cranial R 0°/T 110° 3-D image. The R 0°/T -115° was especially useful to visualize the glenoid fossa as in cases of condylar trauma with subluxation (Fig. 1a) or severe hypoplastic ascending ramus of the mandible (Fig. 2a). The dorsal cut section allow a graphical delineation of condylar pathology (Fig. 1b, 2b). The standard lateral view (R ±90°/T −10°) permits the detection of asymmetry as in cases of condylar hyperplasia (Fig. 3).

Mandibular Regions

The coronoid process was difficult to evaluate, especially when there were pathological changes. The time-consuming cut-section based on an oblique 3-D view (R ± 105°/T −7°) allowed the most optimal presentation of the structure. The coronoid process was also adequate visible using the R ±115°/T −10° view. The lingual aspect of the ascending ramus including the mandible foramen was also visualized using the tangential cut section.

The lateral aspect of the mandible angle were best demonstrated on the R ±60° or R ±90°/T −10° view. The dorsal and caudal aspects require respectively the dorsal cut-section (R 180°/T 8°) and the caudal R 0°/T −115° image view.

The mandible body and chin regions were adequately visualized in the R 0°/T −115° (Fig. 1a, b) as well as in the R 0°/T −95°. The alveolar process was displayed satisfactorily in the frontal R 0°/T −25° view as well as in the R ±60°/T −10° lateral rotation.

A general summary of the results are presented in Table 2, on which only the mean values of all observations for each anatomic structure and 3-D image view are listed.

Discussion

Standardization of imaging methods in diagnostic radiology is essential for an adequate comparison of normal and pathological findings. With the introduction of 3-D CT an almost indefinite number of projections, sections, and reformations are technically feasible. Radiologist must therefore search for the maximum of diagnostic information or spatial orientation with the minimum of processing time or number of projections.

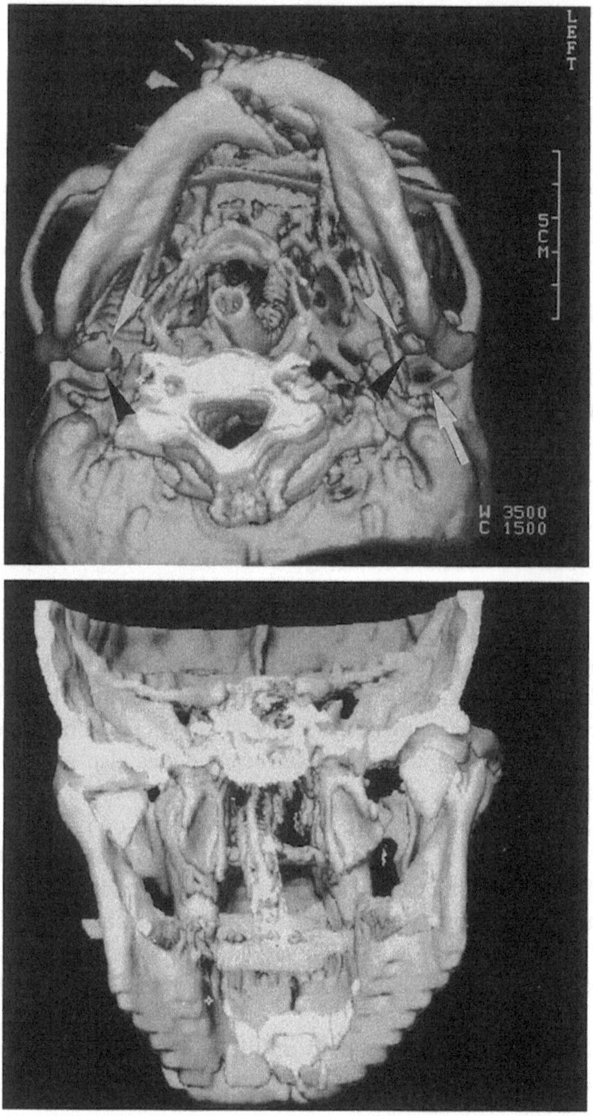

a

b

Fig. 1a, b. Comminuted mandibular fracture. **a** Rotation (R) 0°/tilt (T) –115° 3-D CT view shows the ventral dislocation of the left and inner rotation of the right mandible body. Note also the bilateral displaced condylar fractures (*arrow heads*) with the empty glenoid fossa left (*arrow*) as a subluxation sign. **b** Cut section from a dorsal 3D view (R 180°/T 8°)

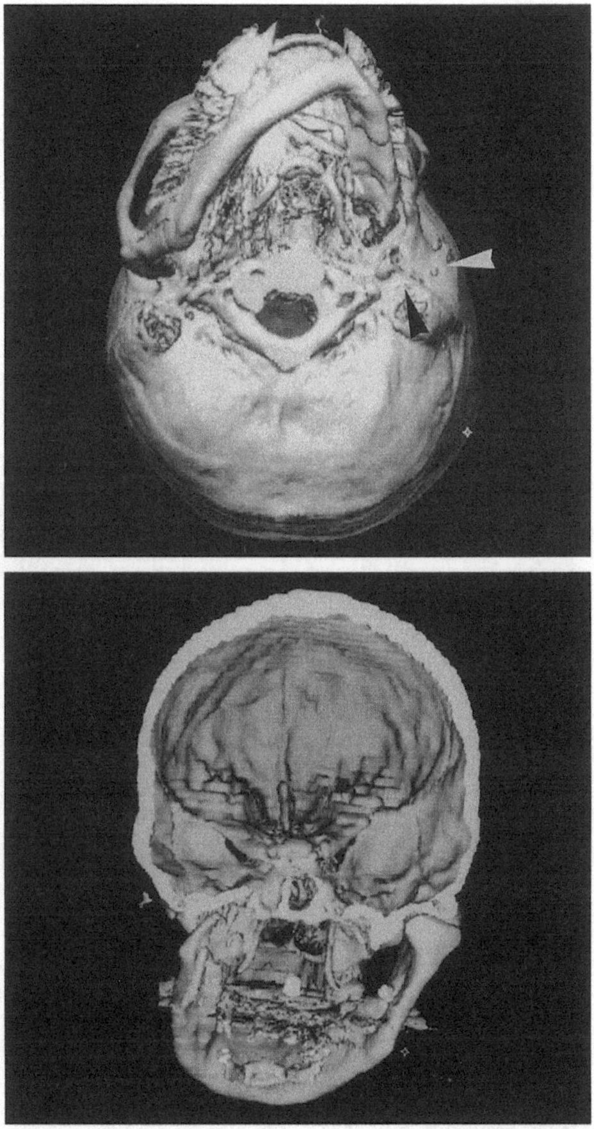

a

b

Fig. 2a, b. Hemifacial microsomia. **a** Rotation (R) 0°/tilt (T) –115° view revealing also an empty glenoid fossa (*arrow head*) on the left, secondary to a severe deformity of the mandible consisting of a hypoplastic ramus and absence of a functional temporomandibular joint. **b** Dorsal cut section (R 180°/T 8°). Note also the deviation of the mandible body and the missing left condylar head

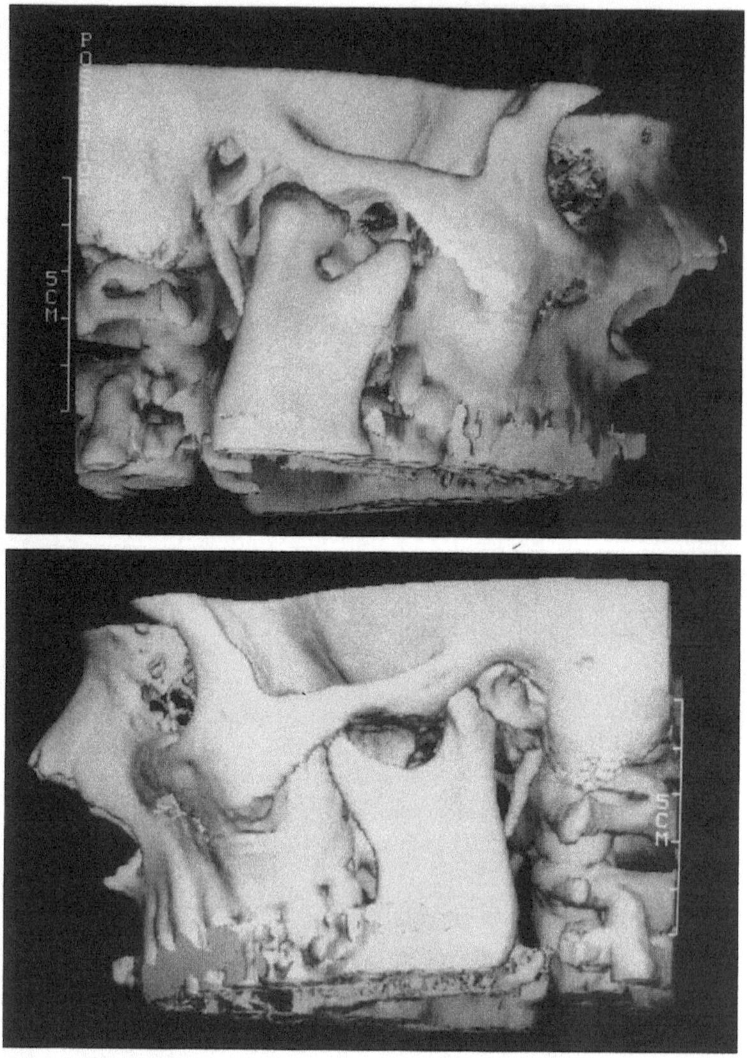

a

b

Fig. 3a, b. Condylar hyperplasia. **a** Rotation (R) 90°/tilt (T) –10°. Note the downward displacement of the enlarged condylar head over the tuberculum. The glenoid fossa is not adequately visible in this projection. **b** R –90°/T –10°. Normal condylar and coronoid processes

The methodical limitation of this retrospective study was the different CT scanning techniques available, which preclude a detailed analysis of the newer developments related to the clinical applications spiral CT [3]. In a single case of ameloblastoma of the left mandible body a spiral CT with a CT angiography emphasizes the possibilities of simultaneous 3-D visualization of vascular and bone structures. The postoperative control CT using the standard 3-D projections allows an adequate assessment of surgical results (Fig. 4a, b). The highest overall score concerning anatomical depiction of mandibular structures was reached by a cut-section

Table 2. Differentiated evaluation of standard 3-D views, cut sections and 2-D reconstructions based on 3-D projections concerning the mandibular and temporomandibular joint regions

Anatomic region	Lateral rotation				Frontal rotation				Cut sections		2-D reconstructions		
	R ±60° T-10°	R ±90° T-10°	R ±115° T-10°	R ±140° T-10°	R 0° T-10°	R 0° T-25°	R 0° T-95°	R 0° T-115°	R 180° T 8°	R ±105° T-7°	R 90° T 0°	R0° T0°	R0° T 110°
Glenoid fossa of temporomandibular joint	2.4	2.8	4.4	4.3	1.0	1.4	3.6	4.5	3.8	3.3	3.4	3.5	4.4
Condylar head	2.5	3.1	4.1	4.8	1.4	2.4	3.3	4.4	4.9	4.1	3.8	3.9	4.6
Condylar neck	2.6	3.1	4.1	4.9	1.4	2.4	3.3	4.5	4.9	4.3	3.8	3.8	4.6
Coronoid process	2.5	3.1	4.4	4.1	1.4	2.6	1.7	1.1	1.3	5.0	1.0	1.6	1.8
Ascending ramus with handible foramen	1.2	1.0	1.0	1.0	1.0	1.0	1.1	2.4	3.9	4.4	1.3	1.1	1.9
Mandible angle – Lateral surface	4.8	4.8	3.3	2.2	1.9	1.8	2.6	3.8	1.0	1.0	1.0	1.2	1.3
– Dorsal surface	1.0	1.0	1.8	3.3	1.7	1.8	2.6	3.8	5.0	1.0	1.3	1.2	1.7
– Caudal surface	1.0	1.0	1.8	2.8	1.0	1.0	3.5	4.6	3.9	1.0	1.1	1.0	1.0
Mandible body/chin	4.9	4.5	3.2	2.2	4.3	4.3	4.9	5.0	4.4	1.8	4.3	1.2	1.2
Alveolar process	4.8	4.4	2.5	1.8	4.6	4.8	1.6	1.1	2.4	2.0	1.0	1.0	1.0
Total score (mean value)	2.7	2.8	3.1	3.2	1.9	2.3	2.7	3.5	3.6	2.9	2.2	2.0	2.5

R, rotation; T, tilt
Score: 1 = not visible; 2 = poor; 3 = moderate; 4 = satisfactory; 5 = optimal image quality

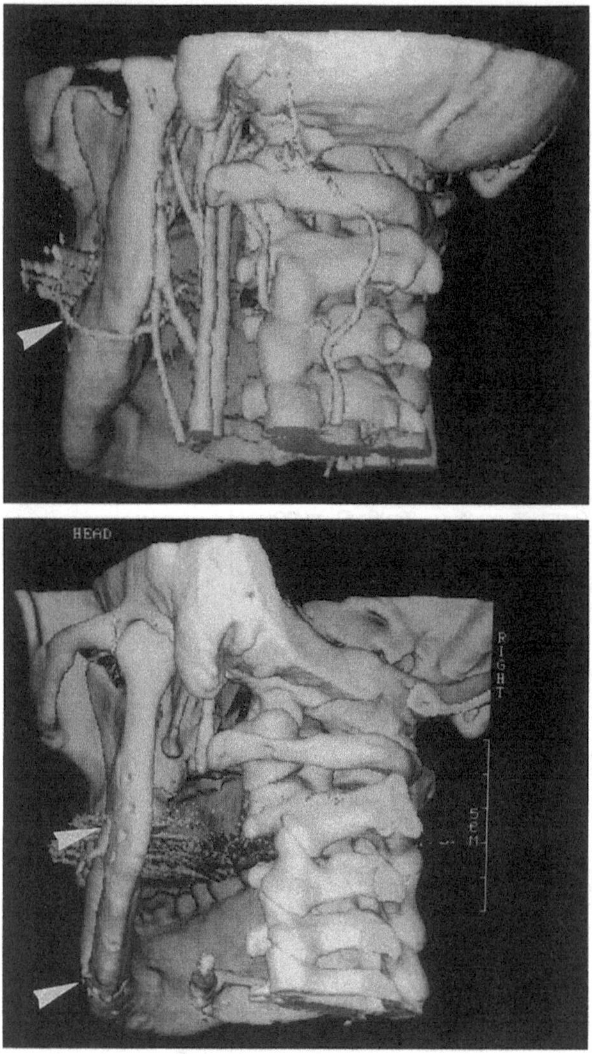

a

b

Fig. 4. Ameloblastoma of the mandible. **a** Rotation (R) –140°/tilt (T) –10° 3-D CT view with simultaneous spiral CT angiography. This projection underlines the expansile lesion of the left mandible body surrounded by the facial artery (*arrow head*). **b** The same view 6 months after tumor resection, fibula reconstruction (*arrow head*) and plate removal in the mandible angle

Table 3. Basic approach to mandibular and temporomandibular joint pathology using 3-D views

Lateral rotation:	R ±140°/T −10°
Frontal rotation:	R 0°/T −115°
Cut-section from a dorsal 3-D view up to the dorsal margin of the glenoid fossa:	R 180°/T 8°
2-D reconstructions (coronal, sagittal, oblique) based upon a cranial 3-D view:	R 0°/T 110°

R, rotation; T, tilt.

Table 4. Additional optimal 3-D views according to specific mandibular structures

Cut-section tangential to the ascending ramus: – Coronoid process – Ramus of the mandible with foramen mandibulae	R ±105°/T −7°
Lateral rotation: – Mandible angle lateral – Alveolar process – Mandible body/chin	R ±60°/T −10°
Frontal rotation: – Alveolar process – Coronoid process	R 0°/T −25°

R, rotation; T, tilt.

up to the dorsal margin of the glenoid fossa of a dorsal 3-D view (R 180°/T 8°). This may result from the adequate reproduction of the symmetrial 3-D nature of the condyles, the depiction of the lingual aspect of the ascending ramus and the mandible body in a single view.

Conclusions

1. A standard basic approach to the diagnosis of bony disorders of the mandible and TMJ is proposed. According to our data, just five 3-D views are sufficient to obtain an adequate overview of osseous mandibular and TMJ structures (Table 3).
2. Special 3-D projections may be additionally added depending on the specifical clinical case or the anatomical structure to be studied (Table 4).
3. The use of a standard 3-D approach guarantees the reproducibility of diagnostic images to detect possible changes intra- and interindividually after growth or surgery.

References

1. Buitrago-Tellěz CH, Wächter R, Ferstl F, Stoll P, Düker J, Langer M (1994) 3-D-CT zur Befunddemonstration bei komplexen Gesichtsschädelverletzungen. Fortschr Röntgenstr 160: 106–112
2. Herman GT (1988) Three dimensional imaging on a CT or MR scanner. J Comput Assist Tomogr 12:450–458
3. Hirschfelder U (1992) Die Spiral-CT-Aufnahmetechnik – erste Erfahrungen für kieferorthopädische Fragestellungen. Fortschr Kieferorthop 53:247–253
4. Mutoh Y, Ohashi Y, Uchiyama N, Terada K, Hanada K, Sasaki F (1991) Three-dimensional analysis of condylar hyperplasia with computed tomography. J Cranio-Max-Fac Surg 19:49–55
5. Ono I, Ohura T, Narumi E, Kawashima K, Matsuno I, Nakamura S, Ohhata N, Uchiyama Y, Watanabe Y, Tanaka F, Kishinami T (1992) Three-dimensional analysis of craniofacial bones using three-dimensional computet tomography. J Cranio-Max-Fac Surg 20:49–60
6. Vannier MW, Marsh JL, Warren JO (1984) Three dimensional CT reconstruction images for craniofacial surgical planning and evaluation. Radiology 150:179–184
7. Whyte AM, Hourihan MD, Early MJ, Sugar A (1990) Radiological assessment of hemifacial microsomia by three-dimensional computed tomography. Dentomaxillofac Radiol 19: 119–125
8. Zwicker C, Langer M, Astinet F, Köhler D, Wolff K-D, Felix R (1990) Wertigkeit der 3D-CT in der kieferchirurgischen Diagnostik und Therapieplanung. Fortschr Röntgenstr 152:393–397

Spiral CT with Three-Dimensional reconstruction – A New Dimension in Diagnosing the Thoracic Outlet Syndrome

K.-A. Lindgren, H. Rytkönen

Introduction

Thoracic outlet syndtome (TOS) is a controversial topic in surgery. TOS is difficult to diagnose using current clinical, radiological or neurophysiological criteria. The diagnosis is almost always based on positional tests of the upper limb that aim to reproduce the patient's symptoms. A positional compression of the neurovascular structures during these tests is a common phenomenon in normal subjects [11].

Certain anatomical anomalies, such as cervical ribs, anomalous first ribs or fibrous bands are said to cause TOS symptoms [13]. These are, however, also seen among asymptomatic individuals and such anomalies found during an operation do not necessarily enable the surgeon to predict the outcome [4]. Arteriography should not be used in the diagnosis of TOS, except in patients with signs of pronounced compression [12]. Non-invasive assessment of the TOS such as Doppler flow studies is of little help in the diagnosis of TOS [14] and is often of no value to the surgeon in establishing a causal link with the symptoms [8]. Panegyres et al. have claimed that magnetic resonance imaging (MRI) of the brachial plexusis is potentially valuable in its diagnosis. They argue that distortion of nerves and blood vessels suggests the presence of radiographically undetectable bands and that these cause the symptoms of TOS [10].

TOS symptoms are most often seen among young females doing sedentary work. Recent studies [7] suggest that a functional disturbance of the upper aperture may cause TOS symptoms. We describe a young woman with a typical history of TOS symptoms, who presented with malpositioned first rib on the symptomatic side which we detected using clinical tests described previously [7]. We could confirm this malposition with a three dimensional computerized scan.

Case History

Our patient was a 38-year-old woman who helped and cared for patients at home. Her work was heavy and included lifting patients and assisting them in their daily activities. Two years ago, she felt gradually increasing pain in her left shoulder which went down her chest and left arm into the medial forearm and hand. Her left arm became weak and clumsy. She could not work with her arms above the horizontal level and suffered from nocturnal pain after a day's work. Ultrasound and massage treatment failed to relieve her symptoms.

On clinical examination she had a normal flexion, rotation and lateral bending of the cervical spine. Lateral flexion of the rotated cervical spine (CRLF test [6]) was severely restricted on the symptomatic side, indicating a malfunction of the first rib and subluxation at the site of the costotransverse joint. The unaffected side was normal. The Roos provocation test was positive and after a few seconds during this test her left arm became pale and pulseless, she felt increasing pain and numbness in the hand and in the segments innervated by the ulnar nerve. Cervical X-ray, X-ray of the shoulder as well as ultrasound studies of the shoulder were normal. Neurophysiological studies were normal as well as an MRI of the cervical spine.

The patient underwent digital subtraction angiography (DSA) (Inficon FC 2000, Italy) with the contrast injected into the aortic arch; this done in the upright position with her hands raised it showed total obstruction of her left subclavian artery at the clavicular level. During this provocation temporary stenosis was induced on the right hand side. The region around the first thoracic vertebra and the first ribs was imaged by spiral computed tomography (spiral CT, Siemens Somatom Plus-S, Erlangen, Germany) with 3-mm slice thickness, 3-mm/s feed rate and standard algorithm. Four different spiral CT examinations were performed: arms in rest position during full inspiration and full expiration, and arms in upright position during full inspiration and full exspiration. All spiral-CT data were reconstructed using 2-mm increments and then transferred to a workstation (Sienet, DRC 2). In the workstation, three-dimensional CT images were created and viewed using what is known as "surface reconstruction". Superfluous information such as soft tissue was eliminated by using threshold values about 150 HU. The optimal 3-D images were then printed by laser imager. This detected an assymmetry of the first ribs at the costotransverse joint (Fig. 1), and the first rib was displaced upwards, causing asymmetry of the upper aperture (Fig. 2).

A treatment program [7] restored the function of the first rib and the symptoms of the patient disappeared.

Discussion

With no significant vascular or neurological abnormalities the diagnosis of TOS is always difficult. Over 90% of patients with TOS do not have any physical findings, only subjective symptoms. These patients, however, are the ones who most often undergo surgery, especially in the United States [2], and the outcome is unpredictable [7].

Transaxillary first rib resection promised relief of symptoms wherever the compression was within the upper aperture [3]. Good results after such resection, however, have ranged from 24% to 100% of patients, depending on who was doing the follow-up examination.

Furthermore, transaxillary rib resection is not as hazard free as was once thought, ad complications such as severe plexopathies,causalgias and even deaths have been reported [9].

In a recent paper Panegyres et al. reported changes in MRI studies indicating the presence of anomalous bands and suggesting a distortion of the vascular and neuro-

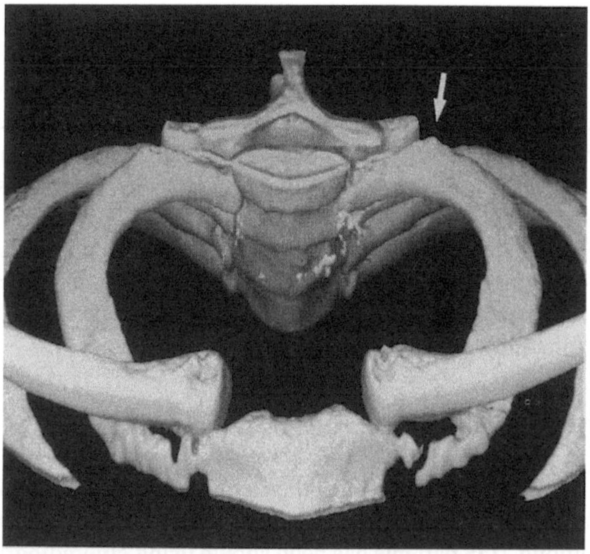

Fig. 1. Computed tomography viewed with three dimensional shaded surface display shows an upward dislocation of the first rib at the costotransverse joint on the left side (*arrow*)

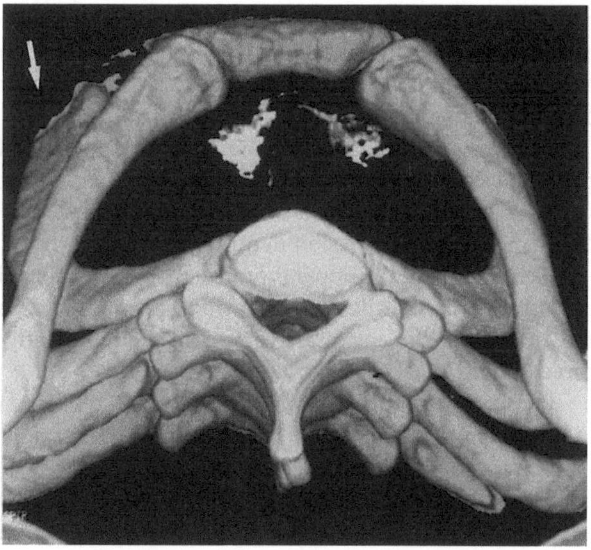

Fig. 2. The upper thoracic aperture viewed from above. The asymmetry of the position of the first ribs can be seen. The left rib is pushed laterally (*arrow*) because of the subluxation of the costotransverse joint

logical structures on the affected side in patients with TOS [10]. In this study a slight distortion of these structures was also found in one asymptomatic patient.

The aetiology of TOS symptoms have been extensively discussed, especially in the surgical literature, but only in terms of possible anatomical abnormalities. Studies recently presented, however, suggest that a functional disturbance in the upper thoracic aperture may cause TOS symptoms as well as explaining the unsuccessful outcome of surgery [7]. TOS symptoms often occur among young women doing sedentary work that stresses the upper limbs. The condition is seldom seen among people above 50 years of age. A functional cause seems to be a more convincing explanation than anomalous structures, which have been present, presumambly, since birth.

Malfunction of Rib Movements

The first ribs, which form the floor of the upper thoracic aperture, should move like birds' wings during expiration and inspiration. Disturbance of this movement among TOS patients has been shown using cineradiography [5], and a test called the CRLF test has proved to be a sensitive and specific test for this malfunction, and we have previously postulated that subluxation of the first rib at the costotransverse joint is associated with this malfunction [7].

In the movement of the first rib is disturbed by a possible subluxation of the first rib at the costotransverse joint, the whole kinesiology of the upper aperture may be affected, and an irritation of the C8 and T1 roots, which emerge in front of the cototransverse joint, may explain the ulnar distribution of the symptoms, perhaps better than more distal irritation of the nerves.

The upward dislocation of the first rib shown by the three dimensional computerised scans in our patient offers a logical explanation of the compression of the vascular structures between the clavicle and the first rib and the DSA angiography confirmed this compression in our patient.

The function of the upper thoracic aperture, especially the first ribs, can easily be assessed by the tests described earlier. This malfunction and possible subluxation of the first rib at the costotransverse joint can evidently also be documented by the three dimenstional CT scan presented here.

If any disturbances are found, either in the movements of the cervical spine or of the first ribs, these should be corrected with conservative non-surgical treatment [7].

The spiral computerized tomography with three-dimensional reconstruction is useful in detecting malfunction of the first ribs that can be corrected with a conservative approach. Before deciding on surgery the surgeon should do a thorough clinical evaluation to detect possible functional disturbances of the upper aperture that may be causing symptoms. Any anatomical structures should not be removed in the treatment of a symptom complex, the cause of which may be functional.

References

1. Carrol RE, Hurst LC (1982) The relationship of thoracic outlet syndrome and carpal tunnel syndrome. Clin Orthop 164 : 149–153
2. Cherington M (1991) Thoracic outlet syndrome: Rise of the conservative viewpoint. Am Fam Physician 43 : 1998–1999
3. Clagett OT (1962) Presidential address. Research and prosearch. J Thorac Cardiovasc Surg 44:153–168
4. Green RM, McNamara, Ouriel K (1991) Long-term follow-up after thoracic outlet decompression: An analysis of factors determining outcome. J Vasc Surg 14 : 739–746
5. Lindgren K-A, Leino E, Manninen H (1989) Cineradiography of the hypomobile first rib. Arch Phys Med Rehabil 70 : 408–409
6. Lindgren K-A, Leino E, Manninen H (1992) Cervical rotation lateral flexion test in brachialgia. Arch Phys Med Rehabil 73 : 735–737
7. Lindgren K-A (1993) Thoracic outlet syndrome with special reference to the first rib. Anales Chir et Gynaecol 82 : 218–230
8. Maisonneuve H, Planchon B, de Fausal P, Mussini JM, Patra P (1991) Vascular manifestation of thoracic outlet syndrome. Prospective study of 104 patients. J Mal Vasc 16 : 220–225
9. Melliere'D, Becquemin J-P, Etienne G, Le Cheviller B (1991) Severe injuries resulting from operations for thoracic outlet syndrome: Can they be avoided? J Cardiovasc Surg 32 : 599–603
10. Panegyres PK, Moore N, Bibson R, Rushworth G, Donaghy M (1993) Thoracic outlet syndromes and magnetic resonance imaging. Brain 116 : 823–841
11. Ribbe E, Lindgren SHS, Norgren L (1986) Clinical diagnosis of thoracic outlet syndrome-evaluation of patients with cervicobrachial symptoms. Manual Medicine 2 : 82–85
12. Roos DB (1976) Congenital anomalies associated with thoracic outlet syndrome. Am J Surg 132 : 771–777
13. Roos DB (1990) The thoracic outlet syndrome is underrated. Arch Neurol 47 : 327–328
14. Sällström J, Thulesius O (1982) Non-invasive investigation of vascular compression in patients with thoracic outlet syndrome. Clin Physiol 2 : 117–125

Abdomen

Chairmen: C. D. Claussen, W. Hruby

The DXP Technique as a New Tool for Abdominal Imaging

M. PROKOP, C. SCHAEFER-PROKOP, N. BAZAK

Introduction

Spiral computed tomography (SCT) is a technique that has gained wide clinical acceptance since its introduction in 1989 (Kalender et al. 1990). The two main advantages of spiral CT are a short scan time and the continuous acquisition of the scan volume. Whole organs such as lungs or liver can be imaged within a single breathhold phase. Injected contrast material can be used more efficiently: either the injected volume can be reduced (Costello et al. 1992) or the intravascular contrast can be increased (Rubin et al. 1993). Due to continuous volume acquisition, more lesions are detected (especially in the chest or liver) than with standard technique and the relation of lesions to surrounding structures can be more easily determined. Depending on the chosen scan parameters and resulting effective slice thickness, multiplanar reformats of excellent quality can be obtained without dose increase (Soucek et al. 1990).

Problems arise from the inverse relationship between scan length and spatial resolution along the z-axis: large scan volumes result in decreased resolution, while a high resolution with small effective slice thickness requires a small scan volume. With contrast application, so far only one perfusion phase could be imaged. Statements about contrast dynamics within particular lesions were not possible.

DXP is a novel technique in spiral imaging that allows for two rapidly succeeding scans in arbitrary direction. The technique can be used to increase the scan length two fold while keeping a good z-axis resolution, or to cover an identical volume at two different times and thus during two separate perfusion phases.

Material and Methods

With the new DXP software on the Somatom Plus S (Siemens, Erlangen), two spiral scans of up to 40 s each can be performed in rapid succession. Scan time, slice thickness and table feed are identical for both scans. Three variants of the DXP mode are available: With the "long" mode, the two spirals head into the same direction and cover twice the volume. In the "shuttle" mode, both scans are performed at identical starting points and have the same direction. In the "commute" mode, the scan direction is inverted and identical scan volumes are covered. The interscan delay varies between approximately 10 and 40 s, depending on the duration of the spiral scans.

Table 1. Examination parameters

	Scan parameters				Contrast administration			Patients (n)
	DXP mode	SL (mm)	TF (mm/s)	RI (mm)	V (ml)	F (ml/s)	D (s)	
Abdomen	Long	5	8	4/8	150	2	40	8
Liver	Commute	5	8	4	150	4	20–30	11
CTAP	Commute	5	8	4	90	2	20–30	8
Kidney	Shuttle	3–5	5–8	4	120	4	30	3
Pancreas	Shuttle	3	5	4	150	4	20–30	2

SL, slice thickness; TF, table feed/s; RI, reconstruction interval; V, volume; F, flow rate; D, start delay; CTAP, CT arteriopartol imaging.

We present our initial experience with 32 patients with various types of abdominal pathology and focus on two main applications: imaging of the whole abdomen at good z-axis resolution, and dynamic imaging of abdominal organs in two perfusion phases (anatomic regions and imaging parameters, Table 1). The interscan delay was chosen as small as possible.

DXP spiral scans of the abdomen were compared to conventional dynamic incremental CT scans. These "standard" CT scans were performed with the dynamic screening mode (5-s interscan delay) during a biphasic injection of 150 ml i.v. contrast (50 ml with 2 ml/s, 100 ml with 1 ml/s).

Images were subjectively evaluated with respect to liver contrast, contrast of the abdominal vessels and presence of artifacts. For each scan it was noted whether the second spiral provided additional diagnostic information.

Results

Routine Abdominal Imaging with DXP

As compared to the standard technique, DXP (first scan) provided an improved parenchymal contrast in the liver, excellent visualization of portal veins, liver veins and the branches of the coeliac trunc. In the second scan the vascular contrast markedly decreased but was still superior over conventional images. This difference was least at the beginning of the scan but increased when the small pelvis was reached. With regard to a differentiation between abdominal vessels and lymph nodes, the performance with the DXP technique was superior over that with standard CT.

Imaging of Abdominal Organs in Two Perfusion Phases

With DXP, parenchymal organs can be scanned in an arterial and a later venous or parenchymal phase. The later phase is thought to capture the organ parenchyma during maximum enhancement with high contrast in the venous structures (portal, liver or renal veins).

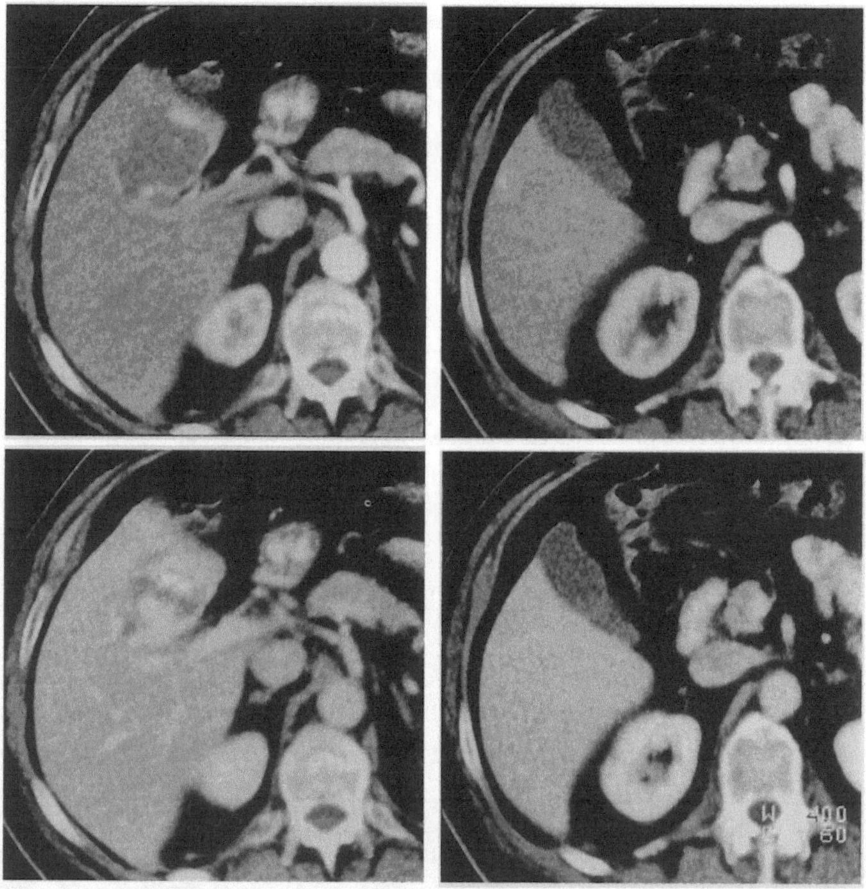

a b c d

Fig. 1a–d. Male patient with multiple hemangiomas. For the larger lesion, images in the arterial phase (**a**) and the mixed phase (**c**) show the typical enhancement pattern, while the small lesion (**b, d**) "vanishes" in the later scan

With our protocol, arterial contrast was excellent during the first scan in all patients. In the second scan, enhancement of the protal vein, the liver veins or the renal vein was less pronounced than arterial enhancement during the first scan but appeared superior to stadard CT. For the liver and the pancreas, parenchymal enhancement was low during the first scan and increased in the second scan (Figs. 1, 2). There was a trend that liver enhancement was better with shorter interscan delay. The renal cortex was clearly identified in the arterial phase, while on the later scan, enhancement of the whole parenchyma occurred.

Hypervascularized lesions in the liver, the pancreas or the kidneys were best seen in the first scan. In 6/11 patients, the second scan yielded additional information including those cases with hypovascularized lesions, with thrombi in the portal or renal veins, and with benign lesions such as hemangioma or focal nodular hyperplasia (FNH) which demonstrated characteristic patterns on the two scans. In

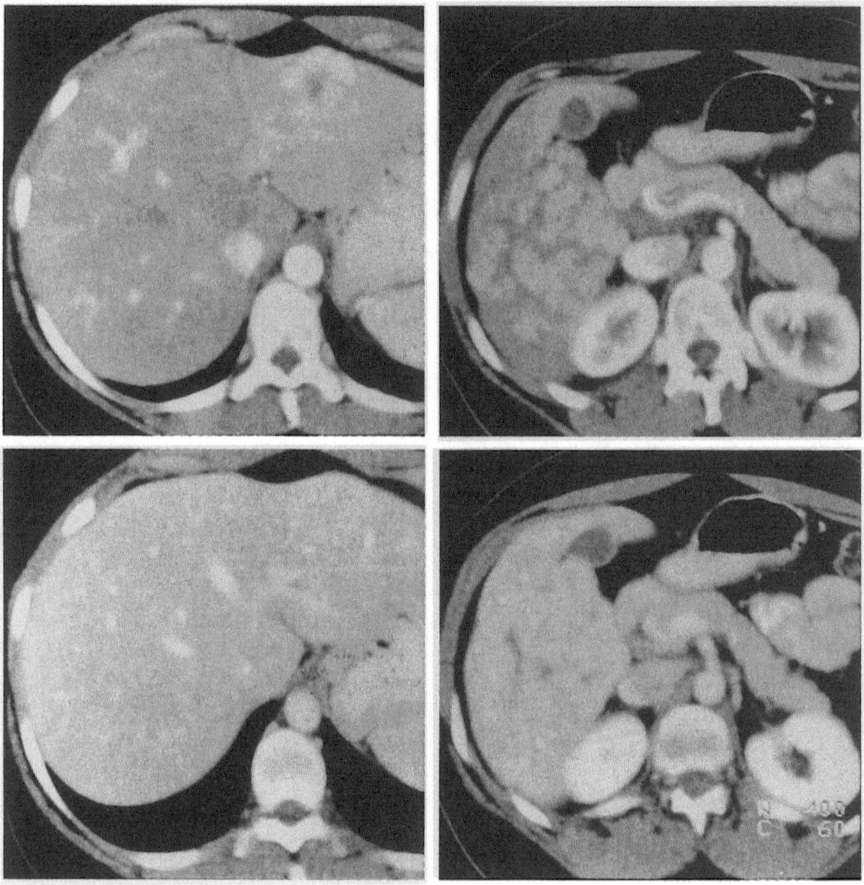

a b c d

Fig. 2a–d. Female patient with two lesions of focal nodular hyperplasia confirmed at surgery. Images in the arterial phase (**a, b**) and the mixed phase (**c, d**) display a typical enhancement pattern

hemangioma, vascular lacunae in the tumor periphery could be seen that are highly contrasted in arterial phase and appeared more ill-defiend and larger in the later phase. Small lesions may "vanish" on the second scan (Fig. 1). FNH presented as a strongly enhancing multi-nodular tumor in the arterial phase that appeared isodense relative to liver parenchyma in the second phase (with the exception of central scars that remain hypodense in both scans, see Fig. 2). In the five patients with hemangioma or FNH that we examined we found multiple lesions (up to five) in four cases, six of which were not previously known and were smaller than 2 cm.

CT Arterioportal Imaging

When applying DXP to arterioportal imaging (CTAP) of the liver, the first scan is performed during contrast injection into the splenic or superior mesenteric artery. It therefore corresponds to a conventional CTAP. The second scan is performed

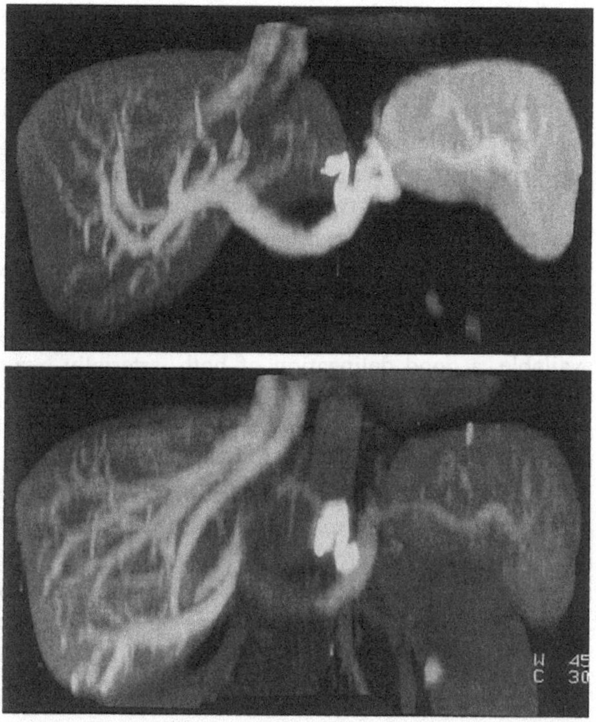

Fig. 3 a, b. Maximum intensity projection images of the portal venous system (a) and the liver veins (b) obtained from a CT arterio portal imaging examination using the DXP technique obtained during the portal phase (a) and during reperfusion (b)

20–30 s later (post-contrast scan), thus already representing a phase in which contrast reaches the liver not only from the portal veins but also from the arteries. The number of flow-related, tumor-related or periportal artifacts is markedly reduced in the post-contrast scan.

Maximum intensity projection (MIP) images of early and late scans of CTAP preferentially displayed the anatomy of the portal veins or liver veins, respectively. In some patients, nearly selective images of these vascular systems could be obtained (Fig. 3). For pre-operative planing, lesions could thus be reliably attributed to the various liver segments.

Discussion

Standard CT protocols for the abdomen may suffer from moderate contrast in the liver and from low vascular contrast in the lower abdomen and pelvis. DXP imaging of the whole abdomen allows for an optimized use of the contrast bolus for both, the parenchymal organs and for the differentiation of vascular and non-vascular structures (lymph node staging) in the lower abdomen and pelvis. In comparison to standard protocols, image quality is increased in most cases. Problems occurred with increased noise in adipose patients.

In our experience, however, the main diagnostic advantage of DXP lies in the ability to scan organs in an arterial and a parenchymal phase. According to our (limited) experience, benign tumors in the liver (hemangiomas, focal nodular hyperplasias) appear to have a distinct enhancement pattern in the arterial and the parenchymal phase. These two phases may allow for a discrimination between benign lesions and those that require further workup and treatment (adenomas, carcinomas, metastases). Due to volume acquisition, even multiple or small lesions can be evaluated that are usually hard to detect and classify using conventional techniques. Further studies, however, are warranted. Besides, as two perfusion phases are available, a good delineation of both, arterially hyper- or hypoperfused lesions, could be demonstrated (cf. Katayama et al. 1993). In our experience, however, shorter interscan delays between the two spiral scans appear preferable to capture peak liver enhancement with the second scan.

When applying DXP to CTAP of the liver, an improved discrimination between perfusion artifacts and real lesions can be shown. Equilibrium effects with "vanishing lesions" are not pronounced because the time span between the end of contrast injection and the second scan is short owing to a contrast bolus of 45-s duration.

MIP images of early and late scans of CTAP provide as superb display of portal veins or liver veins, respectively. Segmental anatomy can be better assessed prior to surgery.

Conclusion

DXP promises to be a valuable tool for abdominal imaging that allows for superior quality of routine images as well as for improved preoperative assessment of the liver and other parenchymal organs.

References

Costello P, Dupuy DE, Ecker CP, Tello R (1992) Spiral CT of the thorax with reduced volume of contrast material: a comparative study. Radiology; 183 : 663 – 666

Kalender WA, Seissler W, Klotz E, Vock P (1990) Spiral volumetric CT with single-breathhold technique, continuous transport and scanner rotation. Radiology; 176 : 181 – 183

Katayama N, Tsukioka T, Oishi T, Fukunaga J, Sasagawa M, Ozawa I (1993) Double-phase helical CT: diagnosis of hepatocellular carcinoma in preoperative patients. Radiology; 189(P) : 426

Rubin GD, Dake MD, Napel SA, McDonnel CH, Jeffrey RB Jr (1993) Three-dimensional spiral CT angiography of the abdomen: initial clinical experience. Radiology; 186 : 147 – 152

Soucek M, Vock P, Daepp M, Kalender WA (1990) Spiral-CT: Eine neue Technik für Volumenaufnahmen. II. Klinische Anwendungsmöglichkeiten. Röntgenpraxis; 43 : 365 – 375

Fast Consecutive Double Phase Spiral CT of the Liver and Pancreas: Benefits for Evaluation of Hypervascular Tumors and Vascular Lesions

L. Van Hoe, G. Marchal, S, Gryspeerdt, A. L. Baert

Introduction

With spiral computed tomography (SCT) relatively large organs such as the liver can be scanned entirely during the phase of maximal parenchymal enhancement, which improves the detection of hypovascular lesions. Hypervascular lesions and vascular anomalies however can be missed if they become iso-attenuating at the time of scanning.

Double phase (DXP) spiral CT allows repeated scanning of the same organ(s) both in the vascular (arterial) phase and in the parenchymal phase after contrast injection. Between October 1993 and March 1994, we applied this technique in 60 patients. The benefits of double phase scanning were analyzed retrospectively in 22 patients with proven hypervascular tumors or vascular (predominantly arterial) lesions.

Materials and Methods

Patient, Population and Scan Technique

Double phase spiral CT images of 22 patients with hepatic ($n = 8$) or pancreatic ($n = 5$) hypervascular tumors and benign ($n = 3$) or malignant ($n = 6$) arterial lesions were retrospectively reviewed. There were 12 men and 10 women whose ages ranged from 25 to 82 years and averaged 53 years. In nine patients with hypervascular tumors, a histological diagnosis was available. Lesions studied were: focal nodular hyperplasia (FNH; $n = 2$), hepatocellular corcinoma (HCC; $n = 1$), insulinoma ($n = 3$), gastrinoma ($n = 1$), metastases of carcinoid tumor ($n = 1$), microcystic adenoma of the pancreas ($n = 1$). Benign vascular lesions studied were an aneurysm of the hepatic ($n = 1$) and splenic ($n = 1$) artery and a hepatic AV malformation ($n = 1$). The other arterial lesions studied were caused by invasion by hepatic ($n = 2$) or pancreatic ($n = 4$) tumors.

All examinations were performed with a Somatom Plus S (Siemens, Erlangen). Contrast was injected in a cubital or antecubital vein. A mechanical power injector (Medrad Mark IV) was used for biphasic contrast administration. Depending on the quality of the vein injected and the age, weight and global cardiovascular status of each patient, an amount of 50 – 100 ml 38% iodinated contrast (Telebrix 38 – Guerbet) was injected with injection rates between 2.5 and 3.5 ml/s, followed by a rapid infusion (rate between 0.8 and 1.5 ml/s). The total amount of contrast medium administered varied between 100 and 150 ml. An attempt was made to start the first scan in the phase of selective arterial opacification. Therefore, a 12-ml test bolus was injected IV prior to patient scanning at the same injection rate as for the spiral tudy (between 2.5 and 3.5 ml/s). Beginning at the moment of contrast injection, single level scans at the level of the liver or pancreas were obtained each three seconds. A ROI was placed in the aorta and time density curves were generated. The length of the interval between the initiation of contrast injection and peack aortic enhancement was measured and was used for individual optimization of the injection-scan delay time for spiral scanning.

Once the injection-scan interval had been determined, the length of the consecutive spiral scans and the acquisition parameters were selected. Technically, the table feed direction could be selected indepedently for the first and second scan; all patients included in this study were scanned twice in the cephalocaudad direction ("shuttle" DXP). The acquisition parameters were identical for both scans: 180 or 210 mAS, 120 or 137 kV, collimation 5–8 mm and pitch 1. The length of each acquisition varied between 20 and 32 s. The delay between the first and second scan (inter-spiral delay) varied between 16 and 21 s (depending on the length of the first scan). This time interval was used for patient respiration. Patient preparation consisted of administration of oxygen prior to scanning and explanation of the scan technique and breathold requirements. Images were always calculated at 8 mm increments. If required, (multiplanar or 3D imaging, densitometry) image calculation at low table increments (1–2 mm) was performed retrospectively.

Data Analysis

The postcontrast images obtained with the first and second scan were reviewed independently by two radiologists (sg, lvh).

For evaluation of the benefits of double phase scanning, the diagnostic information obtained with the second spiral scan ("parenchymal phase" images) was assessed first and was used as reference. Next, the images obtained in the arterial phase were analyzed and their contribution for lesion detection and characterisation was scored on a three- or four-point scale (Table 1). Interobserver agreement was assessed by a kappa index.

Results

The double phase study was well tolerated in all patients. One patient was unable to maintain breathold during the length of both acquisitions; resulting image quality was satisfactory for diagnostic purposes. The optimal contrast injection-scan delay as determined with the test bolus injection varied from 10 to 32 s. The scores for the two reviewers are given in Table 2.

There was a high level of interobserver agreement (kappa-index 0.82).

Table 1. Benefits of arterial phase images: scoring system

Score	Description
	Hypervascular tumors: detection
0	No benefits
1	Improved delineation of lesions without detection of new lesions
2	Detection of new lesions
	Hypervascular tumors: characterisation
0	No benefits
1	Additional information leading to increased diagnostic confidence
2	Additional information leading to a change in diagnosis
	Vascular lesions
0	No benefits
1	Improved display of anatomical details
2	Detection of new lesions, without change in diagnosis
3	Detection of new lesions, leading to a change in diagnosis

Table 2. Benefits of arterial phase images: scores for two reviewers

	Score	Reviewer 1 (*n*)	Reviewer 2 (*n*)
Hypervascular tumors: detection	0	5	6
	1	5	4
	2	3	3
Hypervascular tumors: characterisation	0	6	6
	1	3	2
	2	4	5
Vascular lesions[a]	0	2	
	1	5	
	2	2	
	3	0	

[a] Numbers are for both reviewers

Hypervascular Tumors: Detection

In three patients, arterial phase images allowed detection of new hepatic lesions (one hypervascular metastasis, one FNH and one small HCC). All pancreatic tumors detected on arterial phase images were also visible on parenchymal phase images, but some were less well defined; one small (3 mm) gastrinoma was significantly better displayed on arterial phase images. One insulinoma that was well visible before contrast administration became iso-attenuating both an arterial and parenchymal phase images. Another insulinoma was isodense on arterial phase images and hyperdense on parenchymal phase images.

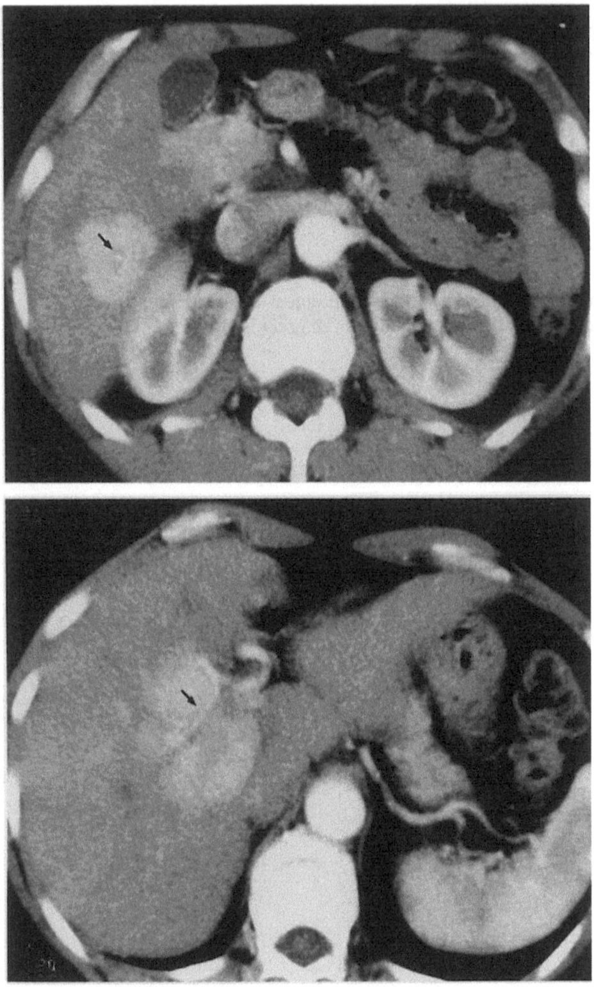

a

b

Fig. 1a–d. Improved detection and characterisation of hepatic focal nodula hyperplasia (FNH). **a, b** Arterial phase images. Well-defied hypervascular liver tumors are visible in the right liver lobe (**a**) and near the porta hepatis (**b**). The centrally located feeding artery is well visible in both lesions (*arrows*). **c, d** Parenchymal phase images. While the FNH in the right liver lobe appears as a hyperdense mass (**c**), the lesion located near the porta hepatis is almost invisible

Hypervascular Tumors: Characterisation

In most patients, arterial phase images improved the delineation of the tumors. In two patients with FNH, arterial phase images showed a central feeding vessel (Fig. 1). One pancreatic microcystic adenoma showed peripheral hypervascularity, which was visible only on arterial phase images (Fig. 2).

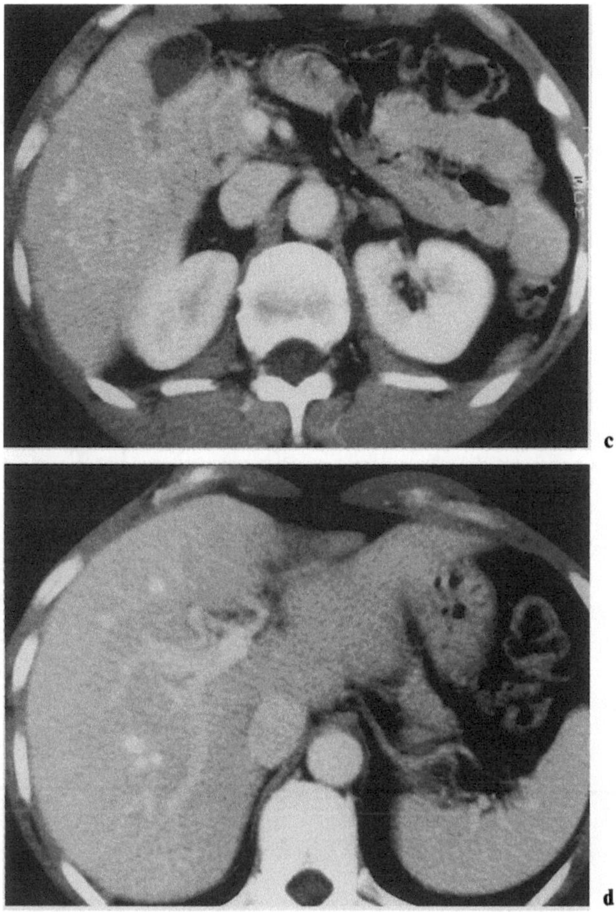

Fig. 1c, d

Vascular Lesions

Arterial phase images improved the display of two aneurysms and one hepatic AV malformation. Surface shaded 3D images led to a better understanding of the anatomy in two patients.

In two patients with pancreatic adenocarcinoma, arterial phase images showed narrowing of the splenic artery involved in the tumor; the diagnosis of vascular tumor invasion could also be suspected with study of parenchymal phase images alone, because of the location of the vessel in the tumor mass.

In one patient with angiographically proven tumor invasion of the proximal gastroduodenal artery, maximum intensity projections calculated from the arterial phase images failed to reveal any abnormality because of partial volume effects.

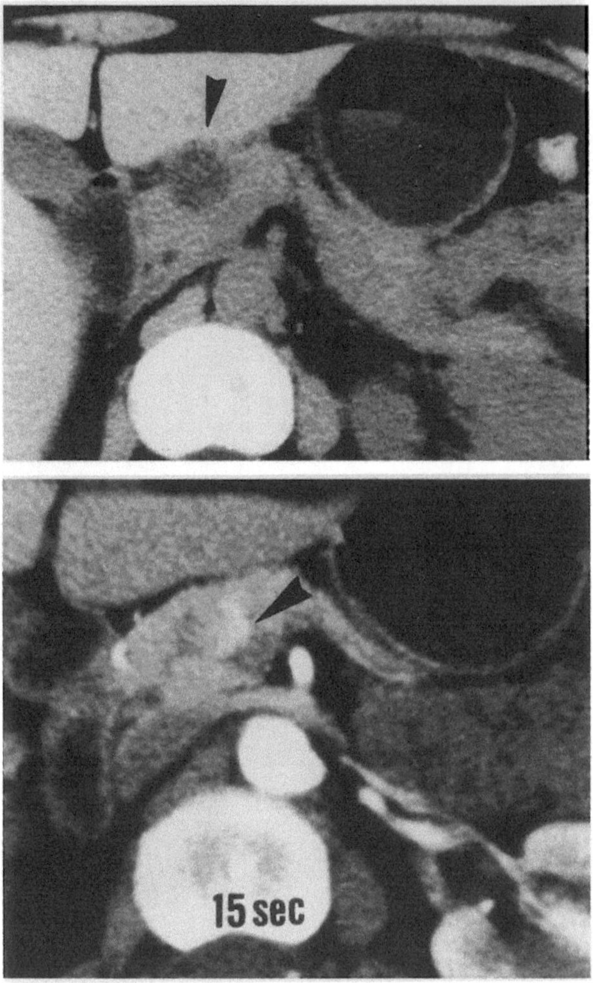

a

b

Fig. 2a–d. Improved characterisation of pancreatic microcystic adenoma. **a** Plain CT: a hypodense lesion is seen in the pancreatic body (*arrowhead*). **b** Arterial phase images show peripheral enhancement (*arrowhead*), which excludes the diagnosis of pancreatic (pseudo) cyst. **c** Parenchymal phase images. The tumor appears as a hypodense mass (*arrowhead*). **d** Angiography confirms peripheral tumor enhancement (*arrow*)

Discussion

The advent of spiral data acquisition has greatly enhanced the speed, quality and clinical applications of CT (Heike et al. 1993).

Rapid consecutive double phase CT opens new perspectives for the detection of hypervascular hepatic tumors (Marchal and Baert 1992; Ohashi et al. 1993).

In comparison with parenchymal phase images, images obtained during the phase of selective arterial enhancement improved the detection and/or characteri-

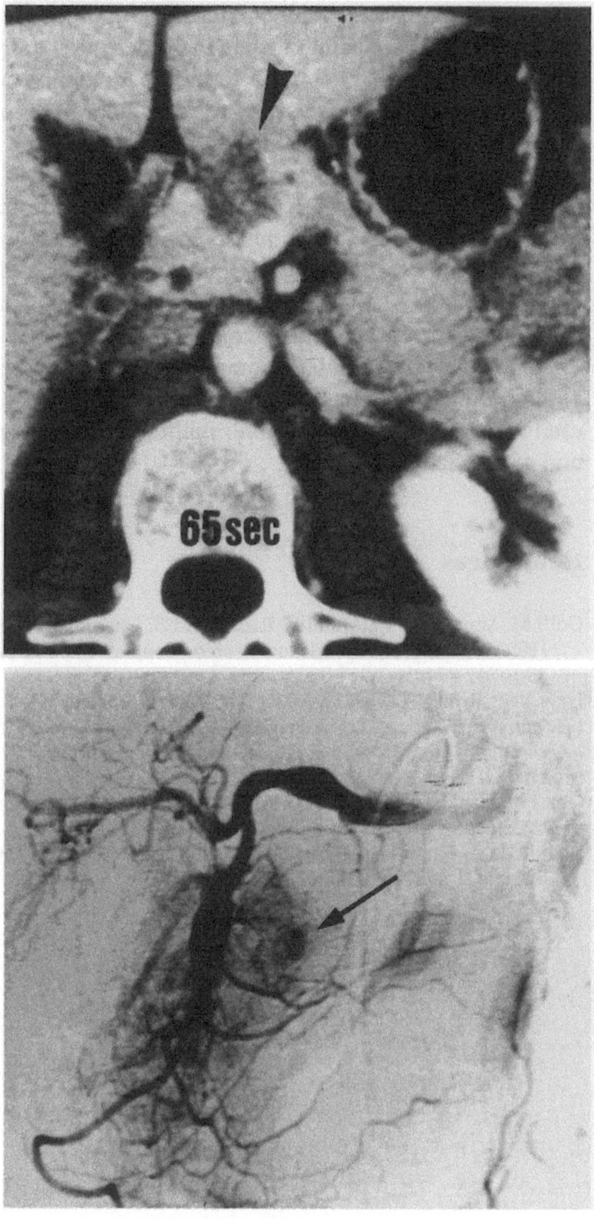

c

d

Fig. 2c, d

sation of a significant number of lesions in our patients. The main diagnostic advantage of the DXP technique lied in the detection of hypervascular liver tumors and the demonstration of central arterial blood supply in hypervascular liver tumors, which suggests the diagnosis of focal nodular hyperplasia (Shirkhoda et al. 1994) and virtually excludes adenoma (Golli et al. 1994). Our preliminary experience suggests that the introduction double phase spiral CT will improve both the sensitivity and specificity of CT for detection of these lesions.

In the pancreas, double phase scanning aided in the detection of endocrine tumors. Because of the wide variability in density and contrast captation pattern of these tumors, we consider the combination of unenhanced CT with double phase spiral CT the preferred CT technique.

For display of vascular anomalies, thin-section spiral CT and catheter angiography remain the imaging modalities of choice. Double phase spiral CT can be used to demonstrate arterial abnormalities in patients primarily referred for evaluation of parenchymal disease.

References

Golli M, Van Nhieu JT, Mathieu T, Zafrani ES, Cherqui D, Dhumeaux D, Vasile N, Rahmouni A (1994) Hepatocellular adenoma: color doppler US and pathologic correlations. Radiology 190:741–744

Heiken JP, Brink JA, Vannier MW (1993) Spiral (helical) CT. Radiology 189:647–656

Katayama N, Tsukioka T, Fukunaga J (1993) Double phase helical CT: diagnosis of hepatocellular carcinoma in preoperative patients (abstract). Radiology 1993, 189 (suppl): 426

Marchal G, Baert AL (1992) Dynamic CT of the liver. Radiology 32:211–216

Ohashi I, Hanafusa K, Yoshida T (1993) Small hepatocellular carcinomas: two-phase dynamic CT in detection and evaluation. Radiology 189:851–855

Shirkhoda A, Farah MC, Bernacki E, Madrazo B, Roberts J (1994) Hepatic focal nodular hyperplasia: CT and sonographic spectrum. Abdom Imaging 19:34–38

The Optimal Time Window for Spiral CT of the Liver During Arterial Portography

O. GRAF, W.I. DOCK, S. THURNHER, J. LAMMER, A. MAIER, G. LECHNER

Introduction

In hepatic oncology it is generally conceded that normal liver parenchyma is perfused primarily from the portal system whereas liver neoplasms receive their supply mainly from the hepatic artery (Burgener and Hamlin 1983; Bressler et al. 1987). The basic idea of computed tomographic arterial portography (CTAP) is that the liver is scanned during the portal and parenchymal phase of contrast distribution prior to significant tumor enhancement during the phase of systemic recirculation or by diffusion (Bluemke and Fishman 1993; Graf et al. 1993). To determine the optimal time window for scanning the liver using CTAP we created time density curves of the portal vein, liver parenchyma, abdominal aorta and tumors after contrast medium injection into the superior mesenteric artery (Graf et al. 1994).

Materials and Methods

Thirteen patients referred to CTAP were included in the study. CTAP was indicated in the course of preoperative evaluation prior to hepatic resection or preceding embolization of inoperable tumors. Approximately 30 min before a full diagnostic spiral CTAP examination of the entire liver we performed repetitive scans at the single level of the portal bifurcation to evaluate enhancement characteristics of the portal vein, liver parenchyma, aorta and tumors. The complete examination took place in the CT suite as the catheter had been placed into the superior mesenteric artery under fluoroscopic control of a C-arch directly on the CT table.

To increase portal blood flow 10 mg tolazoline hydrochloride were given i.a. immediately before injecting 80 ml iopamidol 300 mg iodine/ml with a flow of 5 ml/s with a power injector into the SMA. With a delay of 3 s after the beginning of the contrast injection CT scanning was started and 21 repetitive scans with an interscan delay of 3 s followed by four scans with an interscan delay of 5 s were performed at the single level of the portal bifurcation. Thus, 25 scans were obtained within 83 s after contrast injection at the level of the portal bifurcation.

After reconstruction data were transferred to a PACS workstation and density was measured in the portal vein, abdominal aorta, in liver parenchyma in both lobes and tumors, if present at the single level scans. All data from every single scan were recorded and time density curves were created. Figure 1 shows for example the enhancement profile in one of our patients.

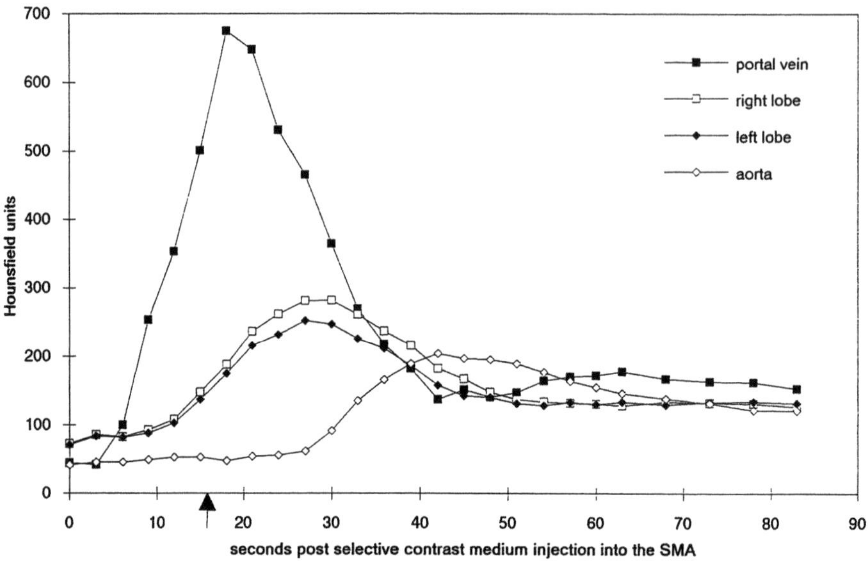

Fig. 1. Typical enhancement profile of portal vein, hepatic parenchyma and aorta contrast medium injection into the superior mesenteric artery (SMA). *Arrow* on x-axis indicates and injection (16 s) (from Graf et al. 1994)

Results

Portal Vein

Base density of the portal vein was 44±4 HU. A few seconds after contrast injection there was a steep increase in portal enhancement with a peak of 668±134 HU after 19 s (±2.6 s) followed by a rapid decline in density. A plateau phase with a density of 144±14 HU occurred after 44±4 s. In 10 patients a second but small increase in portal vein density by 25 HU (±10 HU) occurred after 57±9 s due to a second pass of contrast medium in the phase of systemic recirculation. Three patients showed no significant second increase in portal vein denstiy (<5 HU).

Abdominal Aorta

Base density of the abdominal aorta was 46±5 HU. Enhancement began 25±4 s after contrast medium injection and a peak of 176±26 HU was reached after 44±7 s. Later on density declined slowly and the curve described a relative stable plateau representing the phase of systemic circulation and developing equilibrium.

Liver Parenchyma

In 11 patients parenchymal data were obtained from both lobes, in two patients from the left lobe alone because tumor obstructed the right portal branch.

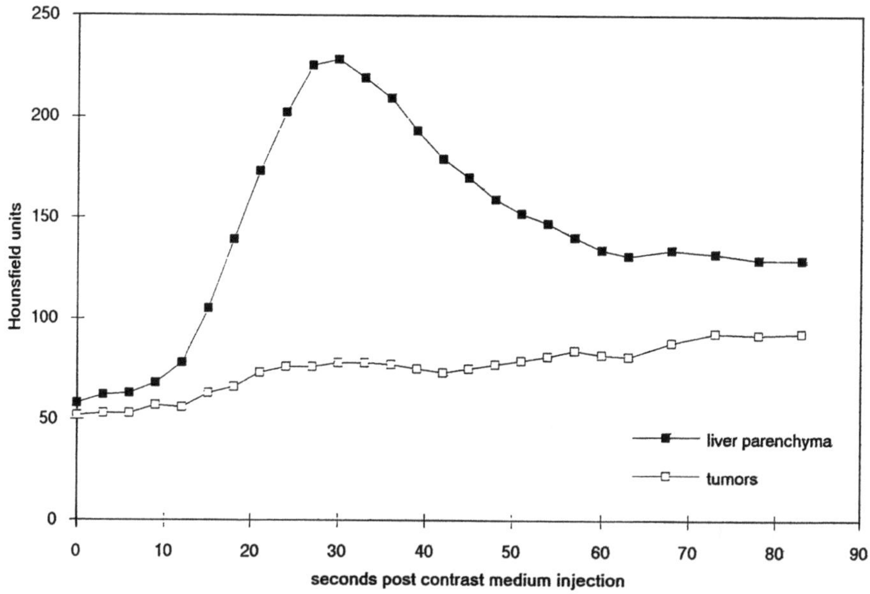

Fig. 2. Averaged time-attenuation curves of liver parenchyma and tumors after contrast medium injection into the superior mesenteric artery (from Graf et al. 1994)

Base density of hepatic parenchyma was 60±6 HU. Eleven seconds (±1.8) post injection hepatic parenchyma began to enhance. After 18±4 s denstiy was higher than 120 HU – approximately twice the base density giving sufficient contrast for lesion discrimination. The highest values (243±54 HU) were reached after 30±4 s. In the following phase parenchymal attenuation declined and after 67±15 s enhancement values were less than 120 HU.

Tumors

In nine patients measurements could be obtained from hepatic lesions as they were located at the level of the scans. If a tumor consisted of necrotic and vital tissue data were obtained from portions of the tumor which showed contrast enhancement.

Base density of tumors was 52±4 HU. After contrast medium injection a significant trend regarding enhancement characteristics of tumor tissues was not present. Regarding the difference in density between regular enhanced liver parenchyma and tumors a difference of more than 50 HU was observed in the time window between 18±3 s and 62±14 s post injection (Fig. 2).

Thus, to scan the liver during high parenchymal attenuation and high parenchyma to lesion contrast we start our spiral CT sequence 20 s after the beginning of the injection and with 8-mm slice thickness and 8-mm table speed per second the entire liver is usually scanned within 45 s. In CTAP performed with conventional CT scanners or when a spiral CT sequence is started too late the selective phase of portal contrast distribution is already missed and contrast between parenchyma and tumors may be diminished or even isoattenuation may occur (Fig. 2).

Conclusion

When using our injection parameters in CTAP high parenchymal attenuation and a high parenchyma to lesion contrast can be achieved within a narrow time window and a spiral CT sequence should be started 20 s after the beginning of the injection.

References

Bluemke DA, Fishman EK (1993) Spiral CT arterial portography of the liver. Radiology 186: 576–579

Bressler EL, Alpren MB, Glazer GM, Francis IR, Ensminger WD (1987) Hypervascular hepatic metastases: CT evaluation. Radiology 162: 49–51

Burgener FA, Hamlin DJ (1983) Contrast enhancement of hepatic tumors in CT: comparison between bolus and infusion techniques. AJR 140: 291–295

Graf O, Thurnher S, Herbst F, Lechner G (1993) Bildgebende Verfahren bei malignen Lebertumoren. Acta Chir Austr 25: 267–271

Graf O, Dock WI, Lammer J, Thurnher S, Eibenberger KL, Wildling R, Niederle B, Lang EK, Lechner G (1994) Determination of optimal time window for liver scanning with CT during arterial portography. Radiology 190: 43–47

Spiral CT During Arterial Portography with Two- and Three-Dimensional Vascular Reconstructions in Hepatic Tumors

F. J. Ferstl, P. Uhrmeister, K. H. Hauenstein, A. Barke, M. Langer

Introduction

Spiral computed tomography (SCT) of the liver performed during the portal venous phase after contrast medium injection into the superior mesenteric artery or splenic artery (spiral CTAP) is currently considered to be the most sensitive method for preoperative assessment of malignant hepatic tumors (Helmberger et al. 1993; Small et al. 1993).

The aim of our ongoing study is to evaluate the image quality and diagnostic value of surface staded display (SSD) and maximum intensity projection (MIP) images of the portal venous system in patients with malignant hepatic disease as an additional information to spiral CTAP.

Material and Method

Study Group

Fifteen patients with histologically proven primary or secondary malignant hepatic tumors were examined prior to surgery. Nine patients had liver metastases from colorectal cancer (7), gastric cancer (1) and malignant melanoma (1). In the remaining six patients hepatocellular carcinoma (HCC) was diagnosed.

Spiral CT Arterioportography

The same procedure for spiral CT arterioportography (CTAP) was used for each patient. After transfemoral placing of a 5 French-Cobra catheter in the splenic or superior mesenteric artery the patient was transferred to the CT scanner (Somatom Plus S, Siemens, Erlangen). A baseline unenhanced CT scan was obtained to detect hepatic cysts. The spiral CT of the liver was performed during transcatheter injection of 45 ml of nonionic contrast material (CM) (Imagopaque 300, Fa. Nycomed, Munich) which was given by an injector machine (Fa. Medrad) in two different flow rates: 15 ml CM with a flow rate of 1.5 ml/s and 30 ml CM with a flow rate of 1.1 ml/s. The first slice was imaged 13 s after the beginning of the injection of the CM. The slice thickness and table feed were 8 mm with 6 mm incrementation. Data were reconstructed with a 360° linear interpolation algorithm.

After completion of spiral CTAP, the patient was re-transferred to angiography and an indirect splenoportography or mesenterico-portography was carried out.

SSD images of each patient were generated with unedited images by using the scanner software. On the basis of vascular enhancement an average threshold level of 150 HU was selected. As only one threshold can be chosen with the implemented software, all structures with CT numbers above the threshold selected, including opacified liver parenchyma, may, therefore, be displayed on 3D images. Three standard projections (front, top, bottom) were created for each patient.

Dependent on the tumor extension, additional oblique views were performed.

The MIP technique, known from magnetic resonance (MR) angiography, projects the maximum intensity voxel along a ray onto a 2D plane. MIP images were reconstructed in two steps:

1. Elimination of bony structures from axial CT sections by using a prototype 3D edit programme (Siemens, Erlangen).
2. Reconstruction of MIP images from these edited CT sections by applying a prototype MIP programme (Siemens, Erlangen).

Thirty MIP images were generated for each patient about the z-axis at 6° intervals. Additional axial MIP images were produced about the x- and y-axis.

As the MIP technique creates 2D images, the cine mode was routinely used for three dimensional presentation.

Results

The images of spiral CTAP, indirect portography, MIP and SSD were visually analyzed with respect to vascular anatomy and tumor infiltration of the portal venous system. The results of image analysis are summarized in Tables 1 and 2. Spiral CTAP revealed a total of 27 liver tumors with an average size of 6.5 cm. In 11 patients the malignant hepatic tumors had spread out in both liver lobes. The intra- and extrahepatic portal venous system showed no abnormalities in all nine patients with metastatic disease. In the remaining six patients with HCC, the central and peripheral portal venous branches were affected either by tumor compression ($n = 2$) or vascular infiltration ($n = 4$, Fig. 1).

The MIP images yielded a clear demonstration of the portal venous system, including the peripheral branches, in 11 patients. In three patients the diagnostic value was reduced because of blurred vessel margins. The MIP images of one patient were insufficient for diagnostic evaluation. The portal venous pathology depicted on the indirect portography of five patients with HCC were completely documented on the corresponding MIP images. Only in one patient with invasion of the peripheral portal branches in the right lobe by HCC, as demonstrated on spiral CTAP, both the indirect portography and the MIP images were normal (Table 2).

SSD images with frontal view proved to be of minor diagnostic value due to blurring in all patients. SSD images with view from top or bottom revealed clear pictures of the vena portae and its branches in 12 of 15 patients. In three of four

Table 1. Comparison of the image quality of spiral CTAP, indirect portography, MIP and SSD

Method	Image quality ($n = 15$)	
	Diagnostic	Non-diagnostic
Spiral CTAP	15	–
Indirect portography	15	–
MIP	14	1
SSD		
Frontal view	–	15
View from top or bottom	12	3

CTAP, computed tomographic arterioportography; MIP, maximum intensity projection; SSD, surface shaded display

Table 2. Comparison of spiral CTAP, indirect portography, MIP and SSD with regard to detection of portal venous infiltration

Method	HCC ($n = 6$)	Metastasis ($n = 9$)
Spiral CTAP	4	0
Indirect portography	3	0
MIP	3	0
SSD (views from top or bottom)	4	0

CTAP, computed tomographic arterioportography; MIP, maximum intensity projection; SSD, surface shaded display; HCC, hepatocellular carcinoma

patients with HCC, SSD images were even superior to MIP. The selected threshold of 150 HU proved to be a reasonable compromise between vessel overlap by perfused liver parenchyma and reduction of anatomic detail.

Discussion

For processing of spiral CTAP data sets to 3D vascular reconstructions, two different 3D rendering techniques are currently available on CT: SSD and MIP (Magnusson et al. 1991; Napel et al. 1992; Rubin et al. 1993).

The SSD algorithm produces surface rendered images of structures with CT numbers above an arbitrary chosen threshold value. Voxels with lower CT numbers are, therefore, eliminated from reconstruction, which can lead to significant loss of information. SSD images are based on the computed reflection of a hypothetical light source from the surface. As the SSD algorithm does not reflect CT attenuation, differentiation between structures of high attenuation is infeasible. The MIP algorithm creates two-dimensional images which preserve CT attenuation. This enables

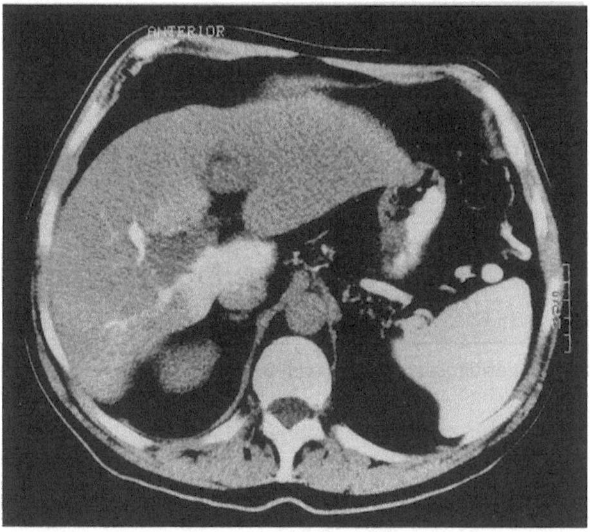

a

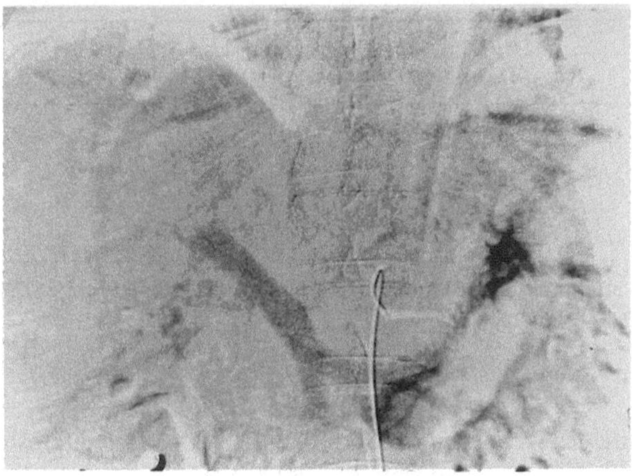

b

Fig. 1a–d. A 65-year-old patient with large hepatocellular carcinoma in the left liver lobe, extending to the liver hilus with infiltration of vena portae. **a** Axial spiral computet tomographic arterioportography section shows tumor lesion in liver hilus with infiltration of vena portae. **b** Indirect portography reveals subtotal occlusion of vena portae with faint opacification of peripheral portal venous branches in both liver lobes. **c** Maximum intensity projection about z-axis clearly displays invasion of vena portae. In comparison to indirect portography peripheral portal venous branches are better visualized on MIP. **d** Surface shaded display with view from bottom depicts filling defect in vena portae, but the site of vessel infiltration is partially obscured by area of enhanced liver parenchyma

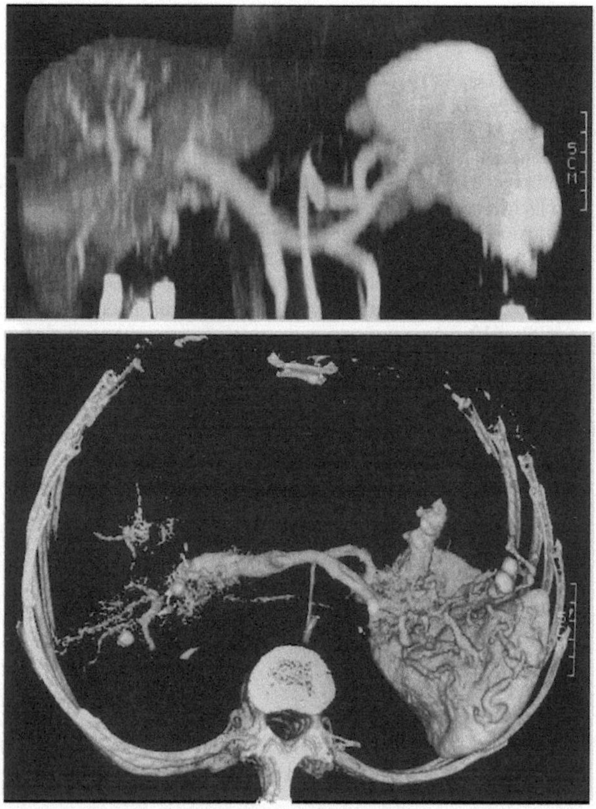

c

d

a differentiation between structures of high attenuation. However, MIP does not convey depth relationship nor does it depict overlapping vessels. The lack of 3D information can be overcome by using the cine mode. The results of our ongoing study indicate that the axial sections of spiral CTAP are superior to indirect portography and 3D vascular images in detecting portal venous system pathology (Table 2).

The comparison of the two 3D rendering techniques with each other confirms the findings of Costello et al. (1993) and Galanski et al. (1993) that the MIP images are overall more informative than SSD images, particularly due to the diagnostic insufficiency of the frontal view SSD images. The evaluation of the portal venous branches was equal or even better on MIP images than on indirect portography. This was particularly noticeable in the liver periphery. A major advantage of MIP over angiography is the capability to view the 3D vascular images from any possible angle. Consequently, the relationship of a tumor to the major vessels can be more precisely determined. A significant disadvantage of the MIP technique is the current consumption of time for generating vascular images.

References

Costello P, Gaa J (1993) Spiral CT angiography of the abdominal aorta and its branches. Eur Radiol 3:359–365

Galanski M, Prokop M, Chavan A, Schäfer CM, Jandeleit K, Nischelsky JE (1993) Renal artery stenoses: Spiral CT angiography. Radiology 189:185–192

Helmberger H, Bautz W, Vogel U, Lenz M (1993) CT-Arterioportographie in Spiraltechnik zum Nachweis von Lebermetastasen. RöFo 158:410–415

Magnusson M, Lenz R, Danielsson PE (1991) Evaluation of methods for shaded surface display of CT volumes. Comput Med Imaging Graph 15:247–256

Napel S, Marks MP, Rubin GD, Dake MD, Mc Donnell CH, Song SM, Enzmann DR, Jeffrey RB (1992) CT angiography with spiral CT and maximum intensity projection. Radiology 185: 607–610

Rubin GD, Dake MD, Napel S, Mc Donnell CH, Jeffrey RB (1993) Three dimensional spiral CT angiography of the abdomen. Initial clinical experience. Radiology 186:147–152

Small WC, Mehard WB, Langmo LS, Dagher AP, Fishman EK, Heiken JP, Bernadino ME (1993) Preoperative determination of the resectability of hepatic tumors: Efficacy of CT during arterial portography. AJR 161:319–322

Spiral CT of Liver Tumors: Comparison with CTAP

W. Dock, S. Puig, J. Liskutin, O. Graf, K. Eibenberger, N. Farres,
F. Grabenwöger, G. Lechner

Introduction

Spiral computed tomography (SCT) offers many advantages compared to conventional CT such as the possibility of administration of a much higher contrast bolus, the reduction or elimination of motion artefacts, the absence of gaps between the reconstructed images [1] and the evaluation of two different phases of contrast enhancement of liver parenchyma after application of one single contrast bolus.

Today the method with the highest sensitivity for detection of liver tumors is CT during arterial portography (CTAP) [2, 6] or spiral CTAP [1], respectively. This modality is followed by contrast-enhanced CT [5, 9], magnetic resonance imaging (MRI) and ultrasound. The aim of our study was to determine the sensitivity of detection of liver tumors by contrast-enhanced spiral CT compared to spiral CTAP.

Materials and Methods

Between November 1992 and December 1993, 31 patients were examined with spiral CTAP and spiral i.v. contrast-enhanced CT (spiral CT). The mean age of the 19 female and 12 male patients was 61.4 years, the range from 35 to 81 years. All examinations were performed with a Somatom Plus S scanner for determination of tumor extent before embolization therapy or surgery.

The patients were administered with following diagnoses: 11 hepatocellular carcinomas (HCC), five metastases of carcinoid tumors, three metastases of malignant insulinoma, three metastases of thyroid carcinoma, seven metastases of colon carcinoma, one metastasis of melanoma, and one metastasis of breast carcinoma.

Spiral CT was performed in three series: one native scan with a slice thickness and a table feed of 8 mm, 120 kV and 250 mAs. The first spiral scan (slice thickness and a table feed 8 mm, 120 kV, 210 mAs) was started 25–30 s after beginning the contrast injection. Nonionic contrast agent (120 ml) was administered over an antecubital vein with a power injector with a flow rate of 4 ml/s. The second spiral scan was initiated as quickly as technically possible after the first spiral scan, which was between 120 and 215 s after the beginning of contrast injection. For the spiral scans a picture reconstruction increment of 4 mm [8] was chosen. Measurement and counting of the lesions was performed on a picture archiving and communication (PACS) workstation.

Spiral CTAP was performed in the following manner [3]: After sterilization of the inguinal regions as for a surgical procedure a 5-F sidewinder catheter was inserted over a femoral artery and the tip of the catheter was positioned into the superior mesenteric artery. Over this catheter 80 ml of nonionic contrast agent was injected with a flow rate of 5 ml/s. The spiral scan (slice thickness and a table feed 8 mm, 120 kV, 210 mAs) was started with a delay of 20 s. Pictures were reconstructed using an increment of 4 mm. Again measurement and counting of the lesions was performed on a PACS workstation.

Results

Spiral CTAP revealed 110 discernible lesions (27 patients) with a range of one to 20 lesions within a single liver. More than 20 lesions per liver were defiend as inumerable (four patients).
Spiral CT counted 103 lesions. Some 64 lesions were already apparent on the native scans, 100 during the early contrast enhanced spiral scan and 79 lesions still were differentiable on the second spiral CT. Three lesions were additionally detected with the third series, therefore the total number of 103 lesions.

In 17 examinations the lesions were predominantly hyperdense on the first spiral scan. The histology of those lesions was HCC in nine, metastases of carcinoid in three, of insulinoma in three, and of colon carcinoma in two patients. In these cases spiral CT detected 74 lesions, spiral CTAP revealed 70 lesions. Thus for those lesions i.v. enhanced spiral CT seems to be at least as sensitive as spiral CTAP.

In 14 examinations the lesions were predominantly hypodense on both the native scans and the spiral CT scans. The histology of those lesions was HCC in two, metastasis of colon carcinoma in five, of thyroid carcinoma in three, of carcinoid in two, of breast carcinoma in one and of melanoma in one patient. In these cases spiral CTAP detected 40 lesions and spiral CT discerned 29 lesions. Thus a sensitivity of 0.78 is calculated for detection of hypodense lesions with spiral CT compared to spiral CTAP.

Discussion

With such a study a lot of problems should be discussed. First of all the problem of determination of the sensitivity of an imaging modality. Only in rare cases is comparison of an in vivo examination and a histological work up of a liver possible. Thus, a newly establishing method may only be compared to the best existing method, which is CTAP. Sensitivity of CTAP is reported to be around 90% [2, 6, 7] for detection of primary or secondary liver tumors. Spiral CTAP – as used in our study – even may be more sensitive, but this must be confirmed by further studies.

Our study clearly confirms the value of spiral CT for the detection of hypervascular lesions such as HCC [4] (Fig. 1), metastases of malignant insulinomas or of malignant carcinoid tumors. Since the examination time lasts only around 20 s, a higher flow rate for contrast medium injection may be chosen as it was possible with

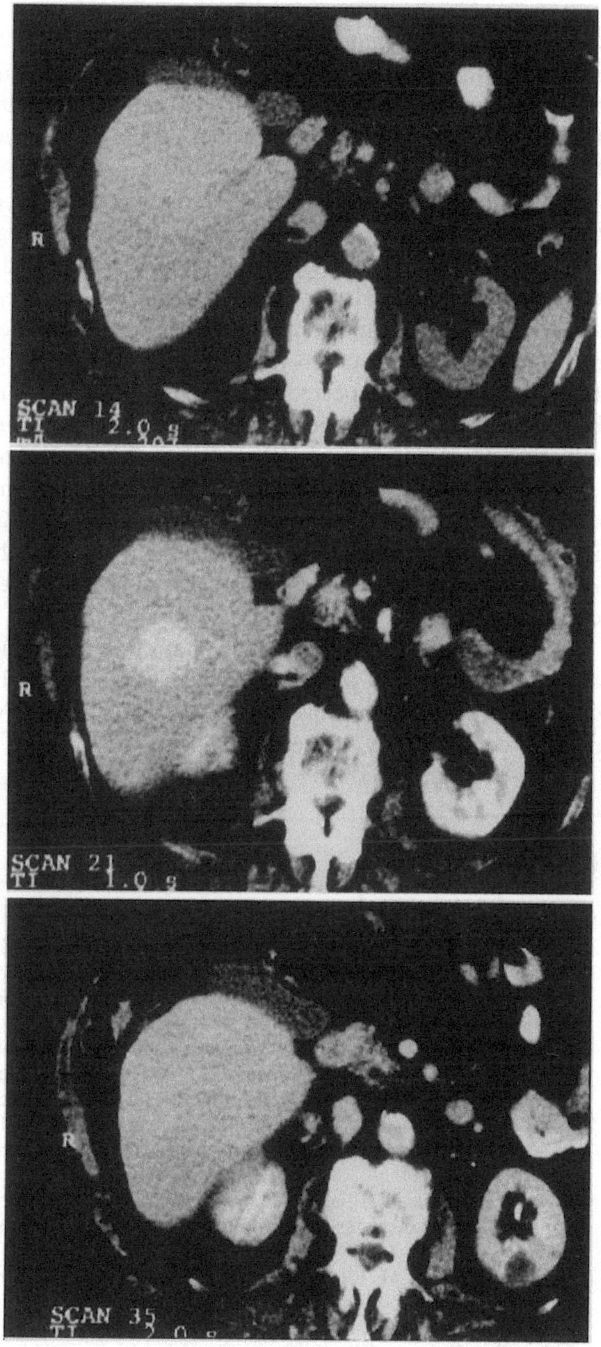

a

b

c

Fig. 1a–c. a Patient 2 years after left hemihepatectomy because of hepatocellular carcinoma (HCC). The unenhanced scan shows a homogeneous liver parenchyma. **b** Same patient. Early spiral CT (120 ml contrast medium i.v.) shows contrast uptake of a lesion measuring 4 cm within the right lobe of the liver, which was confirmed to be recurring. HCC. **c** Same patient. During the second spiral scan the lesion connot be detected any more conventional CT scanners. Thus we administered 120 ml of nonionic contrast medium with a flow rate of 4 ml/s. This regimen provides a dense contrastation of the hepatic artery and of hypervascular tumors. Using this technique the sensitivity for detection of hypervascular lesions seems to be even higher than that of spiral CTAP.

For hypovascular lesions the situation is completely different. The optimal contrast for such lesions is achieved during the phase of highest tissue contrastation of liver parenchyma. Thus a second spiral scan was started as quickly as possible after the first spiral scan. However, the waiting time between the first and the second spiral scan has been too long and in most cases the beginning of the equilibrium phase of tissue contrastation was already reached. Therefore the second spiral scan failed to provide the expected additional information. However, this problem should be solved by the introduction of the so called double spiral (DXP), which allows the initiation of a second spiral CT scan 18 s after the end of the first spiral scan.

A further problem under discussion is the radiation dose with three CT scans during one single examination. However, the dose with 210 mAs for the spiral scans is relatively low. Additionally especially if only pretherapeutic assessment of a known tumor is demanded, the native scan seems to be unnecessary and might be omitted.

The information provided by our study allows the conclusion that spiral CT clearly improves detection of hypervascular lesions of the liver. Detection of hypovascular tumors may be improved by the introduction of DXP. This statement, however, must be confirmed by further investigations.

References

1. Bluemke DA, Fishman EK (1993) Spiral CT of the liver. AJR 160 : 787 – 792
2. Ferrucci JT (1990) Liver tumor imaging: Current concepts. AJR 155 : 473 – 484
3. Graf O, Dock WI, Lammer J, Thurnher S, Eibenberger KL, Wildling R, Niederle B, Lang EK, Lechner G (1994) Determination of optimal time window for liver scanning with CT during arterial portography. Radiology 190 : 43 – 47
4. Honda H, Ochiai K, Adachi E, Yasumori K, Hayashi T, Kawashima A, Fukuya T, Gibo M, Matsumata T, Tsuneyoshi M, Masuda K (1993) Hepatocellular carcinoma: Correlation of CT, angiographic, and histopathologic findings. Radiology 189 : 857 – 862
5. Paushter DM, Zeman RK, Scheibler RK, Choyke PL, Jaffe MH, Clark LR (1989) CT evaluation of suspected hepatic metastases: Comparison of techniques for iv contrast enhancement. AJR 152 : 267 – 271
6. Soyer P, Levesque M, Elias D, Zeitoun G, Roche A (1992) Preoperative assessment of resectability of hepatic metastases from colonic carcinoma: CT portography vs sonography and dynamic CT. AJR 159 : 741 – 744
7. Soyer P, Levesque M, Elias D, Zeitoun G, Roche A (1992) Detection of liver metastases from colorectal cancer: comparison of the intraoperative US and CT during arterial portography. Radiology 183 : 541 – 544
8. Urban BA, Fishman EK, Kuhlman JA, Kawashima A, Hennessey JG, Siegelman SS (1993) Detection of focal hepatic lesions with spiral-CT: Comparison of 4- and 8-mm interscan spacing. AJR 160 : 783 – 785
9. Wernecke K, Rummeny E, Bongartz G, Vassallo P, Kievelitz D, Wiesmann W, Peters PE, Reers B, Reiser M, Bircher (1991) Detection of hepatic masses in patients with carcinoma: Comparative sensitivities of sonography, CT, and MR imaging. AJR 157 : 731 – 739

Volume CT in High-Dose Portography: Detection of Liver Metastases of Colon Carcinoma

M. Oudkerk, R.H. Kruyt, B. van Ooijen, I.H.M. Borel Rinkes

Introduction

In Western countries the incidence of large bowel cancer is high and second only to that of lung cancer in men and breast cancer in women [1]. Survival rates have improved since 1950, but only as a result of an increased resectability rate and decreased peroperative mortality [2]. The prognosis of a patient is mainly determined by the stage of the tumor at initial presentation. Most patients die due to disseminated disease in the liver. Already on first presentation 15%–35% of the patients have apparent or occult liver metastases, whereas two thirds of the patients will have them by the time of their death [3]. Treatment of disseminated disease by chemotherapy is disappointing.

Partial hepatic resection is the only curative treatment currently available for colorectal carcinoma metastases of the liver in selected cases. Previous studies suggest the 5-year survival after properly performed partial liver resection is in the range of 20%–50% [4, 5]. The mortality rate for partial hepatic resection is nowadays about 5% [4]. In a study of the records of 859 patients from 24 institutions a number of factors have been identified that influence the prognosis after partial hepatic resection [5]. These include Dukes classification of the colorectal tumor, number of hepatic metastases if >3, presence of extrahepatic disease, especially lymphatic. The number of liver metastases if <4, the type of resection, the size of liver metastases, the sex of the patient, the disease free interval and the value of CEA do not influence the prognosis [6]. The factors considered to be contra-indications to resection are the presence of positive hepatic nodes, the presence of extra-hepatic metastases (even if resectable), or the presence of four or more hepatic metastases. The resection margin of the liver specimen, the stage of the primary tumor and the disease-free interval also seem to effect survival.

It is apparent from the majority of reported series that patients with only a few metastases will survive longer after hepatic resection. The 5-year survival rates range between 21% and 52% for resected solitary lesions but between 0% and 25% for resected multiple lesions [7].

Improvement of detection of metastatic disease and interpretation of diagnostic imaging techniques is of utmost importance in selecting patients for hepatic resection.

In the 1980s detection of liver metastases was focussed on non-invasive modalities. In a lesion by lesion analysis sensitivity rates for ultrasound ranging from 58% to 69% were reported in a population with colon carcinoma [8, 9]. Although CT detection with i.v. contrast administration seemed to be slightly better with reported sensitivities of 61% – 82%, these figures are far from satisfying [8]. Therefore more invasive techniques have been advocated in order to achieve a more accurate preoperative staging. At first intra-arterial CT enhancement (CTA) was advocated and CTA has been proposed as an obligatory measure in the preoperative assessment of potential candidates for liver resection [10 – 13].

Modification of this technique using continuous ratation over 40 s at each slice level during arterial liver enhancement rendered better results with sensitivities up to 98% in correlation with intra-operative ultrasound (US) and histological examination of the resected specimen but the specificity of the intra-arterial approach seems too low mainly from misinterpretation of flow artifacts [14].

Some authors discourage application of CT during arterial portography (CTAP) because of the many false-positive results [15], but the high sensitivity of the procedure, yielding the detection of more metastases than most other imaging techniques, leads to the policy to apply CTAP in the preoperative work up of patients with colorectal malignancies for most authors [16 – 19].

Although according to recent studies CTAP offers a better specificity (91%) [19] the sensitivities Reported vary from 81% to 91% and especially lesions less than 1 cm in diameter are missed with CTAP. Combination of CTA with CTAP has been reported [20] and also seems to increase lesion detection and discrimination.

Implementation of spiral volume CT (SVCT) in combination with arterial portography (SVCTAP) offers a further improvement of the CTAP method [21]. Since CTAP is based on the attenuation difference between the liver parenchyma which is enhanced from the portal vein and the metastatic deposits which are vascularized from the hepatic artery, metastatic detection hampers from arterial contrast recirculation. The attenuation difference will diminish the more contrast recirculation is accomplished. Data collection within 25 s of the whole volume by SVCTAP enables liver metastases detection without or with minimal contrast recirculation, which is a major advantage compared to single slice CTAP. Furthermore no metastases are missed due to in and out of the slice movement. Finally the total amount of contrast volume needed is decreased by at least 50% compared to CTAP.

Material and Methods

In 22 patients referred for liver metastasectomy a catheter was placed under fluoroscopic guidance in the superior mesenteric artery (because of aberrant vascularization in the splenic artery in one patient) and portography was performed. SVCTAP was carried out (with a Siemens Somatom Plus S) in all patients after obtaining a SVCT examination with and without i.v. contrast, 5-mm table feed, 5-mm increment. For SVCTAP, a 180 ml dilution of Ultravist and saline (1:1) was selectively injected in the mesenteric artery in 60-s injection time [2]. After 40 s the volume scan started data collection with a table feed of 5 mm/s. If liver volume length exceeded 15 cm a table feed of 6 mm/s was chosen. Image reconstruction parameters were: standard algorithm, Z-profile 180°, zoom factor 1.5, table increment 4 mm, multiplanar reconstructions. After 4 h a delayed SVCT was performed. Patient data obtained with SVCT and SVCTAP were evaluated separately without knowledge of other data. The results of SVCT with and without i.v. contrast enhancement, together with the 4-h delayed SVCT were compared with the data obtained with SVCTAP. As gold standard were used: histologic analyses of the resected specimen and/or follow up studies with US and SVCT after 1 and 3 months. Initially resection was indicated by the data obtained at SVCT, intraoperative US, palpation and inspection. In the decision to operate, results of SVCTAP were not included since the study was designed to test the value of this technique against the actual policy for these patients. As it became apparent that far more metastases were detected with SVCTAP during the study the policy altered to wait and see, for three patients instead of operation.

Results

Of the 22 consecutive patients referred for liver metastasectomy, 17 patients were eligible for prospective evaluation and analysis, five patients did not meet all criteria for analysis.

Comparison of the Results with the Gold Standard

Of the 17 patients that were eligible for prospective evaluation and analysis, the SVCT and SVCTAP results of two were equivocal and confirmed during a surgical intervention. The extra metastases that were detected on the SVCTAP in 15 patients were confirmed during the surgical procedure in four patients and during follow up after 1 and 3 months in seven patients. In the remaining four patients false-positive findings were present on the SVCTAP examination, all were confirmed during the surgical intervention.

With SVCT 42 true positive metastatic lesions were detected, 38 false negative lesions were established and one false positive of in total 80 metastatic lesions, resulting in a sensitivity of 52% for SVCT.

With SVCTAP all 80 true positive metastatic lesions were detected, but six false-positive lesions were established in four patients resulting in a sensitivity up to 100%. Since patient selection makes it almost impossible to acquire enough negative patients for metastatic disease, it is impossible to get reliable specificity figures. This problem is also reflected in the literature.

Therapeutic Consequences of SVCTAP Versus SVCT

In 15 of the 17 patients more lesions were detected in the liver with SVCTAP. For seven of these patients this would have had no consequences. For the other eight patients the different strategy would include a more extensive resection for two patients, for the other six patients the possibility of curation would have been ruled out on the bases of the findings at SVCTAP. Of these six patients three were operated (Figs. 1, 2) and the other three were evaluated by follow up after 1 and 2 months.

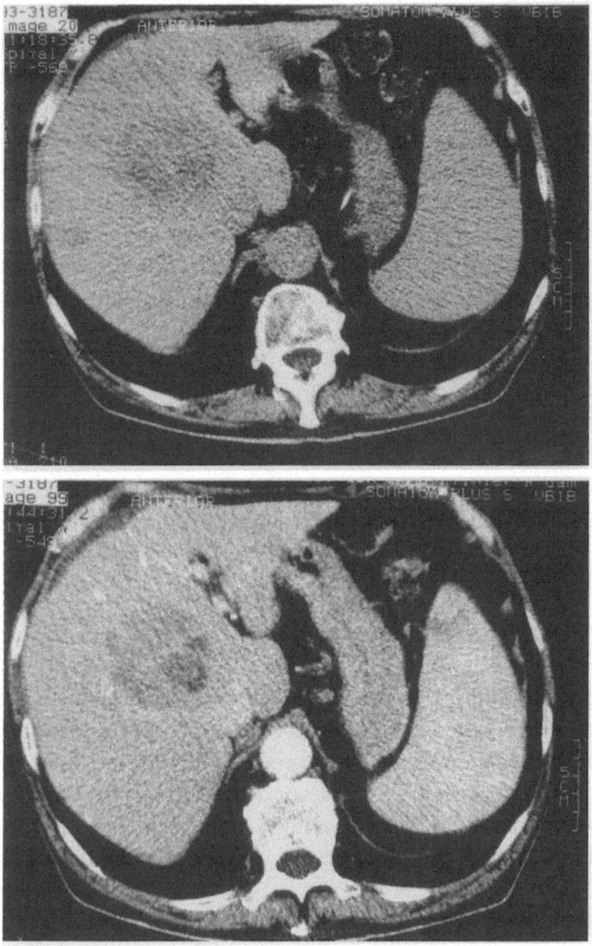

a

b

Fig. 1a – d. Spiral volume computed tomography (SVCT) examination of a patient with suspected liver metastases pre-contrast **a**, during i.v. contrast infusion **b**, after a 4-h delay **c** and during intra-arterial portography **d**. The non-invasive SVCT studies **a – c** show one large tumor mass in segments VIII and V (diameter > 5 cm) together with a second tumor deposit in segment VII (diameter = 2 cm). SVCT during portography (SVCTAP) shows multiple other focal lesions in the right as well as in the left liver lobe. All lesions were confirmed at laparotomy. Patient was classified as inoperable

In the total group there were four patients with false-positive findings on SVCTAP. This would have implied no consequences for one patient, a more extensive resection for two patients and for one patient the policy would have altered from operable to inoperable. In conclusion six patients would have become inoperable from the results of SVCTAP compared to CTAP, but in one patient inoperability would have been unjustified because of a false positive lesion at SVCTAP.

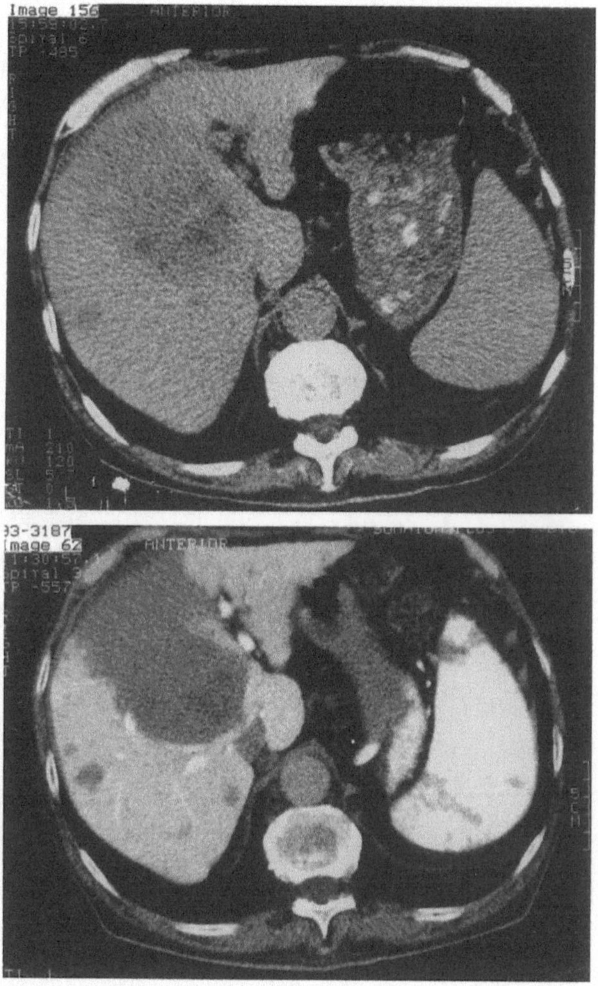
c

d

Fig. 1 c, d

Discussion

Partial hepatic resection has obtained a definitive place in the treatment of (isolated) liver metastases from colorectal cancer [23–25]. The most important parameters predicting success for hepatic resection are whether the number of metastatic deposits do not exceed three or four and whether tumor-free margins can be obtained. Imaging methods must be accurate to provide the information necessary to select patients for successful interventions.

Over the past decade, the standard modalities for preoperative evaluation of hepatic metastases have been CT and US [26, 27].

However, surgical findings in combination with intra-operative ultrasonography (IOUS) have shown that CT and US have low sensitivity for correct diagnosis of all metastatic lesions [28–30]. Combined IOUS and palpation are the most accurate in

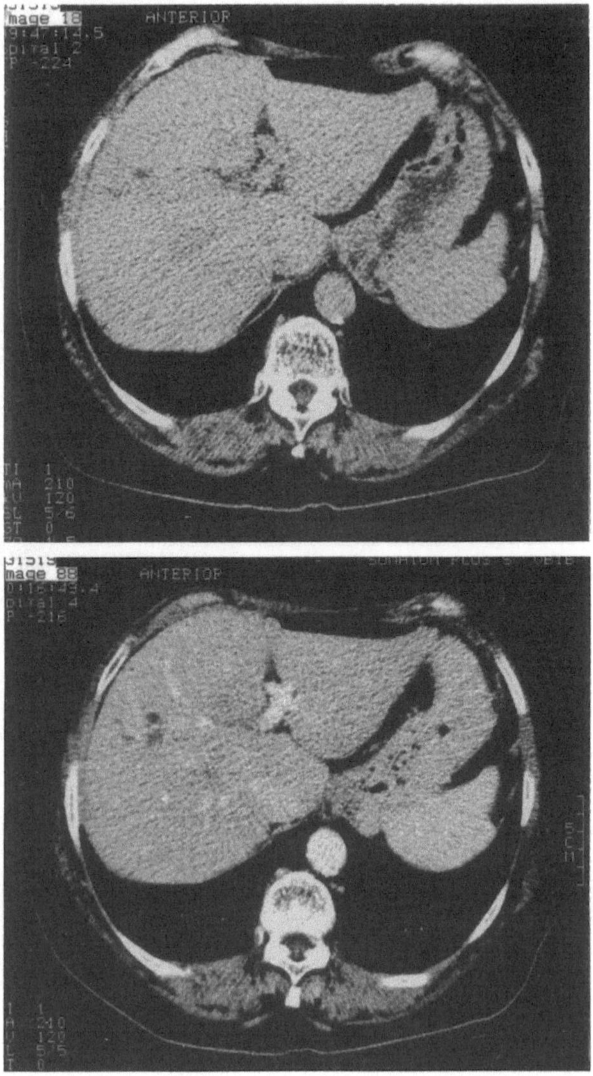

a

b

Fig. 2a – d. Spiral volume computed tomography (SVCT) examination of a patient with suspected liver metastases pre-contrast **a**, during i.v. contrast infusion **b**, after a 4-h delay **c** and during intra-arterial portography **d**. The pre-contrast and i.v. contrast examination **a, b** show two well-defined lesions in segment VII probably cysts and a ill-defined lesion in segment VI, which is also visible at the 4-h delay examination **c**. The latter examination **c** shows two other ill-defined lesions: one in segment VI and in segment VII. The SVCT during portography (SVCTAP) reveals multiple focal nodular lesions highly suspected for liver metastases in all presented liver segments. Special attention for the central hepatic metastases around the liver hilum compressing the portal vein branches. The lesions were confirmed during surgical exploration from which the patient was classified as inoperable

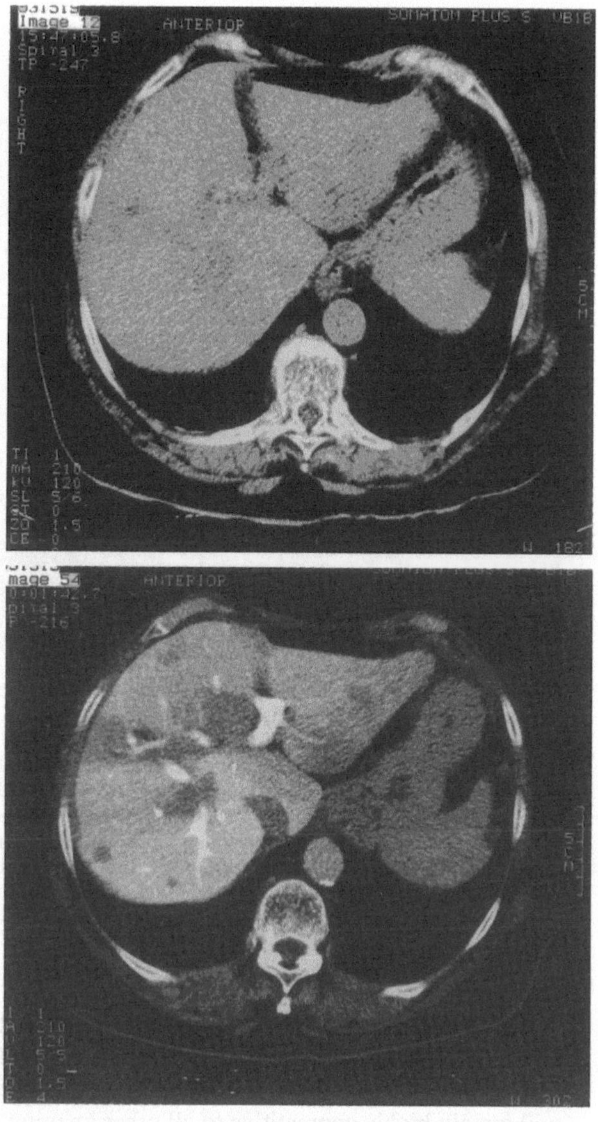

c

d

Fig. 2 c, d

the detection of hepatic metastases [31]. In the present study, a lesion was considered positive at laparotomy only if interpreted as a metastasis by means of intraoperative ultrasound examination by a radiologist or a positive identification by surgical palation. For those patients who did not undergo surgery, lesions were followed at 1 and 3 months.

In the present study application of SVCT leads to sensitivity figures of only 52%. Most of the missed lesions are smaller than 1 cm in diameter. Therefore, to detect small lesions and examine the liver thoroughly when resection of hepatic metastases is being considered, other investigative procedures are needed. In the present study a new diagnostic technique based on CT during arterial portography was used.

a

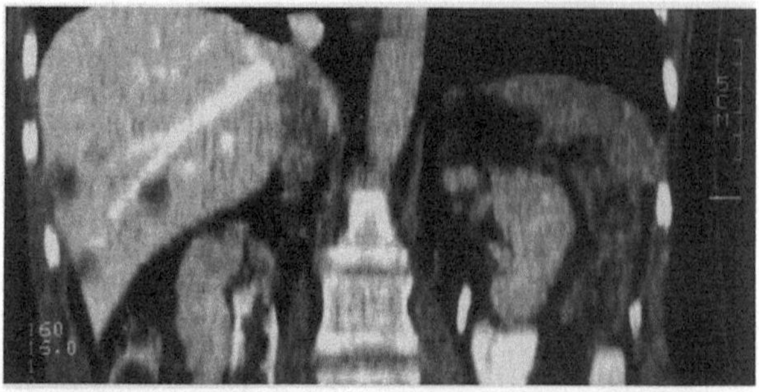

b

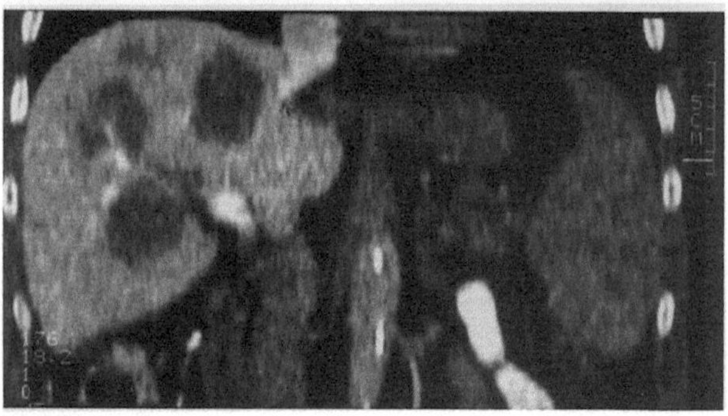

Fig. 3a–d. Multiplanar reconstructions in spiral volume computed tomography in combination with arterial portography (SVCTAP) examinations. **a** Coronal reconstruction through segments VI and VII. Anatomical position of three hepatic metastases in relation to the right hepatic vein is clearly demonstrated. Note the inflow of the hepatic vein in the non-opacified inferior caval vein. **b** Coronal reconstruction through segment I, IV, VI, VII and VIII. The close relationship of the large hepatic mass in segment IV towards the inflow of the hepatic vein in the inferior caval vein is demonstrated. **c** Semi-sagittal reconstruction through segment IV of the same lesion as in **b** shows again the very close relationship of the lesion central to the hepatic vein and inferior caval vein. **d** Oblique reconstruction along the middle hepatic vein showing impression of two separate hepatic tumor masses from both sides. Note the catheter position in the superior mesenteric artery

CTAP has been reported to provide a much higher lesion detection sensitivity. With SVCTAP no false negative lesions were found in this limited series, resulting in a sensitivity up to 100%. In further series this figure will lower down slightly, but will remain highly competitive to all other imaging modalities.

A very high sensitivity (overall 94%) in detection of liver metastases was obtained with C (continuous CT angiography) CTA [14] and even 90% of the lesions with a diameter of 1 cm or less were detected. Conversely, the false-positive rate of this technique was high. Most of the false-positive interpretations were probably caused by perfusion abnormalities. According to recent studies CTAP offers a much better specificity (91%) [19].

Some authors have recommended CT during CTAP. The metastasis detection rate for CTAP is comparable to that of C CTA, but the specificity was better in most studies [16–19] although this is not true in all studies [15]. Magnetic resonance imaging (MRI) also a new imaging technique that is more sensitive than conventional CT scanning, but it does not seem to be as sensitive as C CTA or CTAP [16,

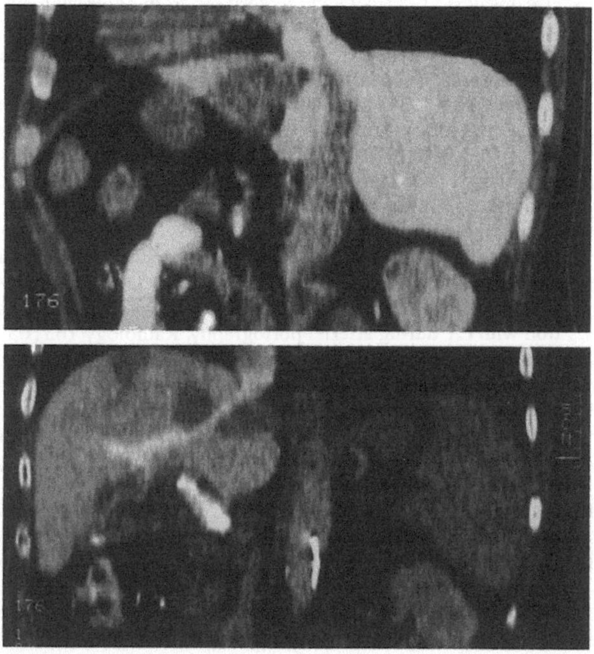

c

d

Fig. 3c, d

32]. In the present study we performed SVCTAP. With SVCTAP more metastases were detected in 15 of 17 patients. As to the indication for liver surgery six patients would have become inoperable and in only one patient inoperability would have been unjustified. Although false positive findigs remain a problem [33] SVCTAP bypasses the limitations of CTAP because one single high dose portography suffices for examination of the whole liver volume. Because of the high contrast differences between normal and abnormal liver tissue at all levels without arterial recirculation, lesion detection increases dramatically which is also reflected in the data we present in this study. No metastases are missed due to out of the slice movements because data collection is performed during one breath hold. An additional advantage of SVCTAP is optimal morphological and attenuation correlation. This guarantees multiplanar reconstructions of high quality for evaluation along surgical resection planes and clear demonstration of anatomical relations to the caval and portal vein (Fig. 3). This extra feature facilitates surgical planning. Therefore SVCTAP is the imaging method of choice if compared to CTAP in the preoperative evaluation of liver metastases from colorectal carcinoma, although one must be aware that false positive findings may be encountered.

References

1. Boyle P, Zaridze DG, Smans M (1977) Descriptive epidemiology of colorectal cancer. Int. J. Cancer 36 : 9
2. Cutlers SJ (1969) Trends in cancers of the digestive tract. Surgery 65 : 740

3. Greenway B (1988) Hepatic metastases from colorectal cancer: resection or not. Br. J. Surg. 75 : 513
4. Ekberg H, Tranberg KG, Anderson R et al. (1986) Determinants of survival in liver resection for colorectal secondaries. Br. J. Surg. 73 : 727
5. Hughues KS (1988) Registry of hepatic metastases. Resection of the liver for colorectal carcinoma metastases: A multi-institutional study of indications for resection. Surgery 103 : 278
6. Sugarbaker PH (1990) Surgical decision making for large bowel cancer metastatic to the liver. Radiology 174 : 621 – 626
7. Cady B, McDermott W (1985) Major hepatic resection for metachronous metastases from colon cancer. Ann. Surg. 204
8. Lundstedt C, Ekberg H, Hederstrom E, Stridbeck H, Torfason B, Tranberg KG (1987) Radiologic diagnosis of liver metastases in colo-rectal carcinoma. Acta Radiologica 28 : 4
9. Matsui O, Takashima T, Kadoya M et al. (1987) Livermetastases from colorectal cancer: detection with CT during arterial portography. Radiology 165 : 65
10. Gothlin J, Gutierrez R, Kurdziel J, Schwartz S (1986) Computed tomographic arteriography (CTA) of the liver. Evaluation of technique, results and indications. Europ. J. Radiol. 6 : 191
11. Lundstedt C, Gotberg S, Lunderquist A, Stridbeck H, Tranberg K (1986) Computed tomographic angiography of the liver via the coeliac axis. Acta Radiol. Diagnosis 27 : 285
12. Prando A, Wallace S, Bernardino M, Lindell M (1979) Computed tomographic arteriography of the liver. Radiology 130 : 697
13. Stack J, Legge D, Behan M (1984) Computed tomographic arteriography in the presurgical evaluation of hepatic tumors. Clin. Radiol. 35 : 189
14. Oudkerk M, Ooijen B van, Mali SPM, Tjiam SL, Schmitz PIM, Wiggers T (1992) Liver metastases from colorectal carcinoma: Detection with continuous CT angiography. Radiology 185 : 157 – 161
15. Miller DL, Simmons JT, Chang R, Ward BA, Shawker TH, Doppman JL, Chang AE (1987) Hepatic metastasis detection: Comparison of three CT contrast enhancement methods. Radiology 165 : 785 – 790
16. Soyer P, Levesque M, Caudron C, Elias D, Zeitoun G, Roche A (1993) MRI of liver metastases from colorectal cancer vs. CT during arterial portography. J. Comput. Assist. Tomogr. 17 (1) : 67 – 74
17. Peterson MS, Baron RL, Dodd GD III, Zajko AJ, Oliver JH et al. (1992) Hepatic parenchymal perfusion defects detected with CTAP: Imaging-pathologic correlation. Radiology 185 : 149 – 155
18. Soyer P, Levesque M, Elias D, Zeitoun G, Roche A (1992) Preoperative assessment of resectability of hepatic metastases from colonic carcinoma: CT portography vs. sonography and dynamic CT. Am. J. Radiol. 159 : 741 – 744
19. Lindberg CG, Lundstedt C, Stridbeck H, Tranberg KG (1993) Accuracy of CT arterial portography of the liver compared with findings at laparotomy. Acta Radiologica 34 (2) : 139 – 142
20. Chezmar JL, Bernardino ME, Kaufman SH, Nelson RC (1993) Combined CT arterial portography and CT hepatic angiography for evaluation of the hepatic resection candidate. Radiology 189 : 407 – 410
21. Bluemke DA, Fishman EK (1993) Spiral CT arterial portography of the liver. Radiology 186 : 576 – 579
22. Graf O, Dock WI, Lammer J, Thurnher S, Eibenberger KL, Wildling R, Niederle B, Lang EK, Lechner G (1994) Determination of optimal time window for liver scanning with CT during arterial portography. Radiology 190 : 43 – 47
23. Adson MA (1987) Resection of liver metastases: when is it worthwhile? World J. Surg. 11 : 511 – 520
24. Steele G, Ravikumar TS (1989) Resection of hepatic metastases from colorectal cancer. Ann. Surg. 210 : 127 – 138
25. Ooijen B van, Wiggers T, Meijer S et al. (1992) Hepatic resections for colorectal metastases in the Netherlands. Cancer 70 : 28 – 34
26. Smith TJ, Kemeny MM, Sugarbaker PH et al. (1982) A prospective study of hepatic imaging in the detection of metastatic disease. Ann. Surg. 195 : 486 – 491
27. Schreve RH, Terpstra OT, Ausema L, Lameris JS, Seijen AJ van, Jeekel J (1984) Detection of liver metastases: A prospective study comparing liver enzymes, scintigraphy, ultrasonography and computed tomography. Br. J. Surg. 71 : 947 – 949

28. Clarke MP, Kane RA, Steele G et al. (1989) Prospective comparison of preoperative imaging and intraoperative ultrasonography in the detection of liver tumors. Br. J. Surg. 76 : 1323 – 1329
29. Machi J, Isomoto N, Kurohiji T et al. (1991) Accuracy of intraoperative ultrasound in diagnosing liver metastases from colorectal cancer: evaluation with postoperative follow up results. World J. Surg. 15 : 551 – 557
30. Knol JA, Marn CS, Francis IR, Rubin JM, Bromberg J, Chang AE (1993) Comparisons of dynamic infusion and delayed computed tomography, intraoperative ultrasound, and palpation in the diagnosis of liver metastases. Am. J. Surg. 165 : 81 – 88
31. Charnley RM, Morris DL, Dennison AR, Amar SS, Hardcastle JD (1991) Detection of colorectal liver metastases using intraoperative ultrasonography. Br. J. Surg. 78 : 45 – 48
32. Collier BD, Foley WD (1993) Current imaging strategies for colorectal cancer. J. Nucl. Med. 34 : 537 – 540
33. Soyer P, Lacheheb D, Levesque M (1993) False-positive CT portography: Correlation with pathologic findings. Am. J. Radiol. 160 : 285 – 289

Spiral CT After Intravenous Cholangiography – Can It Replace Plain Film Cholangiography, Diagnostic PTC and ERC?

W. Anzböck, M. Wassipaul, H. Mosser, W. Krampla, G. Pärtan, W. Hruby

Introduction

The aim of the study was to evaluate the clinical use of spiral computed tomography (SCT) after i.v. Cholangiography compared to conventional cholangiography, including conventional tomography, in order to perform this noninvasive investigation instead of diagnostic endoscopic retrograde cholangiography (ERC) or percutaneous transhepatic cholangiography (PTC), which are both invasive methods.

Spiral CT after i.v. cholangiography gives more and better information of the intrahepatic biliary system, the common bile duct, cystic duct and gallbladder and therefore in our opinion has the potential to replace diagnostic PTC and ERC.

Patients and Method

From March 1993 to March 1994 130 patients underwent i.v. cholangiography mainly prior to laparoscopic cholecystectomy or for detection of biliary duct stones suspected in ultrasound prior to ERC or in case this method had failed.

In 24 patients (12 male and 12 female with an age from 24 to 92; mean 69.5 years) spiral CT of the biliary system was performed.

Conventional cholangiograms and tomograms were performed on a Siregraph D with a 33 cm Image Intensifier or a Siregraph D40 with a 40 cm Image Intensifier combined with a Flurospot H using a 1024 × 1024 matrix. The biliburin level was below 2 mg%. A precontrast image of the right upper abdomen was taken in a supine position.

Then 100 ml of Meglumin-Jodoxamat (Endobil) 45 mg I/ml (Gerot, Austria; Licence by Bracco, Italy) were administered over a period of at least 30 min [13].

AT 30, 60 and 120 min after contrast administration images were taken in a slightly LAO position.

Conventional tomograms were performed in the same position (Fig. 1). At 60 min p.i. spiral CT was performed on a Somatom Plus S.

Slices ranged from 1 to 2 cm below the right diaphragm to the caudal endplate of the second lumbal vertebra enabling the visualisation of the biliary system to the papilla vateri. The scan data were 5 mm/s table speed at a slice thickness of 5 mm with an interslice increment of 2 mm using a standard algorithm.

Multiplanar reconstructions were done on the Plus S in "Quick Mode" coronal, sagittal or paraxial orientation at convenient sites (Fig. 2).

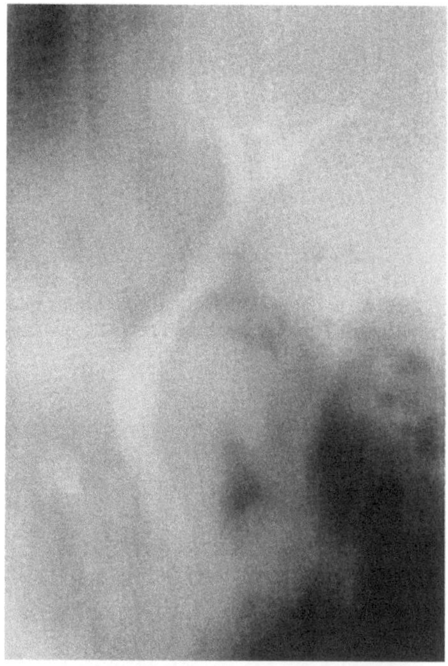

Fig. 1. Conventional tomogram in a slightly LAO position

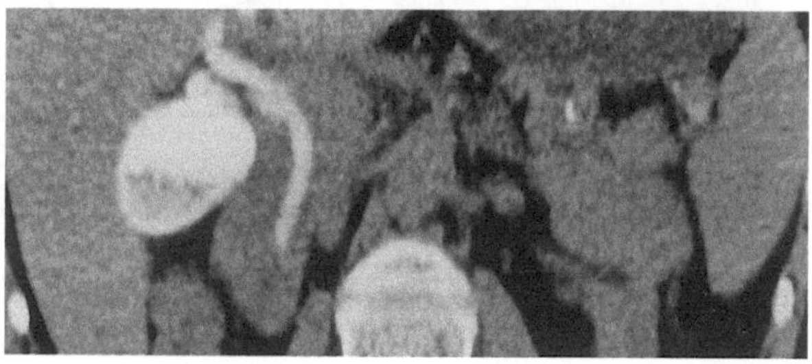

Fig. 2. Spiral CT: oblique "quick mode" reconstruction

3D MIP (maximum intensity projection) (Fig. 3a) and 3D surface reconstructions (Fig. 3b) were performed on a DRC 102 (diagnostic reporting console), in 12 projections after the bony structures were cut off.

Contrast densities were measured of the biliary system and of gallbladder or biliary duct stones.

Data aquired on conventional cholangiograms and spiral CT were studied and correlated.

Results

Of the stones 25% were radioopaque on the precontrast image.

Gallbladder stones were found in 41.7% on conventional i.v. cholangiography in and in 75% with spiral CT.

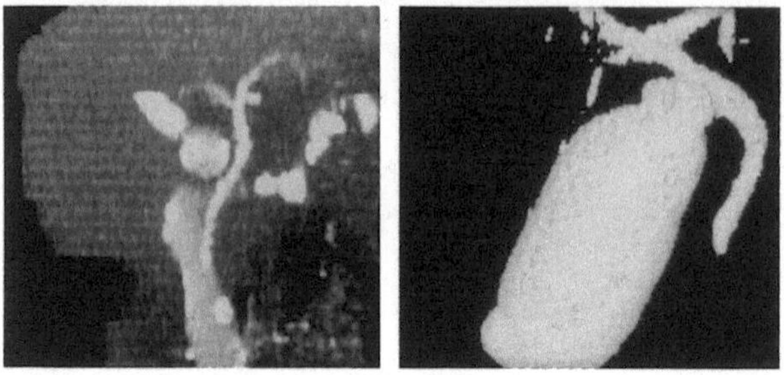

a b

Fig. 3. a Three-dimensional maximum intensity projection reconstruction with doudenogastral reflux. b Three-dimensional surface reconstruction

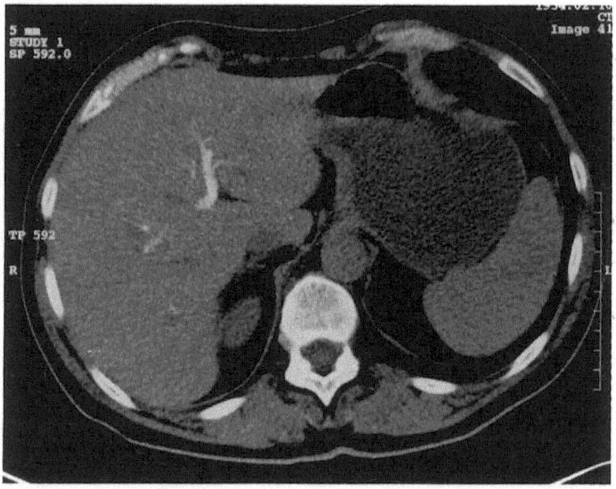

Fig. 4. Peripheral intrahepatic nondilated intrahepatic bile ducts with axial spiral CT

Calculi of the common bile duct were found in four patients (16.7%) on conventional i.v. cholangiography, of which two were false positive, with spiral CT in three patients (12.5%), all of which were true positive.

Calculi of the intrahepatic bile ducts were detected only in one patient on spiral CT (4.2%).

The intrahepatic ducts could be demonstrated to the first division in 100% to the second division in 91.7%, to the third division in 41.7% and to the four division in 4.7% on conventional i.v. cholangiography (Fig. 1).

With spiral CT up to the first division in 100%, to the second division in 100%, to the third division in 95.9%, to the fourth division in 70.9% and to the periphery in 37.5% (Fig. 4). The cystic duct could be demonstrated in 49.9% of the patients in conventional i.v. cholangiography and 83.3% with spiral CT (Table 1; Fig. 5).

Cystic duct calculi could only be demonstrated with spiral CT in two patients (8.3%).

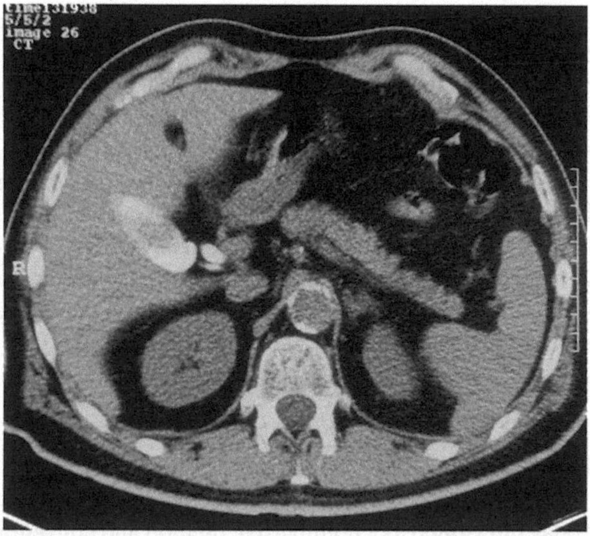

Fig. 5. Spiral CT: cystic duct inosculation with the choledochus

Table 1. Visibility of intrahepatic bile ducts and cystic duct

	Conventional i.v. cholangiography (%)	Axial spiral CT (%)
First division	100	100
Second division	91.7	100
Third division	41.7	95.9
Fourth division	4.7	70.9
Periphery	0	37.5
Cystic duct	49.9	83.3

CT, computed tomography

An aberrant cystic duct was found in none of the patients in conventional i.v. cholangiography but in two patients (8.3%) with spiral CT resulting in an open cholecystectomy.

Contrast media in the gallbladder could be seen in 29.2% on conventional i.v. cholangiography and on 41.7% with spiral CT.

The density of the common bile duct ranged from 134–387 HU/SD 8–70 HU (mean 211/23 HU).

The density of the gallbladder or biliary tract stones ranged from 21–360 HU/SD 9–208 (mean 67/36 HU).

ERC was performed in 29.2% with a failure rate of 28.5%. Doudenogastral reflux of the contrast medium was observed in 20.8% of the patients.

Paradox renal contrast media excretion was observed in 20.8%.

Adverse reactions to the intravenously administered contrast medium were not observed.

The number of axial images accquired ranged from 36 to 79 (mean: 63.58).

The X-ray dosage of spiral CT (tube current 125 kV, 145 mA ranged from 4420 mAs to 8700 mAs (mean: 6676.75 mAs).

Additional findings with CT were four cysts in the kidneys, three cysts in the liver, thickening of the wall of the gallbladder in three patients, two adenomas and two calcifications of the adrenal glands, two distal cystic duct inosculations with the choledochus, two st. p. nephrectomy and one juxtapapillary diverticulum, liver abscess, local peritonitis, right pleural effusion, choledocho-duodenal fistula, dilatation of the pancreatic duct and st. p. splenectomy.

Discussion

Today ultrasound as a noninvasive method and conventional i.v. cholangiography [3] with a complication rate of 1%–9% [4, 11] or three to four times higher than in angiography [13] are performed for diagnostic work up of the biliary system. They are followed by invasive methods like ERC [10] with a complication rate of 5%–7% and a failure rate of 3% and PTC [3] with a technical sucess rate of 50%–95% in nondilated bile bucts and a complication rate from 0.9%–40% [6].

Spiral CT of the biliary system [7] as a noninvasive method was superior to conventional i. v. cholangiography.

Nondilated intrahepatic bile ducts (Fig. 1) could be demonstrated significantly better on axial spiral CT than on i.v. cholangiography [8].

The demonstration of the inosculation of the cystic duct with the choledochus and the presence of biliary common duct calculi is an important feature for planning laparoscopic cholecystectomy (Fig. 5).

Axial spiral CT provided this information in more than 80% of the patients, whereas additional three-dimensional maximum intensity projection (3D MIP) or surface reconstruction were less accurate.

Gallbladder stones could be seen with axial spiral CT and 3D MIP even if the gallbladder did not fill with contrast. The gold standard for diagnostic work up of gallbladderstone still seems to be ultrasound.

The common bile duct could always be demonstrated clearly with spiral CT [1, 5].

Radiolucent stones of the gallbladder or the common bile duct, cystic duct and intrahepatic ducts [12] were seen with axial spiral CT as filling defects in almost equivalent quality to ERC with the advantage that no small air bubble can be misinterpretated as a concrement.

These stones also can be demonstrated in 3D MIP but not in 3D surface reconstruction.

Calcified intraductal stones are masked by the contrast medium but may be suspected when local increase of HU values are noted by scanning the common bile duct with the cursor on the Somatom Plus S or on the DRC.

MRI seems not to be the method of choice for demonstration of a non dilated biliary tract but can give additional spatial information in an obstructed biliary system [9, 14].

In our opinion spiral CT after i.v. cholangiography has the potential to replace diagnostic ERC or PTC as well as conventional i. v. cholangiography.

References

1. Cory DA, West SD and K (1990) CT cholangiography of a choledochocele. Pediatric Radiology 21 : 73 – 74
2. Drexler G, Panzer W, Widenmann L et al. (1985) Organ Doses in X-ray Diagnosis (Hoffmann, Berlin) 33 – 41
3. Feld R, Kurtz AB, Zeman R (1991) Imaging the Gallbladder: A Historical Perspective. AJR 156 : 737 – 740
4. Hald JK (1984) Adverse reactions to intravenous cholangiography with Biligram. European Journal of Radiology 4(3),196 – 197
5. Höglund M, Muren C and Boijsen MW (1990) Computed tomography with intravenous cholangiography contrast: a method for visualizing choledochal cysts. European Journal of Radiology, 10 : 159 – 161
6. Hoevels J (1990) Percutaneous Transhepatic Cholangiography and Percutaneous Biliary Drainage. In: Dondelinger RF, Rossi P, Kurdziel JC and Wallace S. (Editors). Interventional Radiology Georg Thieme Verlag, Stuttgart, New York, 187 – 199
7. Klein H-M, Wein B, Truong S, Pfingsten F-P, Günther RW (1993) Computed tomographic cholangiography using spiral scanning and image processing. The British Journal of Radiology, 66 : 762 – 767
8. Liddell RM, Baron RL, Ekstrom JE, Varnell RM, Shuman WP (1990) Normal Intrahepatic Bile Ducts: CT Depiction. Radiology, 176 : 633 – 636
9. Morimoto K, Shimoi M, Shirakawa T, Aoki Y, Choi S, Miyata Y, Hara K (1992) Biliary Obstruction: Evaluation with Three-dimensional MR Cholangiography. Radiology; 183 : 578 – 580
10. Neuhaus H, Ungeheuer A, Feussner H, Classen M, Siewert JR (1992) Laparoskopische Cholecystektomie: ERCP als präoperative Standarddiagnostik? Deutsche medizinische Wochenschrift 117 : 1863 – 1867
11. Nilsson U (1987) Adverse reactions to iotroxate at intravenous cholangiography. A prospective clinica investigation and review of the literature. Acta Radiologica (Sweden), 28(5),571 – 575
12. Regge D, Debernardi S, Kienle S, Martina MC, Biselli S, Gandini G (1992) CT of intrahepatic lithiasis. European Journal of Radiology, 2 : 520 – 525
13. Schill D (1991) Röntgenkonstrastmittel – Entwicklungen, Substanzen, Einsatzgebiete. Krankenhauspharmazie, 12. Jahrgang, Nr. 1, S 4 – 11
14. Schumacher KA, Wallner B, Weidenmaier W, Friedrich JM (1991) Biliäre Obstruktion: MR-Cholangiographie mit einer schnellen Gradientenecho-Sequenz (2D CE-Fast). Fortschr. Röntgenstr. 155 : 332 – 336

CT Cholangiography with Spiral CT and Three-Dimensional Imaging

R. Dore, L. Preda, L. Storti, G. Di Giulio, E. Di Maggio, C. Villa, R. Campani

Introduction

Even if traditional cholecystectomy remains the gold standard for the treatment of patients with symptomatic cholelithiasis, increasing developments in nonsurgical and in minimally invasive methods are spreading. Laparoscopic cholecystectomy, first performed in 1987, has gained growing acceptance among surgeons. Cholangiography and ultrasonography prior to hepatobiliary surgery are particularly important when minimally invasive laparoscopic techniques are used [2]. In the radiologic evaluation some problems have to be considered:

1. Obstructions or stones in biliary ducts.
2. Abnormal anatomy of the cystic and of the right hepatic duct.
3. Adhesions from previous upper abdominal surgery.
4. Chronic cholecystitis.

Intravenous cholangiography with conventional tomography is usually performed; when biliary opacification is not optimal, in obese or scoliotic patients and in cases of overlap of feces or gas the informations given by radiographic examination decreased.

Endoscopic retrograde cholangiopancreatogram (ERCP) is a reliable but invasive method and involves troubles for the patients; ERCP is not usually performed but it is used to remove stones in the common biliary duct before or after laparoscopic cholecystectomy. Two theoretical considerations point out the reasons of computed tomography (CT) in this clinical approach:

1. For its high contrast resolution CT can visualize both faintly opacified biliary ducts and weakly calcified stones.
2. Single-breath hold volumetric spiral CT provides a good evaluation either of small stuctures than of their spatial relationships such as cystic duct and ductal stones.

The aim of this study is to check the accuracy of spiral CT compared with intraoperative results of conventional surgery, to check the role of spiral CT in the preoperative plan particularly compared with conventional colangiography.

Patients and Method

During a period of 3 months (December 1993 – February 1994) we examined 26 patients (11 male, 15 female, age range 35 – 75 years, average 60 years) who underwent i.v. cholangiography before conventional cholecystectomy. All patients accepted to be submitted to spiral CT before and after, i.v. cholangiography (IVC).

A first spiral CT has been performed prior i.v. infusion of contrast medium in order to evaluate hyperdense calculi in comparison with initial plain image: 5-mm slice thickness and 5 to 8-mm/s table speed were obtaied on total volume thickness previously evaluated on scout view.

After initial plain X-ray, 7.6 g iodosamicmeglumine (Bracco, Italy) were infused in 10 – 15 min and postcontrast images were obtained 20, 40, 60 and 120 min after the start of infusion; in 21 patients conventional tomography was performed in 20 – 40 min in order to improve image quality.

A second spiral CT, cholangio-CT (CCT), was performed 50 – 120 min post-infusion (mean 80 min). During the first phase of IVC and during the transfer to CT room, patients maintained a prone and LAO position but were examined in CT unit in a supine position. Immediately prior to cholangio CT patients drank a glass of water in order to reduce contrast concentration in duodenal loops.

Somatom Plus S was used allowing up to 24 continuous 1-s rotations. Two different slice thickness (5 mm and 3 mm) were used and compared in spiral CCT. In eleven patients the scanning parameters were 24 s, 5 mm/s table feed, 3-mm slice thickness, 165 mA, 120 kV (Protocol A); in ten other patients 5 mm/s, 5 mm, 165 – 210 mA, 120 kV were selected (Protocol B). Five patients, aging over 60, have been examined with both protocols (A + B) for a direct comparison. Image reconstruction was performed with soft resolution algorithm slim 180° reconstruction algorithm, 2-mm interslice increment in both protocols.

Axial images was prior evaluated in cine display, then in multiplanar reconstruction (MPR) and in three-dimensional (3D) imaging. Cine display of axial images

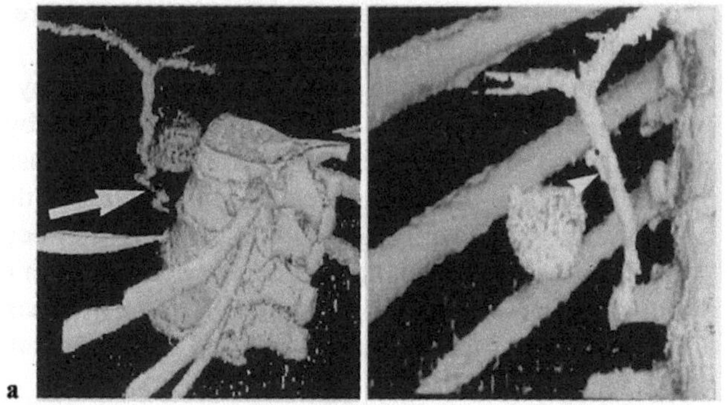

Fig. 1a, b. Lateral **a** and frontal **b** view of three-dimensional reconstructed images: patient breathed in during scanning of terminal choledochus, causing "zig-zag" artifact of the course of the duct (*arrows*). **b** Lateral confluence of cystic in common duct (*arrowhead*)

was first performed to verify the total or interrupted apnea of the patient during volumetric scanning. A sudden movement of the abdominal wall observed in cine display of axial images indicated an interrupted apnea: multiplanar or 3D reconstruction of these images can suffer from zig-zag artifact (Fig. 1). In case of sudden abdominal wall movements we preferred to repeat a new volumetric scan after warning again the patient.

MPR were obtained in coronal, sagittal and especially oblique views (fast and real-time technique) in order to visualize the whole common bile duct, the cystic confluence in the hepatic duct and the distal aspect of choledochus.

At last 3D surface shaded reconstructions (SSD) were performed in all patients using the 3D software of the CT unit: areas of the biliary system and surrounding bony stuctures were extracted using "edit" manual technique, a threshold of 110–140 HU, matrix 512 voxel.

Conventional and CT cholangiographic images (axial, MPR and 3D images) were independentely reviewed by three radiologists and one surgeon. Criteria were: degree of visualization of biliary structures; diagnostic reliability of intra and extra-hepatic intraductal pathology; demonstration of spatial relationship of cystic duct; demonstration of distal choledochal aspect; evaluation of main ducts caliber.

A quality rate was employed using a four point scale (0 = none; 1 = incomplete; 2 = complete but soft; 3 = complete and clear visualization). Imaging data have been correlated with macroscopic and surgical features in 18 patients who underwent open cholecystectomy.

Results

Surgical Results

Eighteen patients underwent conventional cholecystectomy. In 14 cases stones have been found in the gallbladder; diagnostic accuracy of ultrasound (US) was 100%, of non-enhanced spiral CT was 57%, of conventional cholangiography 28% and of plain X-ray 14%. In a patient many microcalculi were evident on non-enhanced spiral CT but were hidden by contrast media in CCT.

All four cases of common duct lithiasis verified by surgery were detected by nonenhanced and cholangio-spiral CT (100%), none by plain X-ray, two by conventional cholangiography (50%), and only one was suspected by US. We have not obtained any false-positive indication of biliary duct lithiasis in spiral CT, while in one conventional cholangiography it was wrongly suspected in common duct.

In ten cases surgery found perivisceral adhesions, in one cholesterolosis, in one a gallbladder neoplasm: two different US examinations misappreciated a neoplastic lesion that was suspect on basal CT and demonstrated by angio-TC, infiltrating surrounding hepatic tissue.

In eight patients we have no surgical data, in one case US diagnosed a stone in common duct not confirmed either by IVC or by non-enhanced and cholangio spiral CT. In another case IVC was false-negative on US and spiral CT.

Table 1. Quality score of visualization of biliary structure

	A	B	C	D
Intrahepatic duct	0.6	2.1	0.7	1.8
Common duct	1.9	2.9	2.6	2.8
Cystic duct	0.7	2.4	1.7	1.6

A, Conventional cholangiography; B, axial cholangio spiral computed tomography (CT); C, multiplanar reconstruction iamges of spiral CT; D, 3D images of spiral CT

Results of Visualization of Biliary duct

The quality scores of biliary duct visualization are summarized in Table 1. *Intrahepatic biliary duct evaluation* is difficult to obtain in IVC. Axial cholangio-CT images demonstrated secondary arborizations in 12 cases, primary in five and only main hepatic duct in nine cases. The 3D images represented intrahepatic ducts as well as axial scan but in a spatial evaluation; MPR were the worse modality for the evaluation of intrahepatic ducts.

Common biliary duct visualization was optimal in 25/26 patients in CCT. Conventional tomography had the same positive marks only in six patients. Two cases with insufficient duct opacification were completely evaluated in spiral CT. There was no differences between the grade of axial and of 3D visualization of common duct; while in five cases (three protocol A, two protocol B) MPR showed some difficulties to visualize completely the common duct.

All ductal calculi have been clearly demonstrated by axial images especially using cine-display; they have been all detected by A and B protocols; nevertheless with protocol B it has been easier to distinguish each stones in multiple lithiasis (Fig. 2). MPR recognized multiple stones too and made easier their localization in a longitudinal section. Only in one case 3D image was altered by the presence of the stone (Fig. 3).

A complete *cystic duct visualization* has been very difficult to obtain with cholangiography and cholangiotomography: scores varied from 0 to 2, in 45% of the cases was 0; only in two cases tomography increased the score. On the other hand, axial images of CT cholangiography dramatically increased diagnostic capacity to visualize cystic duct in an optimal score in 19 patients; only in one patient cystic duct has not been visualized.

Cine display has been always usefull to recognize immediately cystic duct and to distinguish it from common hepatic duct or from the duodenal loop (Fig. 4). In four cases cystic visualization in axial images differed in A protocol versus B one (A > B in three cases, B > A in one case). MPR has been less immediate in the cystic visualization than cine-display of axial images. The 3D images allowed complete visualization of cystic duct only in 29% of cases and in 53% have not improved conventional X ray results. There was no statistically significant difference between A and B protocol in obtaining MPR and 3D images.

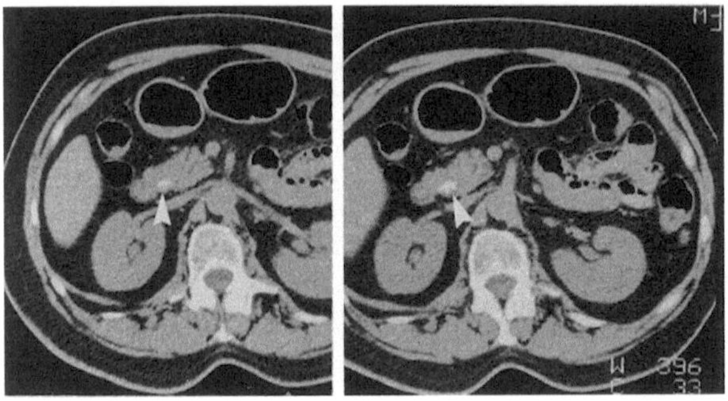

Fig. 2. Choledochal lithiasis. Two small calculi demonstrated during cholangiography spiral CT with 3-mm slice thickness (*arrowheads*)

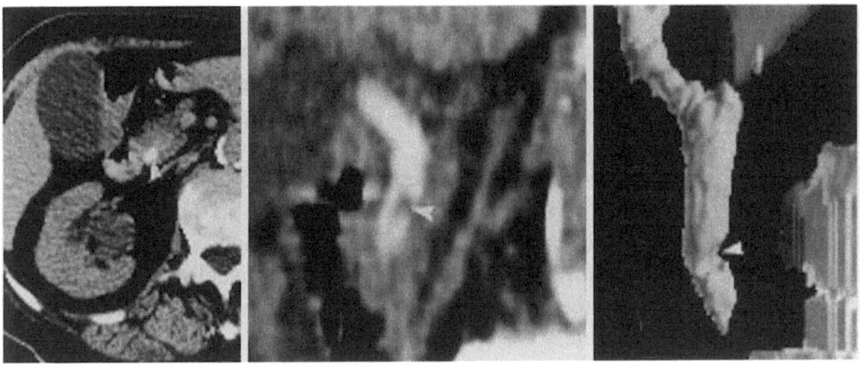

Fig. 3. Choledochal lithiasis. Single stone in opacified duct in the same patients. Axial and coronal images demonstrate the diameters of the stone

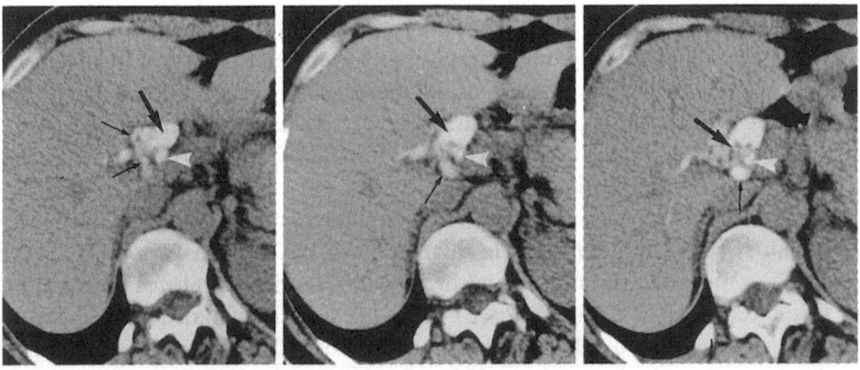

Fig. 4. Overlapped spiral images during cholangiography. Circumflex course of cystic duct (*small black arrows*), common duct (*arrowheads*), and lithiasic cystic neck (*large black arrows*) are well visualized

In single or contiguous axial images we tried to measure *length of cystic duct*. For this purpose 3D images are not useful because they suffer spatial distortions. We distinguished less than 30 mm length from more than 30 mm cystic duct. CT evaluation of cystic lenght underestimated the surgical measurements.

A perfect correlation was obtained in 86% of the cases in the description of spatial relationship between cystic and hepatocholedocal duct (lateral, posterior, medial), especially on the base of axial images. The 3D and MPR images have never corrected axial information about the course and the confluence of cystic in common duct.

Time, Involved and Patient Compliance

Twenty of 26 patients (76%) held their breath perfectly during the whole volumetric scan. Only two patients (7.6%) breathed during spiral CT that has been repeated; four other patients made some movements at the margins of volumetric scan not compromising the quality of reconstructions. Each spiral examination took from 5 to 15 min (for the patient and CT room). The most important time involvement regarded the operator because MPR and expecially 3D display required 30–40 min for each patients.

Discussion

Conventional cholangiography has been extensively used as the gold standard diagnostic method in the presurgical evaluation of biliary tract, second to intraoperative cholangiography [2]. In association with conventional tomography this method gives a good demonstration of intraductal pathology and a worst evidence of the biliary ducts anatomy. Some Authors determined an ovarian dose of 0.01 mGy for a single standard PA X-ray of the gallbladder with common technical parameters, and a total dose of about 0.04 mGy for conventional tomography [3].

US, gold standard for the gallbladder pathology, gives a difficult and inconstant accuracy in ductal stones; moreover, the US description of biliary anatomy is quite difficult and not easily communicable to surgeons [2].

Laparoscopic biliary surgery calls new attentions for an accurate preoperative evaluation, since these new methods allow limited flexibility for intraoperative changes in surgical strategy. Current absolute contraindications are peritonitis and pregnancy, relative ones are extensive adhesions, extreme obesity and choledocolithiasis [1, 5]. A good knowledge of the spatial relationship and of the course of cystic duct is usefull and permitt to gain time in laparoscopic procedures to perform cystic legature. Preoperative ERCP has been evocated but not routinely performed in candidates for laparoscopic cholecystectomy [1]. Volumetric CT has been proposed alternatively to the invasive and uncomfortable ERCT [4].

In our study, axial images obtained by spiral CT after intravenous cholangiography, demonstrated a better quality score compared to the conventional method for the visualization of all biliary structures; differences are more evident for intrahepatic and cystic ducts. These results agree with Klein previous report [4]. CT evaluation of biliary tract overcomes some common conditions that can limit or unable Xray exploration: intestinal gas, scoliosis, hepatic reduced excretion of contrast medium, extreme obesity. In our series also in few cases with invisible cholangiographic Xray opacification, spiral CT has been suitable for an axial imaging; 3D images, in a scoliotic patient gave a good spatial demonstration difficult to obtain in standard X ray projections.

In our experience an accurate evaluation of axial images in cinedisplay allowed the best identification of the critical region of the cystic duct based on the variability of normal common anatomy (Fig. 4). The 3D images obtained with SSD have been less constant in the demonstration of whole cystic duct course, while the region of cystic orifice has been documented in a better spatial view and more suitable for surgeons (Fig. 5). We believe that the poor differences of informations between axial and 3D images don't justify the routine emplojment of a time expensive technique as 3D reconstruction; this modality can be reserved for cases with unusual cystic course visualized or suspected by axial images.

All ductal lithiasis surgically treated during conventional cholecystectomy have been previously diagnosed by axial and MPR images obtained with spiral CT. Contrast enhancement doesn't mask calculi using 3- or 5-mm thickness; small stones about 2–3 mm in diameter have been detected with 3 as well as with 5 mm; nevertheless it seems that 3-mm slice thickness allows a better evidence of each little calculi, a better separation of long and circumflex cystic duct image from common duct in 3D reconstruction and a better demonstration of the aspect of the extremity of choledochus in 3D (Fig. 6).

On the other hand we have not observed any handicap of 3 mm in comparison with 5 mm protocol, neither when volume scanning required Pitch greater than 1 (but less than 1.5). On the basis of these experiences we retain that the problem of thickness slice is not essential, but that 3 mm thickness could be prefered.

Another question we propose in this study regards the convenience of non-enhanced spiral CT. Our data are not definitive and sumarize a poor series; all cases of choledochal stones appeared in non enhanced axial images obtained with spiral CT as little calcifications. This consideration gives importance to non-enhanced study; in addition X-ray exposure seems to be more than 0.01 mGy if spiral CT technique is performed [4], similar to the ovarian dose determined for a single standard PA X-ray film [3]. We think that approximately gonadal dose for whole our cholangio-spiral CT can range from 0.02 and 0.04 mGy maximum; these doses are inferior compared to those indicated for conventional tomographic examination [3]. So we believe that nonenhanced spiral CT is more useful than plain X-ray especially when cholangio-CT is planned.

Spiral CT patterns allow identification of non lithiasic disease that can contraindicate laparoscopic approach: for instance in our series a gallbladder neoplasm.

Klein stated that a time interval of 35 min from the start of contrast infusion and the start of the spiral scan seems to be optimal. Nevertheless we observed sufficient contrast enhancement and good CT results for at least 80–100 min.

In conclusion we believe that spiral CT cholangiography is a good alternative tool to ERCP if laparoscopic surgery is planned: CT allows reduced expense, reduced

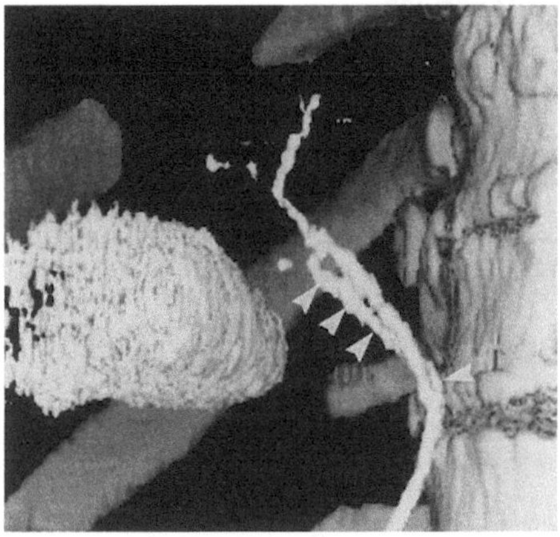

Fig. 5. Three-dimensional reconstruction of spiral computed tomography (3-mm slice thickness) of a long circumflex cystic duct (*arrowheads*)

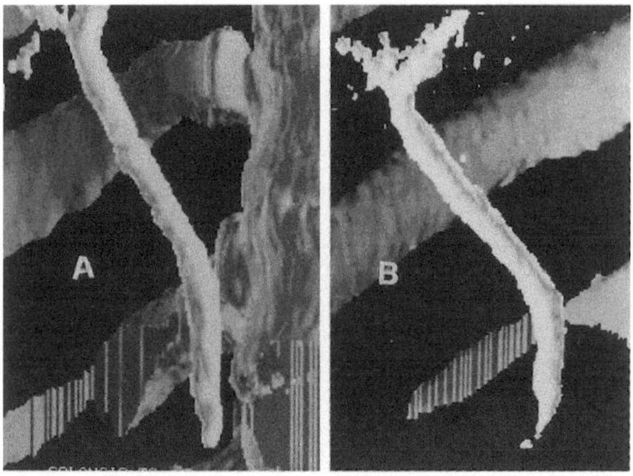

Fig. 6. Different aspects of the extremity of choledochus in the same patient in A and B protocols (5- and 3-mm slice thickness, respectively)

X-ray exposure and disconfort for the patient and for the operators, reduced time examination, have no contraindications, is easily repeatable, and provides constant and clear anatomical and lithiasic information better than conventional cholangiography. Cine display of axial CT images allows quick and precise visualization of critical anatomical zones and of the presence of stones. Time consuming image processings as MPR and 3D are not essential but in few cases make easier spatial anatomical view to the surgeons.

References

1. Brandon JC, Velez MA, Teplick SK, Mueller PR, Rattner DW, Broadwater JR, Lang NP, Eidt JF (1991) Laparoscopic cholecystectomy: evolution, early results, and impact on nonsurgical gallstone therapies. AJR 157 : 235 – 239
2. Calculli L, Caputo M, Papa S, Brusori S, Berardi R, Spagnol A, Totaro C, Mangino S, Gavelli GP (1994) Imaging techniques to assess the indications to laparoscopic cholecystectomy. Ultrasonography versus cholangiography. Radiol Med 87 : 103 – 106
3. Drexler G, Panzer W, Widenmann L et al. (1985) Organ Doses in X-ray Diagnosis. Hoffmann, Berlin pagg 33 – 41
4. Klein HM, Wein B, Truong S, Pfingsten FP, Gunther RW (1993) Computed tomographic cholangiography using spiral scanning and 3D image processing. The British Journal of Radiology 66 : 762 – 767
5. Velez MA, Rays G, Ryan JJ (1991) Laparoscopic cholecystectomy. Contemp Surg 38 : 21 – 25

Dynamic Spiral CT of the Pancreas

R. Kloeppel, S. Lieberenz, H.-G. Schulz

Introduction

The bad prognosis of pancreas carcinoma has been and remains a challenge for imaging diagnostics. Also computed tomography could not solve this problem. In the eighties studies with serial computed tomography were made that examined time density curves of pancreas tumours. As representative the studies of Claussen und Lochner (1983) shall be mentioned. Spiral computed tomography (SCT) (Kalender et al. 1990) gave new hope since on the basis of improved technique and more effective use of contrast medium diagnostic information increased, e.g. by 3-D display of vessels, by high contrast of pancreas and careful marking of the duodenum with negative contrast medium (Bautz et al. 1990; Fishman et al. 1992; Rigauts et al. 1992; Zwicker et al. 1993).

Similar to biphasic liver studies the methodic aspects of dynamic spiral CT of the pancreas are presented.

Material and Methods

A total of 85 patients between 23 and 75 years were examined with the SOMATOM PLUS S (Siemens) in the following way:

- 5 mm slice thickness, 5 mm/s table speed, 12×1 s scan time, 210 mAs, 4 mm increment
  - precontrast
  - Three spiral examinations after i.v. bolus injection of contrast medium (3×60 ml, flow 4 ml/s)
  - postcontrast

The first spiral examination with contrast medium should start with a 15- to 18-s delay, the second with a 25- to 28-s delay, and the third with a 35- to 40-s delay.

The contrast medium Iopamidol (Solutrast 370/Byk Gulden) is injected into the cubital vein by a computer controlled injector (XD5500/Ulrich).

Results

Of the 85 examinations 80 could be evaluated. But only with half of these cases the slices reconstructed from multiple spiral examinations were exactly comparable. In this way 55 pictures were generated besides topogram and scans of upper abdomen for orientation. Starting from the precontrast examination slices at the same position showed the arterial, parenchymal and venous phases and the phase of contrast medium equilibrium (Figs. 1 – 3). Separation of the single phases was of different quality. The arterial phase could be most clearly distinguished. At the end of each spiral scan with increasing enhancement of background the single phases became more indistinguishable. The equilibrium phase gave no new information.

Discussion

Functional spiral CT combines topographic information and as our results show functional information in a diagnostically useful way. Spiral scans at identical positions represent a contrast medium distribution as found with serial computed tomography in normal pancreas tissue and in tumours of the pancreas and as it is used for differentiation of lesions. The topographic information is the result of volume scanning.

A prerequisite of a successful examination is not only a cooperative patient and an optimal timing of contrast medium application (Claussen und Lochner 1983; Heiken et al. 1993; Dupuy et al. 1992; Rigauts et al. 1992; Zwicker et al. 1993) but also short spiral scans (carefully limited to the pancreas) with 5 mm slice thickness. We consider this compromise between spatial resolution and scan time to be acceptable in order to get the contrast medium distribution in all phases with sufficient perception of details. The postcontrast scan can be dispensed with. Spiral CT of the venous phase could be combined with a portal venous examination of the liver (Table 1). It can be expected that the double spiral technique will influence the strategy of contrast medium administration.

We conclude that the chance of early detection of pancreas carcinoma will justify the high expense of dynamic spiral CT examination with special contrasting of the bowels (Bautz 1994) and time consuming image evaluation and that a broader appli-

Table 1. Dynamic spiral CT procedure in the pancreas

	Volume and flow of contrast medium		Delay (s)	CT	Situation
	(ml)	(ml/s)			
1				Upper abdomen	Precontrast
2	60	4	10–18	Pancreas 5/5/4	Arterial
3	60	4	25–28	Pancreas 5/5/4	Parenchymal
4	60	4	35–40	Pancreas 5/5/4 (Upper abdomen)	Venous

CT, computed tomography

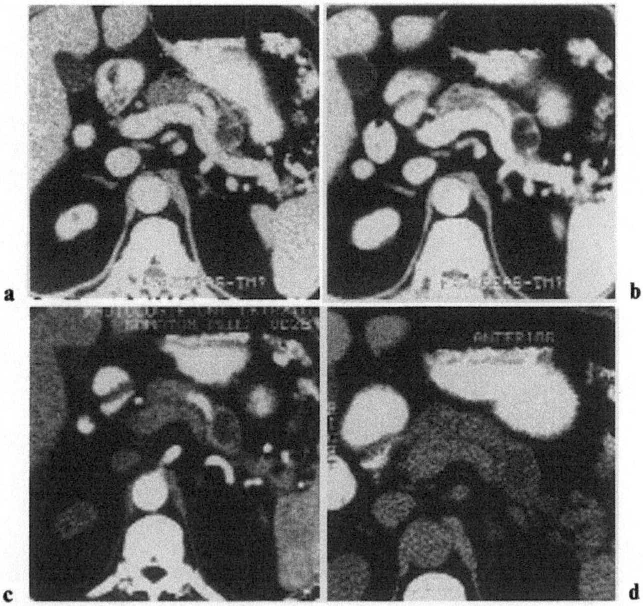

Fig. 1. A 57-year-old man with acinar cell tumour of cauda pancreatis: image selection precontrast, arterial, parenchymal-venous, and postcontrast

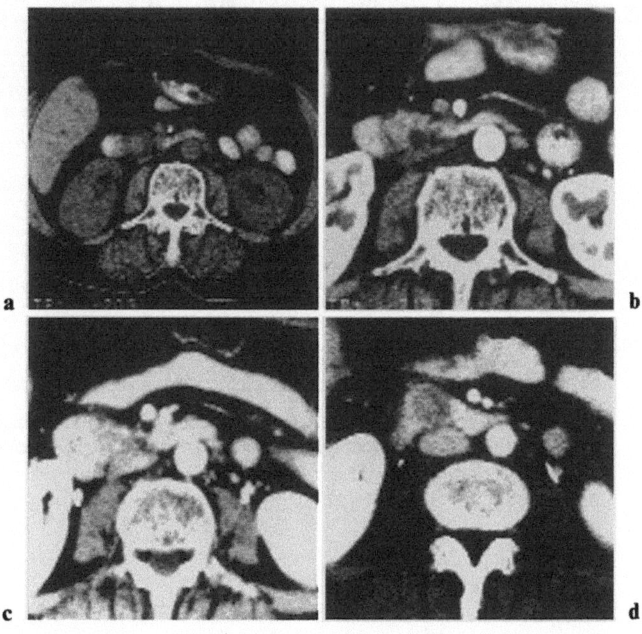

Fig. 2. A 67-year-old woman with early cancer of caput pancreatis: image selection precontrast, arterial, parenchymal, and venous

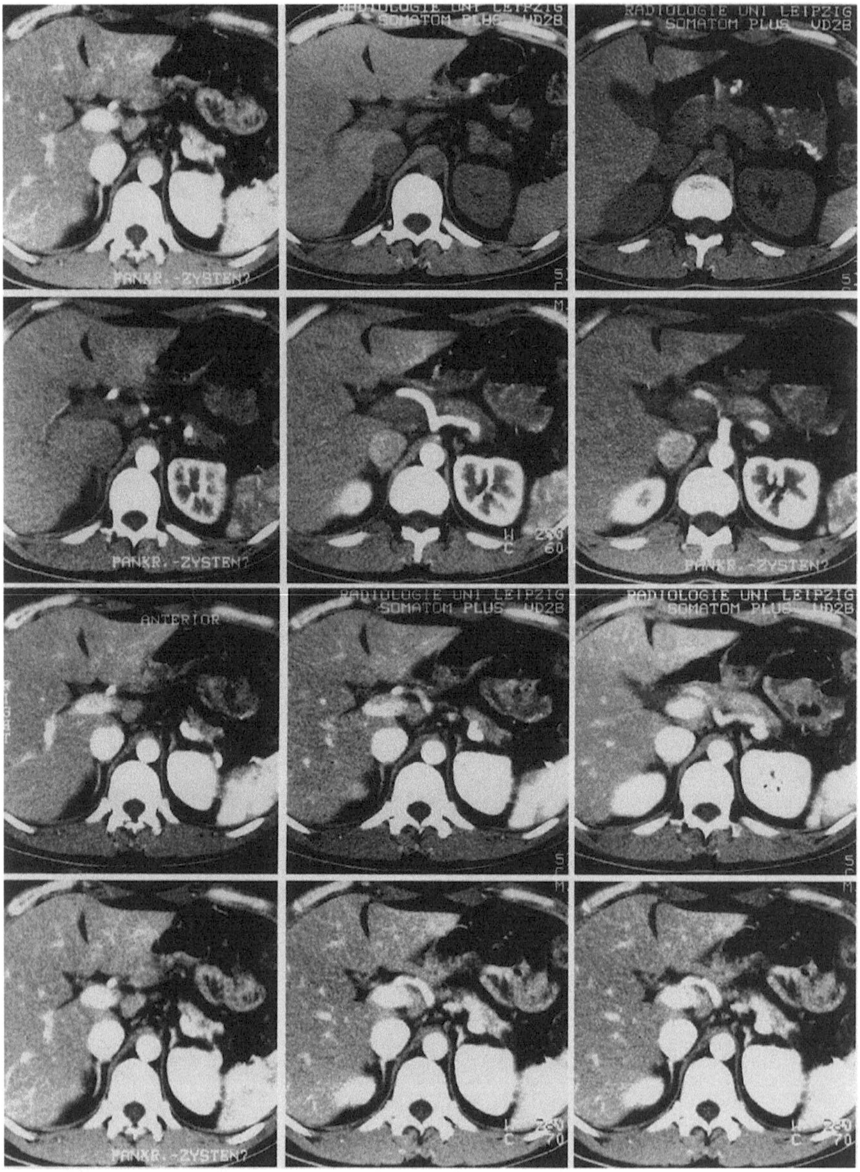

Fig. 3. A 23-year-old man with small pseudocyst of cauda pancreatis: image selection of every spiral CT (horizontal): precontrast (*top row*), arterial (*second row*), parenchymal (*third row*), and venous (*fourth row*)

cation of this method should be taken into consideration. We are well aware of the fact that the growth of tumours without clinical evidence in a patient without pain will not be influenced by improved imaging diagnostics.

References

Bautz W, Skalej M, Kalender WA (1990) Diagnosis of pancreatic disease: clinical impact of spiral CT. Radiology 177 (P): 154

Bautz W (1994) CT und MRT des Pankreas (Vortrag) Symposium für Radiologen, Berlin 3.–6.2.94

Claussen C, Lochner B (1983) Pankreaskarzinomdiagnostik durch Einsatz der dynamischen CT. Fortschr. Roentgenstr. 139 : 266–268

Dupuy DE, Costello P, Ecker CP (1992) Spiral CT of the Pancreas Radiology 183 : 815–818

Fishman EK, Wyatt SH, Ney DR, Kuhlman JE, Siegelman SS (1992) Spiral CT of the pancreas with multiplanar display. AJR 159 : 1209–1215

Heiken JP, Brink JA, Vannier MW (1993) Spiral (Helical) CT Radiology 189 : 647–656

Kalender WA, Vock P, Polcin A, Soucek M (1990) Spiral-CT: Eine neue Technik für Volumenaufnahmen. I. Grundlagen und Methodik. Röntgenpraxis 43 : 323–330

Rigauts H, Marchal G, Baert AL (1992) Enhancement of the pancreas after single bolus combined with spiral scanning: a comparative study with conventional incremental scanning after biphasic contrast injection. Fortschr. Roentgenstr. 156 : 471–474

Zwicker C, Langer M, Langer R, Keske U (1993) Bolusapplikation in der Spiral-CT des Oberbauches. Act. Radiol. 3 : 172–176

Three-Dimensional Display Techniques in the Evaluation of Urinary Pathology Excluding Native Kidney Artery Stenosis

A. Blum, J. Hubert, M. Deneuville, F. Delfau, E. Renoult, M. Claudon, D. Regent

Introduction

Spiral computed tomography (SCT) allows high quality performance three-dimensional (3D) surface reconstruction and maximum intensity projection (MIP) images of vessels [1, 5, 7]. These techniques should also be suited for the analysis of the opacified urinary tract and of renal calcifications. Therefore, they could produce in a single examination a complete morphological evaluation of the urinary system.

The purpose of this study is to illustrate the relevance of 3D display techniques in the evaluation of the urinary system.

Materials and Methods

A total of 70 patients with urological pathology underwent spiral CT with a Somatom Plus S machine (Siemens, Erlangen). Afterwards, 3D surface reconstruction images (3D SSD) and MIP images were obtained.

There were 24 renal transplants, 15 staghorn calculi, nine congenital anomalies of the urinary tract, seven ureteral obstructions or hydronephrosis, 12 pretransplantation evaluations and three renal aneurysms. Renal transplants were evaluated with color duplex ultrasound (US). All vascular lesions were assessed with angiography and urinary tract lesions with intravenous urography and sonography.

Spiral CT were performed with a 20- to 40-s acquisition time and the parameters indicated in Table 1. In recent studies, a pitch of 1.67 or 2 were used, resulting in a larger imaging volume or a shorter imaging time. Therefore, in these cases, a higher injection rate of contrast media could be used. Contrast media, meglumine ioxitalamate (Telebrix 30, Guerbet) or ioversol (Optiray 300, Guerbet) was injected into an antecubital vein with the parameters indicated in Table 2. The renal functions in all patients with renal graft were kept under close control.

Results and clinial applications

Depending upon the type of examination, the anomalies are classified into six categories: renal artery aneurysms, urinary tract lesions, mixed (vascular and urinary tract) anomalies, pretransplantation evaluation, renal transplant evaluation and staghorn calculi.

Table 1. Parameters used for spiral computed tomography

	Nominal slice thickness (mm)	Table speed (mm/s)	Increment (mm)	Interpolation algorithm
Renal artery Nephrolithiasis	2 or 3	2 or 3	1 or 2	360°
Renal transplant	3	5 or 6	2	180°
Hydronephrosis or ureteral obstruction	5	5	3	360°
Urinary tract anomaly	3	6	2	180°
Pretransplantation evaluation	3	6	3	180°

Table 2. Contrast media injection paramters

	Delay between injection and acquisition	Rate (ml/s	Volume (ml)
Nephrolithiasis	0	0	0
Urinary tract disease	15 min–2 h	–	60
Urinary tract and vessels	15–30 min 25–35 s	– 2–3	30 120–130
Pretransplant evaluation	30–40 s	2	100
Renal artery kidney, renal transplant	25–40 s	2–5	120–160

Renal Artery Aneurysms. Axial slices, 3D SSD and MIP images all demonstrate the aneurysm but the 3D display techniques document precisely the vascular supply and surrounding vascular anatomy before surgical treatment [6].

Urinary Tract Lesions. When kidney function impairement is severe, the nephrogram is faint on intravenous urography. There may be no recognizable opacification of the pyelocalicial system, even on later films. In these cases, CT clearly shows the anatomical structures and often demonstrates the specific obstruction cause (Fig. 1) [6].

Mixed Anomalies. In mixed anomalies, when the urinary tract is opacified, spiral CT produces in a single examination a complete morphological evaluation of the urinary system. Therefore, urinary obstruction due to vascular prosthesis or congenital anomalies such as pericaval ureter are well documented (Fig. 2) [4].

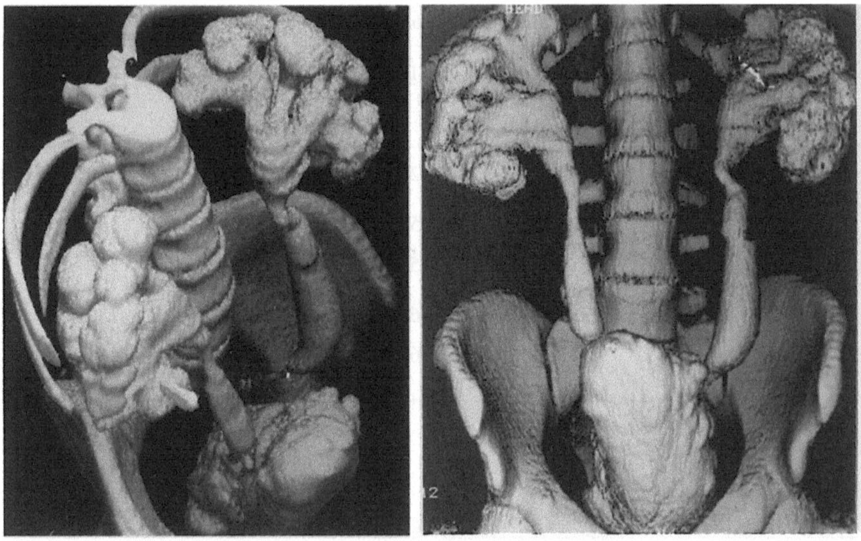

a b

Fig. 1a, b. Control after corrective surgery of vesico-ureteral reflux in a patient with neuropathic bladder. Three-dimensional surface reconstruction images show a grossly trabeculated bladder with small diverticula, bilateral hydroureterohydronephrosis but pelvic ureters with normal caliber

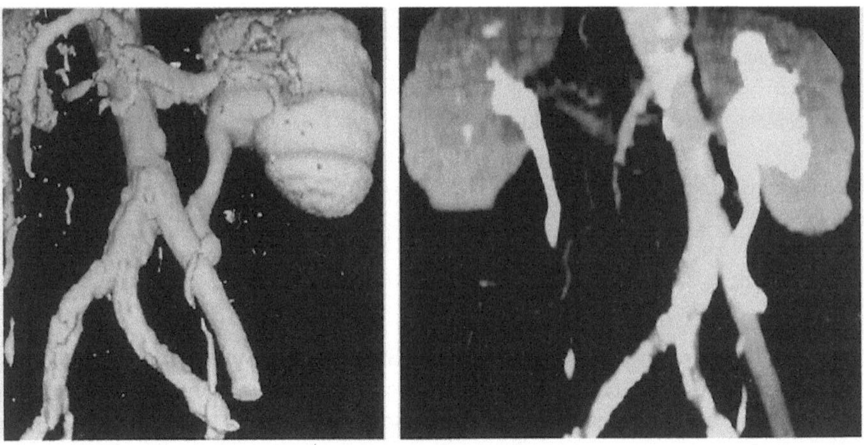

a b

Fig. 2a, b. Aorto-femoral graft responsible for ureteral obstruction. **a** Three-dimensional surface reconstruction image; **b** maximum intensity projection image

Evaluation Before Renal Transplantation. Stenosis and calcifications of the recipient arteries must be detected in order to select the best location for anastomosis. Calcifications are often very important in patients with renal insufficiency and can make the surgical anastomosis difficult. MIP reconstruction is more accurate than angiography and plain films to demonstrate which arterial segment is free of calcification. When calcifications are not significant, the detection and the grading of

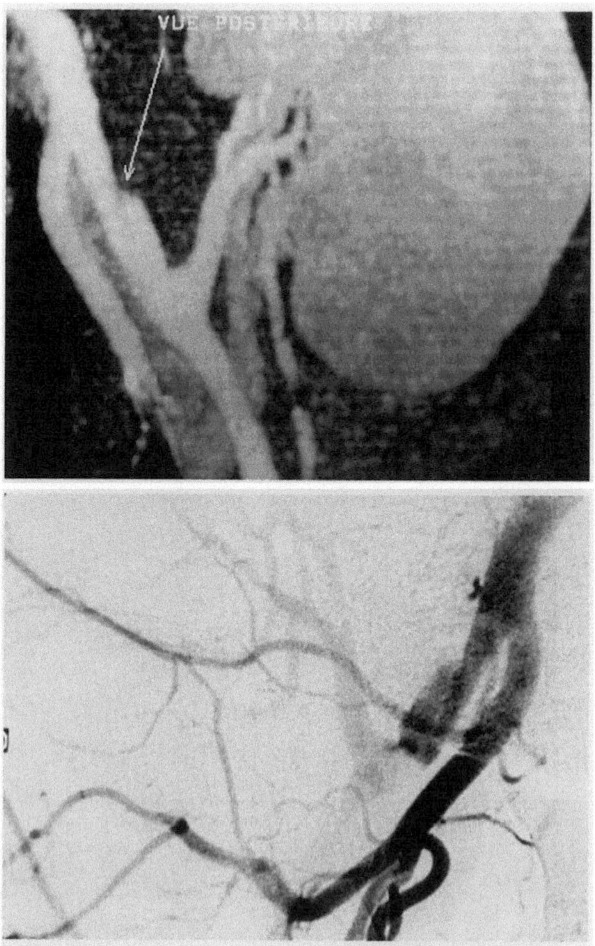

a

b

Fig. 3a, b. Dissection (*arrow*) of the right external iliac artery dure to technical difficulties with surgical anastomosis. **a** Maximum intensity projection image; **b** angiography (antegrade injection)

stenosis of iliac arteries on MIP images is well correlated with angiography. In other cases, axial slices are required to evaluate stenosis.

Renal Transplant Evaluation. Although it is minimally invasive, CT evaluation of vascularity requires a volume of 120–160 ml of contrast media, therefore, it is unadvisable as a screening method for patients with impaired renal function. However, when surgery is required, spiral CT with 3D display techniques procure a precise location of the artery stenosis and of the surrounding vascular and urinary tract structures. Detection of accessory renal arteries requires an injection rate of at least 4 ml/s. External iliac artery lesions, usually related to the surgical procedure, are well depicted (Fig. 3). During the same procedure, urinary tract obtruction and perinephric fluid collections are also identified. CT is useful in differentiating

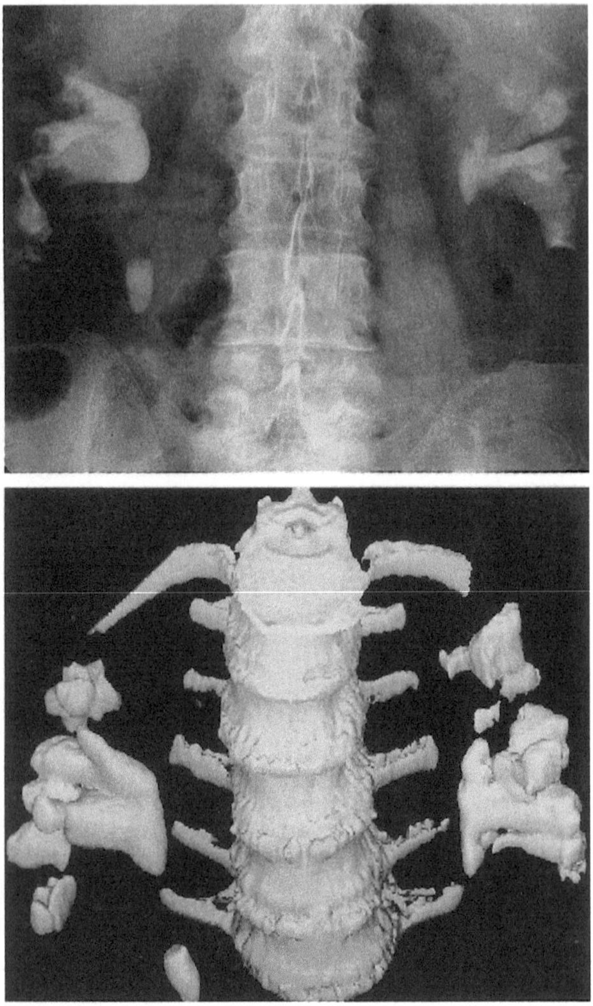

a

b

Fig. 4a, b. Staghorn calculi. **a** Plain film; **b** Three-dimensional surface reconstruction image

lymphocele from abcess or hematoma [2]. With spiral CT, their eventual consequences on the urinary tract or the vessels are well demonstrated.

Staghorn Calculi. Percutaneous nephrolithotomy is the best known treatment for large staghorn calculi. Therefore, the location of the calculi in the calyces precisely demonstrated with 3D surface reconstruction images is important for the determination of the kidney puncture site (Fig. 4) [3].

Conclusion

The 3D surface reconstruction images and MIP images are complementary in many situations and need to be confronted for analysis. In no case, however, should they replace the axial slices but constitute a valuable additional diagnostic tool. Therefore, while taking a CT scan, the examination performance would be in many cases enhanced with spiral acquisition permitting high quality 3D display. In the above-studied pathology, spiral CT provides a unique vision of the vascular and urinary tract anomalies. The obtention of more specific and complete information should develop the applications of these techniques in the urinary system.

References

1. Galanski M, Prokop M, Chavan A, Schaefer CM, Jandeleit K, Nichelsky JE (1993) Renal arterial stenoses: spiral-CT angiography. Radiology 189 : 185 – 192
2. Halvorsen RA (1991) Computed tomography and magnetic resonance imaging of renal transplants. In: Letourneau JG, Day DL, Ascher NL. Radiology of organ transplantation, Mosby Year Book, S 121 – 134
3. Hubert J, Blum A, Six A, Pertek JP, Claudon M, Guillemin P (1992) Intérêt de la reconstruction tomodensitométrique 3D dans le traitement de la lithiase coralliforme. Prog. Urol 2 (suppl 4): A41
4. Hubert J, Fournier G, Blum A, Punga-Maole ML, Mangin Ph. Uretère rétro-cave associé à une ectopie rénale pelvienne contralatérale. A propos d'un cas et revue de la littérature. Progrès en urologie (under press)
5. Napel SA, Marks MA, Rubin GD et al. (1992) CT angiography with spiral CT and maximum intensity projection. Radiology 185 : 607 – 610
6. Pollack HM (1990) Clinical urography. WB Saunders Company, Philadelphia
7. Rubin GD, Dake MD, Napel SA et al. (1994) Spiral-CT of renal artery stenosis: comparison of three-dimensional rendering techniques. Radiology 190 : 181 – 189

Lung

Chairmen: R. Rienmüller, D. Hahn

Minimum and Maximum Intensity Projections for Evaluation of Spiral CT Data of the Chest

C. Schaefer-Prokop, M. Prokop, M. Galanski

Introduction

Spiral computed tomography (CT) allows for complete examination of the lungs within one breathhold. A continuous data acquisition eliminates discontinuities of the examined volume due to inconstant inspiration depth that otherwise lead to missing of small lesions. To fully utilize the advatages of spiral CT, however, a considerably larger number of (overlapping) images has to be evaluated than in standard CT. On the monitor display, these axial images can be reviewed in an interactive cine mode. We examined properties of maximum (MIP) and minimum (mIP) intensity projections as film display modalities for evaluation of spiral CT data of the chest.

Diagnostic value of MIP and mIP was examined with respect to various kinds of pulmonary and bronchial pathology. The impact of slab thickness, degree of overlap and volume of interest on the quality of MIP and mIP were studied.

Material and Methods

Study Group

Thirty patients were selected for the study group in such a way that a large range of pulmonary and bronchial pathology of various degree of conspicuity was covered (Table 1).

Table 1. Study group

Pulmonary lesions								Bronchial lesions ($n = 10$)	
Increased density ($n = 13$)				Decreased density ($n = 7$)					
Nodules	*n*	Interstitial	*n*	Cystic disease	*n*	Emphysema	*n*		*n*
								Strictures	2
Miliary	2	Long lines	1	Bullae	1	Subpleural	2	Intraluminal tumor	1
Multiple	4	Reticular	2	Honeycombing	2	Centroacinar	1	Wall infiltration	2
Singular	4					Diffuse	1	Bronchiectasis	2
								Dehiscences	1
								Fistula	2

Scan Parameters

All patients underwent spiral CT of the chest using 2- to 5-mm slice thickness and 2- to 9-mm table feed/s depending on the desired scan range. All data were reconstructed using the "slim" slice profile and a standard or high resolution filter kernel.

Standard examinations, e.g. for screening for metastatic disease, were carried out with the scan parameters 5/8 – 9/4 [nominal slice thickness (SL, mm)/table feed (TF, mm/s)/reconstruction interval (RI, mm)] in order to cover both lungs within one breathhold phase of up to 32 s. The table feed was adjusted to the required scann-length.

The z-axis resolution was increased for the evaluation of circumscribed pathology of known location, for pulmonary fibrosis or for bronchial lesions using scan parameters of 1 – 2/2 – 3/1 – 2 (SL/TF/RI).

Examinations were routinely performed in inspiration. To improve patient compliance, the need for a long period of apnoea was carefully explained and a trial 30 s breathhold was performed. Immediately before the scan the patients were instructed to hyperventilate. The spiral scan was started at the lower level and carried out towards the apex of the lung to reduce potential breathing artifacts that would be more pronounced closer to the diaphragm.

Maximum and Minimum Intensity Projections

MIP and mIP are three-dimensional (3D) volume rendering techniques. They build up two-dimensional images from a given perspective by displaying the minimum or maximum CT numbers encountered when projecting a 3D volume of interest (VOI) into the view plane at arbitrary projection angles. The underlying data volume used for computation of a MIP or mIP is called slab. VOIs of only a few nominal slice thicknesses are called "thin" slabs. Usually MIPs or mIPs are computed from multiple perspectives (using the VRT software on the Somatom Plus) and displayed in a rotating cine-loop to convey 3D structure.

For parenchymal disease, we focused in this examination on the reduction of the total number of images to be evaluated by producing ("axial") MIP and mIP images of 3, 5 and 10 axial slices only in a caudocranial projection (180° rotation around x-axis) that is comparable to the usual axial planes. Table 2 lists scan and reconstruction parameters. Projections were computed with no overlap and an overlap of one and two reconstruction intervals. MIP and mIP images of larger data volumes and rotation around the z-axis were created only in selected cases. MIP images of this kind required the prior removal of the chest wall and the mediastinum using image editing tools.

For bronchial disease we computed mIPs in five views in a.p. projection with rotation angles around the z-axis of –20° (i.e. 340°) to +20° in 10° steps. The width of the VOI was varied from 2 cm to 5 cm. A centrally located VOI was chosen that included the main bronchi and as many bronchi as possible down to the segmental level. In patients with bronchiectasis that also were located more anteriorly or posteriorly, VOIs were chosen to include the affected segments.

Table 2. Scan and reconstruction parameters

	Pulmonary lesions			Bronchial lesions
	Nodules	Interstitial	Cystic/Emphysema	
SL/TF/RI	5/8–9/4	1–2/2/1	2/2/1 5/8/4	2/2/1
Effective SL	7.5–8	1.7–2.4	2.4–7.5	2.4
MIP	×	×		–
MIP	×	×	×	×
Slab (mm)				
2 slices		2.7–3.4	3.4–11.5	
3 slices	16	3.7–4.4	4.4–16	
5 slices	24	5.7–7.4	6.4–24	
10 slices	34	10.7–11.4	11.4–34	>10 slices: 60 mm
Overlap (mm)				–
1 RI	4	1	1–4	1
2 RI	8	2	2–8	2

SL, slice thickness (mm); TF, table feed (mm/s); RI, reconstruction interval (mm); MIP, maximum intensity projection; mIP, minimum intensity projection

Axial MIP and mIP images were compared to axial images reviewed in the cine mode ("gold standard") with respect to complete depiction of pathology in order to study the effect of slab thickness, degree of overlap and volume of interest.

Results

Maximum Intensity Projections

Nodules

For screening of metastases in ten patients we used scan parameters of 5/8/4 (SL/TF/RI) that provide a sufficient volume coverage at an adequate effective slice thickness of 7.5 mm. Differentiation between nodular and micronodular opacities, and tubular vasculature was simplified in axial MIPs. For diffuse nodules (>20 nodules) rather thick slabs (40 mm) were advantageous to show extent and distribution of disease. MIPs were found to increase the conspicuity of very subtle, yet diffuse disease by "summing up" the lesions of several axial slices into one projection (Fig. 1). For singular nodules of 2–6 mm in diameter a slab 25 mm thick appeared to be the optimum for differentiation of pathologic and anatomic structures. This was true for perihilar and peripheral nodules. In thicker slabs the vasculature appeared too dense, while in thinner slabs the tubular character of the vessels was not yet sufficiently established.

For the detection of singular nodules, an overlap of the slabs was obligatory. An overlap identical to the table feed/s appeared adequate. A smaller overlap was found to be insufficient, a larger overlap produced too many ad too similar images. Especially small singular nodules (2–3 mm) could be obscured by overlying tubular

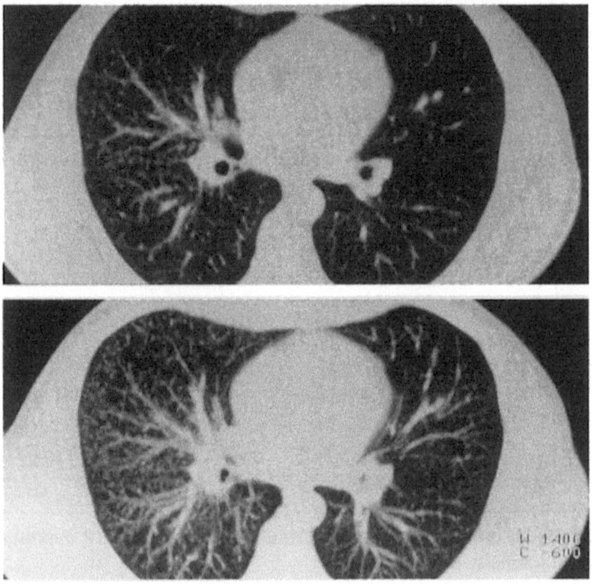

a

b

Fig. 1a, b. Sarcoid with bilateral, asymmetric pulmonary disease that is more easily appreciated in the slab (24 mm; **b**) than in the single slice (5 mm; **a**)

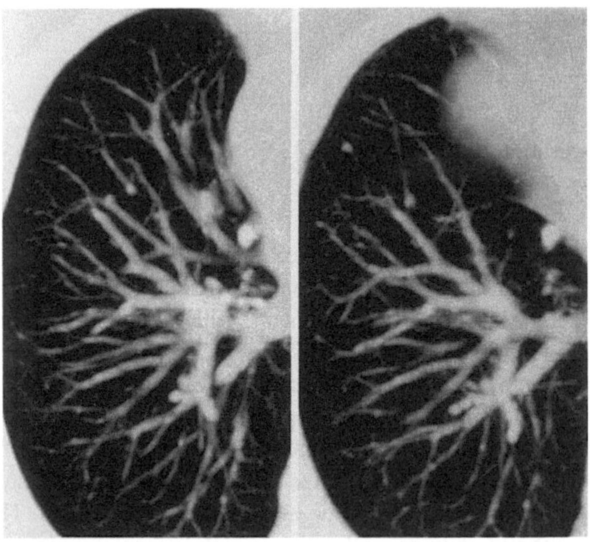

Fig. 2. Overlapping construction (8 mm) of MIPs (24 mm) is obligatory for the detection of singular nodular lesions (*arrows*)

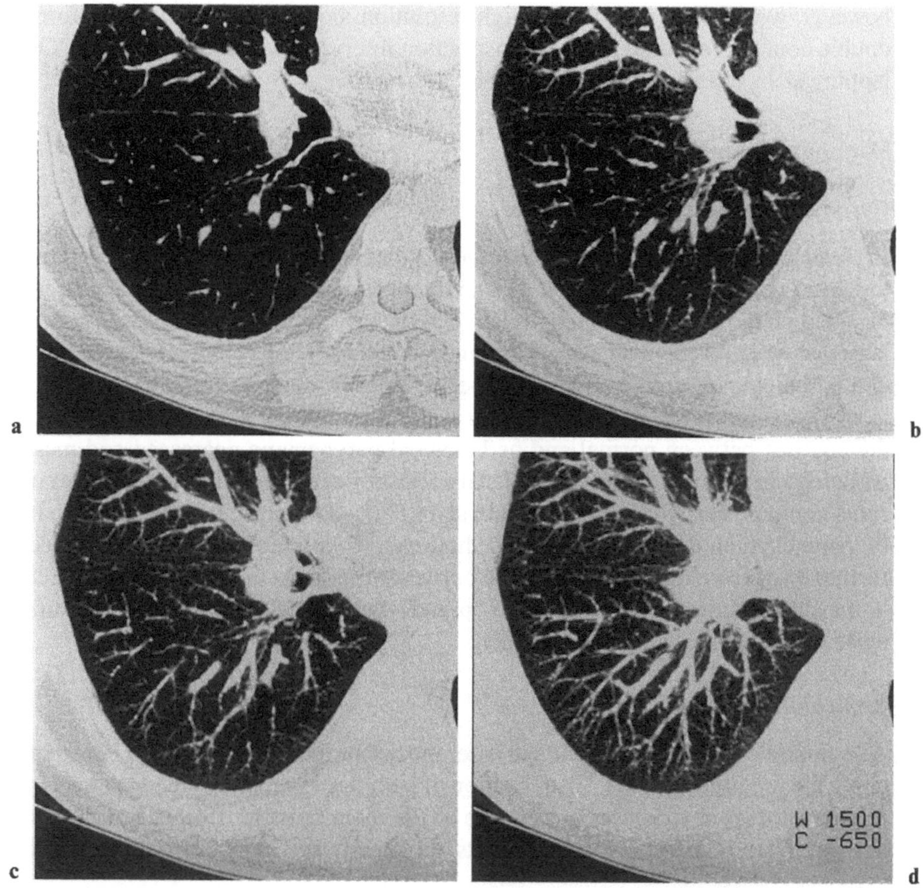

Fig. 3 a–d. Initial fibrosis with subtle thickened interlobular septi: **a** 1-mm single slice; **b** 3.7-mm slab; **c** 5.7-mm slab; **d** 10.7-mm slab

vessels in one slab, however, were readily appreciable in the overlapping slab due to a different view of the vascular architecture (Fig. 2).

Linear and Reticular Disease

For screening of reticular disease in three patients we applied scan parameters of 1–2/2/1 (SL/TF/RI). Visualization of subtle reticular opacities and long lines caused by thickened interlobular septa were found to be more obvious in thin slabs (2.7–3.4 mm) as compared to single axial planes. By collating the data of two or three thin slices in one MIP, long lines were imaged over a longer course and subtle reticular disease was seen to a greater extent (Fig. 3). In patients with severe fibrotic changes parenchymal distorsion was readily appreciable in slabs of three to five slices (4–6 mm). Thicker slabs appeared to be inadequate because of superposition of parenchymal structures. For all linear and reticular opacities, their presence and extent could be more easily appreciated in thin slabs, contour sharpness and detail, however, were better with single high resolution axial slices. Artifacts in form of double contours occured if the reconstruction interval was larger than 1 mm. Overlapping slabs did not provide additional information.

Minimum Intensity Projections

Cystic and Emphysematous Disease

In cystic and emphysematous disease ($n = 7$), due to the high susceptibility of mIPS to partial volume effects, impact of slab thickness and diagnostic efficacy strongly depeded on the size of pathology relative to the effective slice thickness. For pathology that was present in all slices combined in one slab, the contrast between normal and pathological parenchyma was superior in mIP images as compared to single axial slices. However, as soon as slices without pathology were included in a slab, the contrast between normal and pathological parenchyma decreased and masked pathology in the mIP. An overlap of slabs was not necessary. The extent of emphysema could be easily visualized in thin slabs (2.7 – 3.4 mm) due to the accentuation of parenchymal density differences; however, subpleural emphysema projected further away from the chest wall if the border of the lungs did not run perpendicular to the slab. Caution had to be paid to "pseudo-bullae" caused by pulsation artifacts close to vessels near the cardic border.

Bronchial Pathology

As compared to axial scans mIPs in anteroposterior direction improved information along the longitudinal axis. Visualization of pathologic situations in ten patients was facilitated, e.g. in strictures or pouches of the main bronchi. Because of their high susceptibility to partial volume effects mIPs provided only relative information

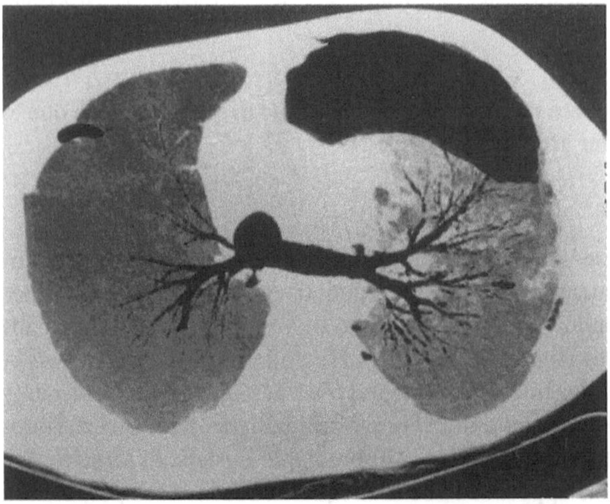

Fig. 4. Minimum intensity projection of the tracheobronchial tree in a patient with anastomotic dehiscenses after bilateral lung transplantation

about bronchial diameter and shape; absolute measurements were not possible. This was especially true for strictures: high grade strictures could appear as pseudo-occlusions depending on the size of the underlying VOI.

mIPS were excellent to demonstrate the extent of peribronchial mediastinal air collections in 3 patients, one with a broncho-esophageal fistula, one with a broncho-pleural fistula, and one with bronchial dehiscences at the anastomoses after lung transplantation (Fig. 4). mIPs did not appear to be useful for imaging of intraluminal bronchial tumors or of wall irregularities caused by infiltrating bronchial tumors or of wall irregularities caused by infiltrating bronchial or esophageal tumors. Limitations of spatial resolution, dependance on projection angle and susceptibility to partial volume effects were to high.

mIPS were able to demonstrate bronchi down to the segmental level. Prerequisite was a narrow VOI (maximum width 2 cm). Cylindrical bronchiectasis appeared as irregularly shaped tubular strcutures on the mIPs that could be followed further into the periphery than the normal bronchi. The spatial resolution of mIPs was poor, and did not add diagnostic information to the axial scans. Placement of the VOI over a particular lung region with local bronchiectasis did not improve diagnostic efficacy of mIPs. Bronchiectasis filled with mucus escaped demonstration on mIPs.

Discussion

Objective of the study was to evaluate the diagnostic efficacy of MIP and mIP for various pulmonary and bronchial lesions. Thick slabs (40 mm) nicely demonstrated distribution and extent of diffuse disease. Slabs 20 mm thick appeared to be adequate for nodule screening and 2.7 to 3.4-mm slabs were suitable for subtle reticular and emphysemateous disease if thin section scans (scan parameters 1 – 2/2/1) were performed. Nodule detection was facilitated in MIPs due to an improved differentiation of nodular disease and tubular vasculature. The presence of subtle reticular, nodular or emphysemateous disease appeared to be accentuated in thin slab MIPs or mIPs, respectively, by "summing up" subtle abnormalities of several slices into one projection. Detail and contour sharpness was lower in MIPs or mIPs as compared to single axial slices. Anteroposterior mIPs improved diagnostic information in the longitudinal axis and facilitate the understanding of the bronchial anatomic situation. However, they did not add diagnostic information with respect to localized intraluminal tumors, wall infiltration or peripheral bronchiectasis. In conclusion we found that MIP images and to a lesser degree mIP images are a valuable additional tool for the evaluation of spiral CT of the chest.

References

Napel S, Rubin GD, Jeffrey RB (1993) STS-MIP A new reconstruction technique for CT of the chest. Journ of Comp Ass Tomogr 17(5): 832 – 838

Polacin A, Kalender WA, Marchal G (1992) Evaluation of section sensitivity profiles and image noise in spiral CT. Radiology 185 : 29 – 35

Prokop M, Schaefer C, Kalender WA, Polacin A (1993) Gefäßdarstellungen mit Spiral CT: Der Weg zur CT-Angiographie. Radiologe 33 : 694 – 704

Spiral Volumetric CT in Patients with Clinical Suspected of Pulmonary Embolism

A.B. VAN ROSSUM, G.J. KIEFT, F.E.E. TREURNIET, S.J. SMITH, R. SCHEPERS-BOK, A.M.C. WITTE

Introduction

The clinical diagnosis of pulmonary embolism (PE) is unreliable, therefore varius diagnostic tests are advocated [1]. Lung scintigraphy is a non-invasive diagnostic method, which however lacks specificity. Pulmonary angiography, which is considered the reference method for the detection of PE, is the usual approach to this patient group. But this is a invasive diagnostic method with a certain morbidity (4%) and mortality (0.2%), and is not routinely used in daily practice [2]. We describe the use of spiral volumetric CT (SVCT) in patients with clinical suspicion of PE. The aim was to evaluate the role of SVCT in the diagnostic workup for PE.

Material and Methods

Eighty-nine patients with clinical suspicion of PE were prospectively evaluated with lung scintigraphy and SVCT. SVCT and lung scintigraphy was performed within 24 h of each other and only in those cases where results of these two were contradictory, pulmonary angiography was performed to estabish the final diagnosis. The lung scan and SVCT scan were interpreted by two separate radiologists, without knowledge of the results of the other imaging studies. Patients with positive results for PE had a control scan 4–6 weeks after the start of anticoagulants.

^{99m}Tc-labeled macroaggregated albumine was used for perfusion lungscanning. Six views were obtained. Equilibrium-ventilation was simultaneously performed with Krypton-81 m. V/Q scans were reported as normal, non-high probability or high probability according to a clinical oriented classification suggested by Hull and associates [3].

CT scans were performed with a Somatom Plus S scanner, using the SVCT technique with intravenous contrast enhancement. If possible scanning was performed during a single breath hold, inability to suspend respiration was not considered a criterion of exclusion. Scanning time was 32 s, with a 5 mm/s table feed, resulting in a scanning volume of 16 cm. Scanning parameters were 210 mA and 120 kV. SVCT was started at the aortic arch, the position of which was obtained from the topoview. Five mm slices were reconstructed with a 4 mm increment. A bolus injection of 100 ml intravenous contrast material (a concentration of 30% iodine) was administered in an anticubital vein. We used a bifasic contrast injection with a flow of 3 ml/s during the first 15 s, the remaining with a flow of 2 ml/s, with a 15-s scanning delay. Direct signs of PE were intraluminal filling defects, partial or complete, wich form the basis of the diagnosis of PE. Indirect signs were such as a wedge-shaped pleural-based parenchymal consolidation. SVCT scan were scored as negative or positive for PE. Other abnormalities, such as emphysema were separately scored.

Pulmonary angiography was performed using the femoral-vien Seldinger technique with a 7-F Grollman catheter (Cordis, Roden, the Netherlands). Pulmonary arterial pressure >50 mm Hg served as a contraindication for further angiographic evaluation. Multiple projections were obtained of the lung with the greatest V/Q scan abnormalities.

Results

Eighty-nine patients, 26 men and 63 women, ranging in age from 19 to 90 (average 60) years, were evaluated. Of these 89 patients, 41 patients (46%) were classified as having a normal V/Q scan, 24 patients (27%) a high probability and 24 (27%) a non-high probability V/Q scan (Table 1). All SVCT scans were made within 24 h of the V/Q scan. With our scanning protocol, pulmonary arteries had a good enhance-

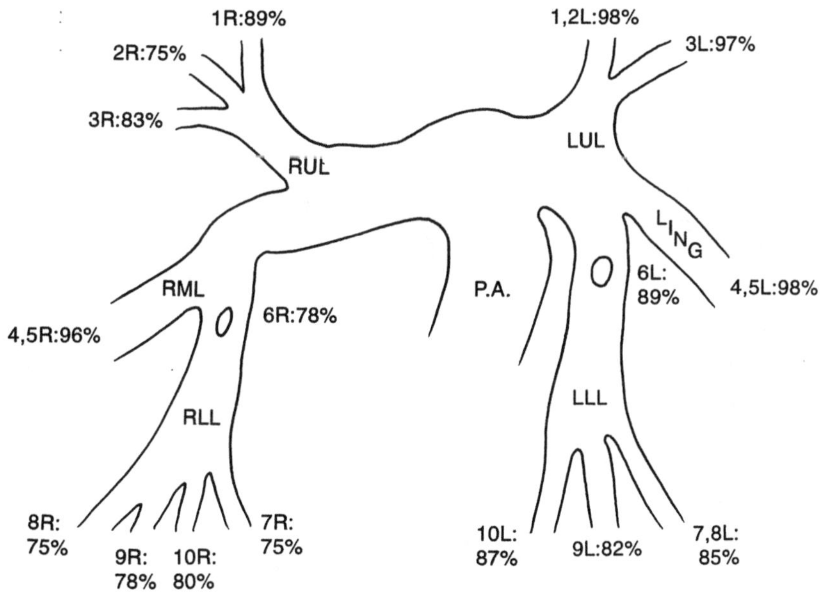

Fig. 1. Visualisation of pulmonary arteries in 61 patients without pulmonary embolism. Abbrevations: *P.A.*, main pulmonary artrey; *RUL*, right upper lobe with 1R apical, 2R posterior and 3R anterior segmental arteries; *RML*, right middle lobe with 4R lateral and 5R medial segmental arteries; *RLL*, right lower lobe with 6R superior, 7R mediobasal, 8R anterobasal, 9R laterobasal and 10R posterobasal segmental arteries; *LUL* and *LING*, left upper lobe and lingula with 1, 2L apicoposterior, 3L anterior, 4L superior and 5L inferior segmental arteries; *LLL*, left lower lobe with 6L superior, 7L mediobasal, 8L anterobasal, 9L laterobasal and 10L posterobasal segmental arteries

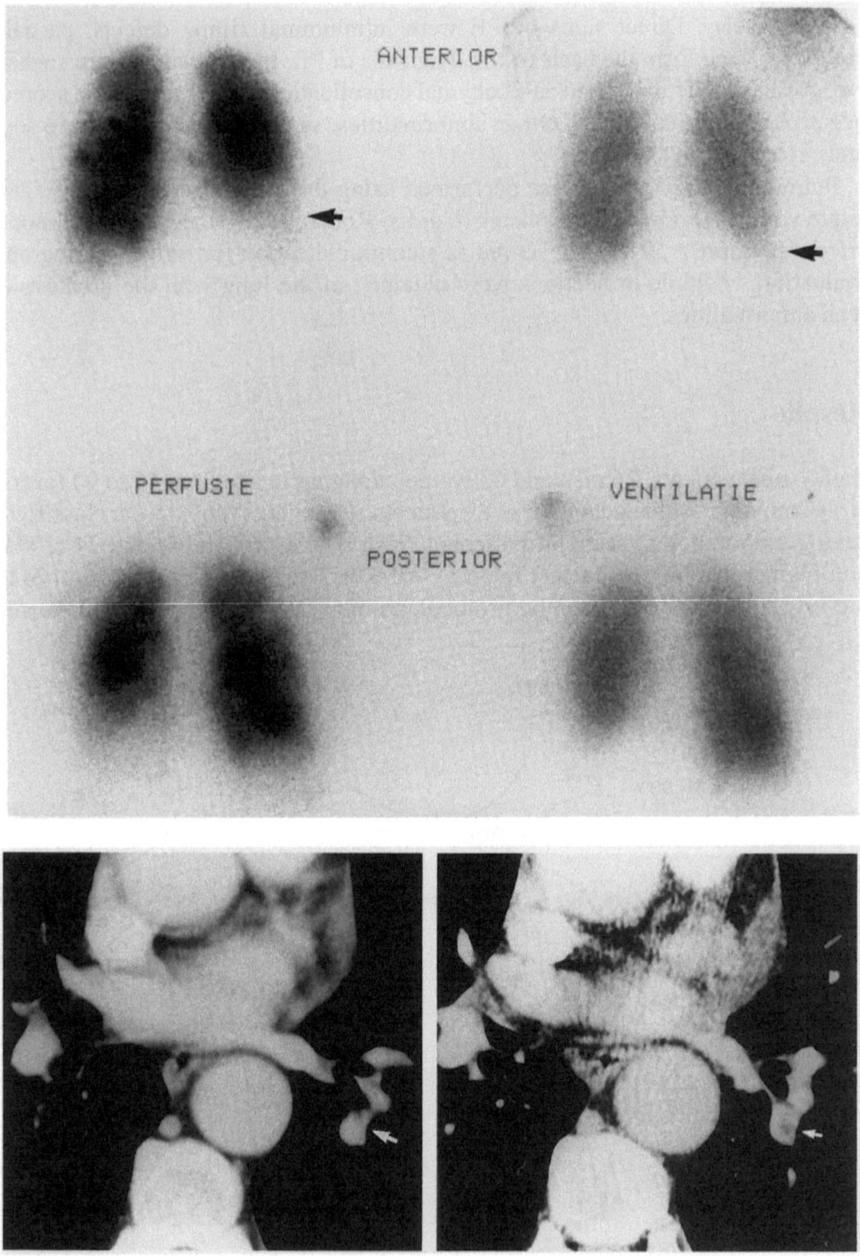

a

b c

Fig. 2a–d. A 72-year-old male with chest pain located at the left side. **a** Two projections of V/Q scintigraphy showed an area of decreased perfusion and normal ventilation in the left lingula area (*arrows*), the scintigram was interpreted as high-probability. **b** A 5-mm spiral volumetric computed tomography (SVCT) scan at the level just below the trifurcation of the left lower lobe artery, possible filling defects in the posterobasal segmental artery (*arrow*). **c** A 2-mm target SVCT scan at the same level showed clear intraluminal filling defect (*arrow*). **d** Pulmonary angiography confirmed the thrombus in the posterobasal segmental artery (*black arrows*), but another thrombus in the lingula artery was found (*white arrows*). This thrombus could not be seen at SVCT

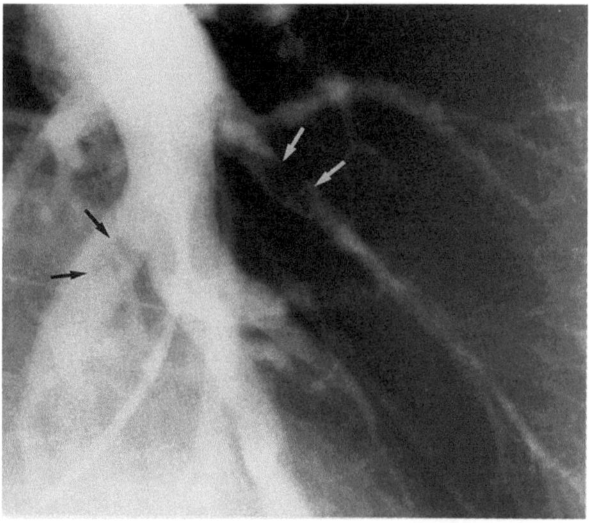

Fig. 2d

Table 1. Spiral volumetric computed tomographic (SVCT) findings versus V/Q scan findings ($n = 89$)

	SVCT		
V/Q scan	Negative	Positive	Total
Negative	41	0	41
Non-high	20	4	24
High prob	0	24	24
total	61	28	89

ment with an average number of 200 HU in the main pulmonary artery. Image quality reduced in obese patients and patients who were unable to hold their breath.

In 61 patients without PE, origin and enhancement of separate segmental arteries of upper and lower lobes could be evaluated in 75–98% of patients (Fig. 1). Right middle lobe and lingular segmental arteries were seldom seen as separate enhancing structures. The origin and enhancement of the right middle lobe artery and the lingular artery were analysable in 59 patients and 60 patients (96% and 98%).

Forty-one patients had a normal V/Q scan, none of these showed signs of PE on the SVCT.

The non-high probability group consisted of twenty-four patients. From these, 18 showed no signs of thromboembolism on SVCT, but they showed a variaty of different abnormalities, at the same location as where the V/Q scan showed defects, so they could serve as an explaination for the V/Q scan defects. The differential diagnosis ranged from consolidation (8), emphysema (2), pleural effusion (4), tumor (2), lymphadenopathy (1), to lung fibrosis (1). These patients were believed to have no PE and no pulmonary angiography was performed. In two patients SVCT showed no signs of PE, but there were also no other abnormalities which could explain the

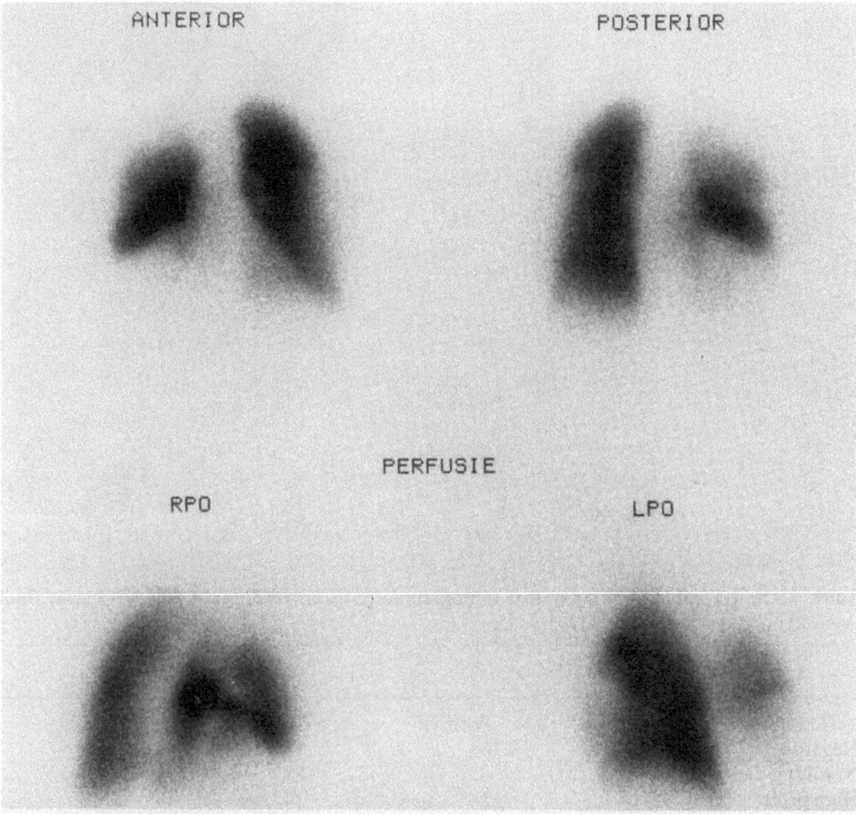

a

Fig. 3a–d. A 73-year-old male with sudden onset of pleuretic chest pain and fever, who recently underwent prostatectomy. **a** Four projections of perfusion lung scan showed multiple perfusion defects in the right lung, ventilation was normal. There was normal perfusion of the left lower lobe. **b–d** Consecutive spiral volumetric computed tomographic scans with 4-mm increment at the level of the right and left lower lobe segmental arteries show multiple emboli in the right lower lobe arteries (*curved arrow*). And a nonobstructing thrombus in the left lower lobe arteries (*straight arrows*) with normal enhancing arteries at the lowest level

V/Q scan matching defects, which were seen on their lung scans. Pulmonary angiography was warrented and no emboli were found. Four, of the 24 patients with non-high probability lung scans, showed signs of PE on SVCT. In three cases PE was confirmed with pulmonary angiography, the remaining one refused angiography, but a control scan 4 weeks after anticoagulantic therapy showed complete lysis of the thrombi. In all 24 patients with a high-probability lung scan, SVCT also showed thromboemblism. In two patients pulmonary angiography was nevertheless performed. In the first patient there was some doubt about the interpretation of the SVCT, and the angiogram confirmed the thrombus in the posterobasal artery. But a thrombus in the lingular artery could not, even in retrospect, be seen on SVCT (Fig. 2). In the second patient SVCT showed much more arterial filling defects then expected on the basis of the V/Q scan. The pulmonary angiogram showed multiple

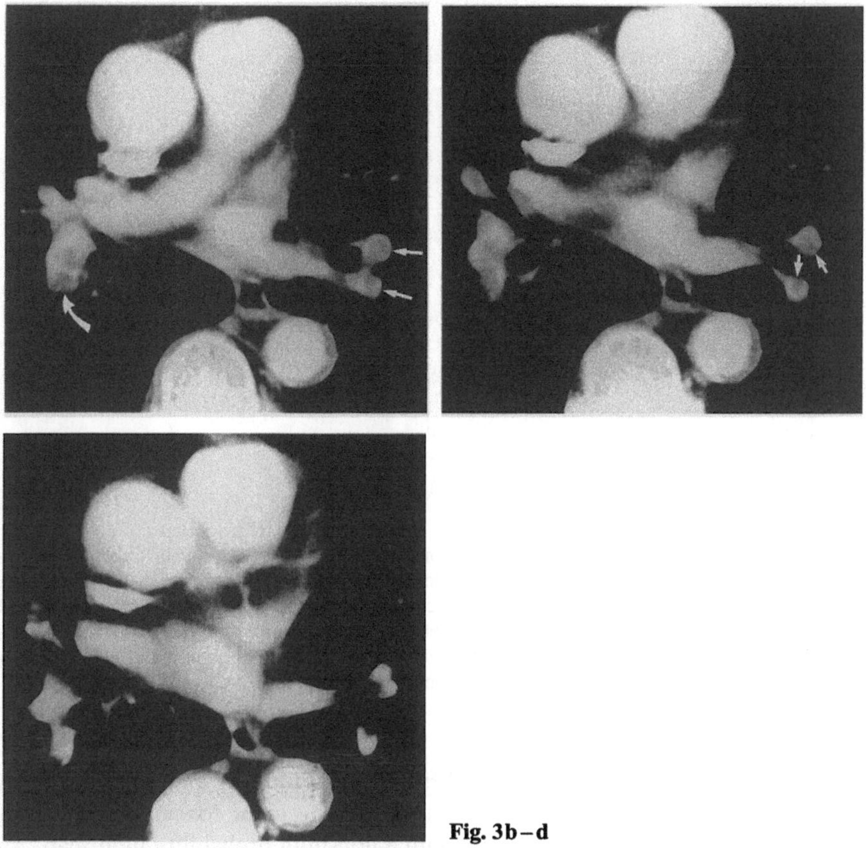

b c d Fig. 3b–d

partially occluding emboli, so perfusion was decreased but not totally blocked (Fig. 3).

The 28 patients with PE had a varying number of emboli ranging from one to fourteen, with an average of seven embolized vessels. Indirect signs of PE, such as pleural-based wedge-shaped infiltrates were seen in 12 patients (43 %).

After 4–6 weeks all patients with PE [28] were asked for a control SVCT, to monitor response to therapy. Five patients refused and one died, in the remaining patients all emboli were dissolved in 17 and five showed definite improvement but some residual thrombi were still found (Fig. 4).

Discussion

Clinical suspicion of PE is a frequent event. However, of these patients only one of the three actually have PE [2]. Our study confirms this finding, 31 % had PE. It is well established that a normal perfusion scan virtually excludes the presence of clinical important PE [3–5]. A high-probaility lung scan result indicates an ap-

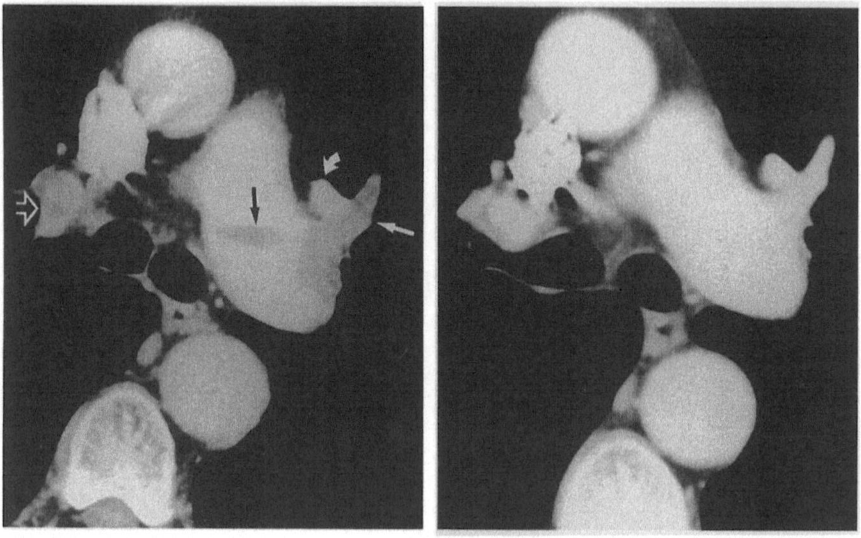

a b

Fig. 4a, b. Spiral volumetric computed tomographic scan of a 66-year-old male shows good vascular opacification. **a** A central filling defect in the main left pulmonary artery (*black arrow*) and complete filling defect in the anterior segment of the left upper lobe (*white arrow*) and at the bifurcation of the apical and posterior segments of the right upper lobe (*open arrow*). Note normal enhancing left superior pulmonary vien (*curved arrow*). **b** Scan obtained after 4 weeks of anticoagulant therapy shows complete resolution of the thrombi

proximal 86–92% probability of PE and institution of anticoagulant therapy is acceptable [2, 3, 6, 8]. However, there is still no clear consensus concerning the appropiate managment of a patient with a non-high probability lund scan. And the majority of patients with a clinical suspicion for PE (40–60%) belongs to this catogery, the frequency of PE in these patients varying from 10% to 40% [2, 3, 6]. The usual approach to these group should consist of performing an angiogram, but nevertheless many clinicians rely on their clinical suspicion of PE and start anticoagulants or withheld them, based on clinical judgement. To date there have been some promising studies concerning the detection of PE by fast scanning technique [8, 9]. Remy-Jardin and Teigen used SVCT and electron beam CT respectively to get good visualisation of the pulmonary vasculature, but they found fewer vessels depicted at CT than at pulmonary angiography [8, 9]. In our study it was also not always possible to view all the vessels, with a visibility of segmental arterial anatomy varying from 75% to 98% there is no doubt that some PE will be missed by SVCT. But usually multiple emboli are present, in our study an average of seven vessels were embolized, and diagnosis of PE requires that only one embolus be detected with confidence [10, 11].

In this study 41 patients had a normal V/Q scan and no PE were found on the SVCT images, hence the outcome of these two tests was the same. There was also no discrepancy between the high-probability lung scans and the SVCT. In the group of patients with a non-high probability lung scan, we found PE with SVCT in 17%, compared to 10–40% found in the literature. In all the other cases we didn't see any signs of PE, but instead fund other abnormalities which could serve as an explaination for the perfusion defects. In this way SVCT aids in the differential diagnosis of PE. In the seven patients with no consensus between the V/Q scan and the SVCT, pulmonary angiography confirmed the SVCT findings.

The control scans, showed resolution of the PE in most patients or definite improvement. SVCT may be used to monitor patients with PE, expecially patients with large central emboli in the first days of therapy.

In summary, our preliminary results show that SVCT represent a fast, non invasive and probably accurate technique to detect acute thromboembolism. Especially for the non-high probability group, if pulmonary angiography is used in all these patients, it would have to be performed in the majority of patients with clinically suspected PE and abnormal perfusion scans; a formidable task in most hospitals and an impractical one in many. Perfusion scintigraphy alone in combination with SVCT may replace V/Q scanning in the diagnostic procedure for PE, pulmonary angiography will only be neccassary in limited cases.

References

1. Hoellerich VL, Wigton RS (1986) Diagnosing pulmonary embolism. Using clinical findings. Arch Int Med 146 : 1699 – 1704
2. PIOPED investigators. Value of the ventilation/perfusion scan in acute pulmonary embolism: results of the prospective investigation of pulmonary embolism diagnosis. JAMA 1990; 263 : 2753 – 2759
3. Hull RD, Hirsh J, Carter CJ et al. (1985) Diagnostic value of ventilation-perfusion scanning in patients with suspected pulmonary embolism. Chest 6 : 819 – 828
4. Hull RD, Raskob G, Hirsh J (1990) Clinical validity of a normal perfusion lung scan in patients with suspected pulmonary embolism. Chest 97(1): 23 – 26
5. Kipper MS, Moser KM, Kortman KE et al. (1982) Long term follow-up of patients with suspected pulmonary embolism and a normal lung scan. Chest 82(4) : 411 – 415
6. Biello DR, Mattar A, Mc Knight RC et al. (1979) Ventilation-perfusion studies in suspected pulmonary embolism. AJR 133 : 1033 – 1037
7. Hull RD, Raskob GE, Carter et al. (1988) Pulmonary embolism in out patients with pleuritic chest pain. Arch Int Med 148 : 838 – 844
8. Remy-Jardin M, Remy J, Wattine L et al. (1993) Central pulmonary thromboembolism diagnosis with spiral volumetric CT with the single hold breath hold technique: comparison with pulmonary angiography. Radiology 188 : 618 – 619
9. Teigen CL, Maus TP, Sheedy PF et al. (1993) Pulmonary embolism: diagnosis with electron beam CT. Radiology 188 : 893 – 945
10. Gurney JW (1993) No fooling around: direct visualisation of pulmonary embolism. Radiology 188 : 618 – 619
11. UPET. Urokinase pulmonary embolism trial: phase 1 results – a coperative study. JAMA 1970; 214 : 2163 – 2172

Evaluation of Pulmonary Fissures by Spiral CT

M.L. Storto, C. Ciccotosto, A. Guidotti, R.L. Patea, L. Bonomo

Introduction

Pleural fissures are important landmarks within the pulmonary parenchyma allowing for accurate localization and distribution of pulmonary disease. Moreover, the assessment of transfissural extension may modify the surgical treatment of patients with lung cancer near a fissure, and require performance of a peumonectomy or bilobectomy rather than a lobectomy [2, 6, 7].

Standard computed tomography (CT), with 8- to 10-mm-thick sections is often sufficient for identifying pulmonary lobes and locating a lesion, but shows low sensitivity (50%) in the evaluation of transfissural tumor spread [6].

High-resolution CT, with thin section scans (1- or 2-mm collimation) provides better delineation of pulmonary fissures thus improving the accuracy of CT in assessing the neoplastic involvement of the major fissure [2, 6, 7].

Because of continuous scanning of anatomic volumes during a single acquisition, spiral CT enables superbe multiplanar reconstructions [3, 8] so that pulmonary fissures can be evaluated in different anatomic planes.

The purpose of this prospective study was to assess whether spiral CT and multiplanar reconstructions can help in the diagnosis of neoplastic involvement of pulmonary fissures.

Material and Methods

Patients with lung cancer near a fissure requiring CT examination of the chest for staging, were considered for inclusion in this study.

After a preliminary standard CT examination of the chest, all patients underwent spiral and high-resolution CT scans through the area of contact between the tumor ad the fissure. CT examinations were acquired on a Siemens Somatom Plus scanner.

High-resolution CT scans were performed with 1-mm slice thickness and 5-mm interscan spacing, 1-s scanning time at 137 kVp and 255 mA, and a high-spatial-frequency ("ultra high") reconstruction algorithm were used.

Spiral CT was performed with 2-mm slice thickness and 2- or 3-mm/s table feed, depending on tumor size, 24-s scanning time at 120 kVp and 165 mA. A standard algorithm was used to reconstruct the axial images at 1-mm intervals. Multiplanar reconstructions in coronal, sagittal and oblique planes were also obtained.

Both high-resolution and spiral CT scans were performed at full inspiration and were viewed at parenchymal window setting (width: 1600 HU; level: −600 HU).

On each CT examination, the presence of motion artifacts and the detection of pleural fissure were evaluated.

In assessing the relationship of lung cancer to a fissure, the following parameters were considered:

- Presence of a solid mass crossing the fissure or neoplastic lobulations extending through the fissure, indicating transfissural spread.
- Presence of dense stripes between the tumor and the fissure.
- Aspect of the fissure that can be normal, thickened, irregular and/or displaced.

The results of both high-resolution and spiral CT were compared with surgical findings.

Results

Twenty-five patients (22 males, three females), mean age 66 years (range 45–80 years) were included in the study; nine of them were secondarily excluded because of general or staging contraindication to surgery. The remaining 16 patients underwent a surgical treatment pneumonectomy ($n=5$), bilobectomy ($n=2$), lobectomy with additional segmentectomy ($n=1$), lobectomy ($n=8$). The tumor was near the major fissure in eight patients and near the minor fissure in seven patients, while in one patient it showed relationship with both fissures. All but one patient were able to hold their breath during the 24-s volumetric acquisition; however, motion artifacts in this patient were minimal and didn't affect image evaluation.

High-resolution CT scans showed transfissural spread of lung cancer near the major fissure in two patients and displacement of the fissure toward the tumor in another patient. The major fissure was normal (Fig. 1) or slightly thickened in the remaining six patients (Table 1). The relationship between the tumor and the minor fissure was not valuable on high-resolution CT scans which never showed clear findings of neoplastic involvement of the minor fissure (Table 2).

Spiral CT and multiplanar reconstructions showed tumor extension across the major fissure in three patients; the fissure appeared displaced in one patient and normal or thick in five patients (Table 1). In four patients with lung cancer near the minor fissure, the spiral CT technique demostrated a mass crossing the fissure (Fig. 2) which was slightly thickened, while in the remaining four patients the minor fissure was normal (Tables 1, 2).

At surgery, the major was involved in four patients and normal in five, while the minor fissure was involved in four patients and normal in four.

Discussion

Assessment of neoplastic involvement of pulmonary fissures is important in the preoperative evaluation of lung cancer, especially in those patients who cannot bear extensive surgical treatments because of impaired pulmonary functions [2, 6, 7].

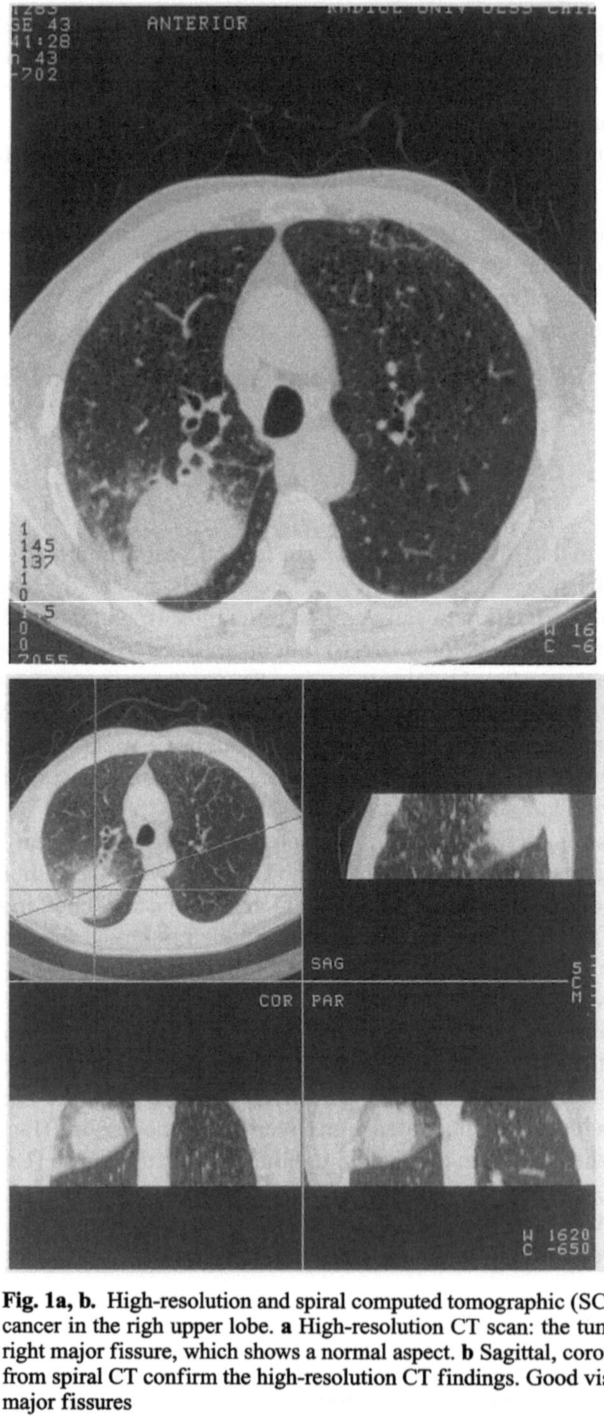

Fig. 1a, b. High-resolution and spiral computed tomographic (SCT) studies in a patient with lung cancer in the righ upper lobe. **a** High-resolution CT scan: the tumor abuts but does not cross the right major fissure, which shows a normal aspect. **b** Sagittal, coronal and paraxial reconstructions from spiral CT confirm the high-resolution CT findings. Good visualization of both right and left major fissures

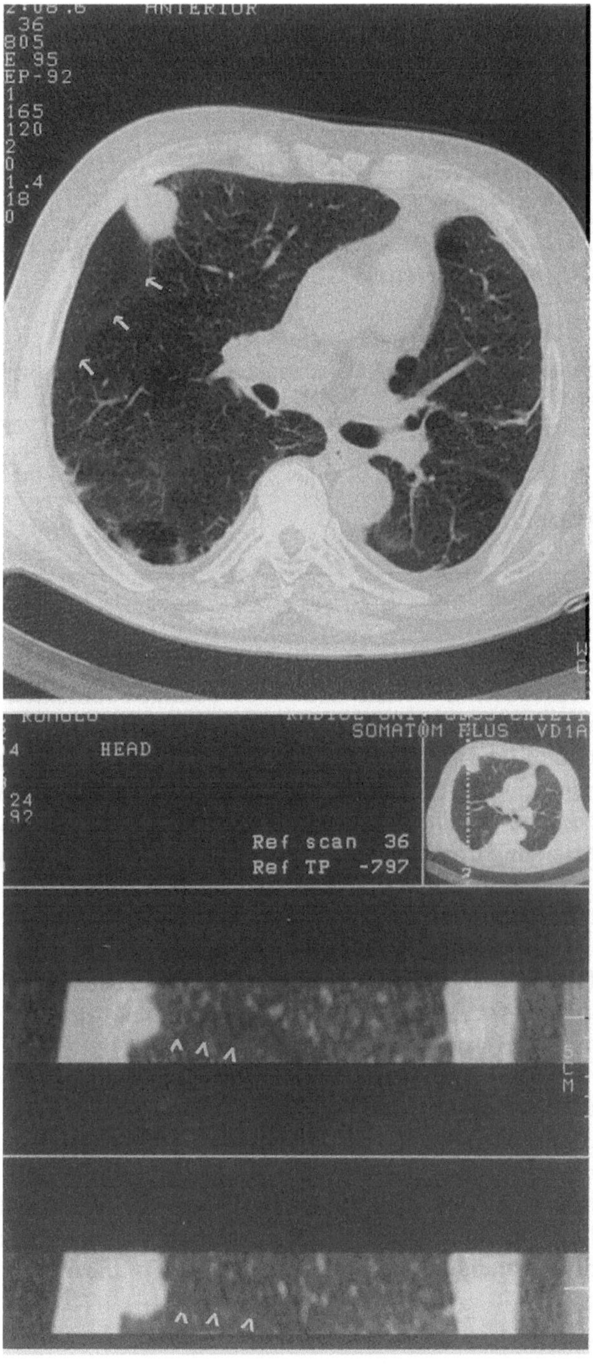

a

b

Fig. 2a, b. High-resolution and spiral computed tomographic (SCT) studies in a patient with a tumor near the minor fissure. **a** High-resolution scan shows the minor fissure as a thin line (*arrows*) but its relationship to the tumor is not clear. **b** Sagittal reconstructions from spiral CT easily demonstrate the extension of the tumor across the minor fissure (*arrow-heads*)

Table 1. High-resolution and spiral CT findings in patients with lung cancer near the major fissure

	High-resolution CT (*n*)	Spiral CT (*n*)
Transfissural spread	2	3
Displacement	1	1
Thickening	2	1
Normal aspect	4	4

CT, computed tomography

Table 2. Correlation of CT and surgical findings in patients with neoplastic involvement of a fissure

	High-resolution CT (*n*)	Spiral CT (*n*)	Surgery (*n*)
Major fissure	3	4	4
Minor fissure	–	4	4

CT, computed tomography

Standard CT scans with 8- to 10-mm collimation may not provide sufficient information about the relationship of a lesion to the fissure, because the visualization of the fissure is often hampered by partial volume averaging of adjacent lung parenchyma [1, 7]. In fact the major fissure is frequently seen as an hypoattenuating band on standard CT scans, while the minor fissure appears as an avascular area extending from the major fissure to the anterior chest wall [4, 5].

On thin-section CT scans (1- to 2-mm collimation) there is less partial volume averaging and the fissures are more frequently visualized as thin lines [1, 2, 7]. As a result high-resolution CT is more accurate then standard CT in assessing transfissural extension of lung cancer. However, because of the horizontal orientation of the minor fissure, the relationship of a tumor near the minor fissure is difficult to assess, even on thin-section CT scans [9].

Spiral CT, allowing multiplanar reconstructions of good quality, can be useful in the diagnosis of neoplastic involvement of pulmonary fissures. Our preliminary results concerning a small number of patients show that spiral CT and multiplanar reconstructions enable visualization of pulmonary fissures and evaluation of lesions near them. Although we didn't observe significant differences between high-resolution and spiral CT in the assessment of the major fissure, spiral CT allowed clear demonstration of neoplastic involvement of the minor fissure.

References

1. Berkmen YM, Auh YH, Davis SD, Kazam E (1989) Anatomy of the minor fissure: evaluation with thin-section CT. Radiology 170 : 647–651
2. Glazer HS, Anderson DJ, DiCroce JJ, Solomon SL, Wilson BS, Molina PL, Sagel SS (1991) Anatomy of the major fissure: evaluation with standart and thin-section CT. Radiology 180 : 839–844
3. Kalender WA, Seissler W, Klotz E, Vock P (1990) Spiral volumetric CT with single-breath-hold technique, continuous transport and continuous scanner rotation. Radiology 176 : 181–183
4. Marks BW, Kuhns LR (1982) Identification of the pleural fissures with computed tomography. Radiology 143 : 139–141
5. Proto AV, Ball JB (1983) Computed tomography of the major and minor fissures. AJR 140 : 439–448
6. Quint LE, Glazer GM, Oringer MB (1987) Central lung masses: prediction with CT of need for pneumonectomy versus lobectomy. Radiology 165 : 735–738
7. Sakai O, Takahashi K, Nakashima N, Furuse M, Takata Y, Ogawa C, Yokoyama H, Ohsawa T (1993) CT visualization of the major pulmonary fissures: value of 25° cranially tilted axial scans. AJR 161 : 523–526
8. Soucek M, Vock P, Daepp M, Kalender WA (1990) Spiral CT: Eine neue Technik für Volumenaufnahmen. II Klinische Anwendungsmöglichkeiten. Röntgenpraxis 43 : 365–375
9. Storto ML, Ciccotosto C, Mucilli F, Sacco R, Bonoma L (1992) Atteinte néoplasique des scissures pulmonaires. Possibilité diagnostique de la tomodensitométrie en haute résolution. J Radiol 12 : 663–668

Reference Values for Lung Density and Structure Measured by Quantitative CT

W. A. Kalender, H. Fichte, W. Bautz, A. Zwick, R. Rienmüller, J. Behr, J. v. Engelshoven, R. Lamers, P. Vock

Introduction

Noninvasive in vivo assessment of lung density and structure by quantitative computed tomography (QCT) has a long tradition in the scientific literature. Early efforts were limited, however, as reproducibility was insufficient due to a lack of respiratory control during scanning and appropriate evaluation software was missing (e.g. Goddard et al. 1982; Gilman et al. 1983; Van Dyk and Hill 1983; Mueller et al. 1988; Rienmüller et al. 1988). We have worked on the respective methodology to improve both accuracy and precision and to provide specific evaluation capabilities. Decisive steps were the design of spirometric control and gating for the CT scan process (Kalender et al. 1990a, b; Rienmüller et al, 1990), dedicated evaluation algorithms (Kalender et al. 1991; Rienmüller et al. 1991) and quality control measures as described below. All these steps were incorporated into the PULMO CT option on the SOMATOM PLUS which meanwhile is in broad clinical use. Reference data on lung density and histograms in a healthy population for comparison purposes are still missing, however. It is the purpose of this paper to present first results of a multicenter study established to gather such data. These results still have to be considered preliminary. An extended publication is intended when all participating centers will have acquired the planned numbers of examinations.

Materials and Methods

All examinations were obtained under spirometric control scanning three representative sections using the SOMATOM PLUS PULMO CT option. The examination parameters are summarized in Table 1. All institutions involved in this study obtained approval from their respective ethic committees. Dose estimates which had to be provided for this purpose were the following: mean organ dose value (lung, breast) are below 1 mSv; effective dose (whole body equivalent) is below 0.1 mSv (Kalender 1993). To put these values into proper perspective, they can be compared to the natural background radiation of 2.4 mSv per year (official value for the Federal Republic of Germany). Before or after each individual study, scans of the anthropomorphic lung phantom which is part of the PULMO CT option were taken and documented for quality control.

Evaluation of all cases was performed centrally in Erlangen, Germany. We used the PULMO CT evaluation package providing automated segmentation of the left

Table 1. Standard examination protocol using the SOMATOM PLUS PULMO CT option

Three representative slices, 5 scans:	
Carina level	50% VC
5 cm cranial	50% VC
5 cm caudal	20/50/80% VC[a]
scan time	1 s
voltage	137 kV
tube current	180 mA
slice thickness	1 mm

[a] Examinations at 20% and 80% vital capacity (VC) were optional

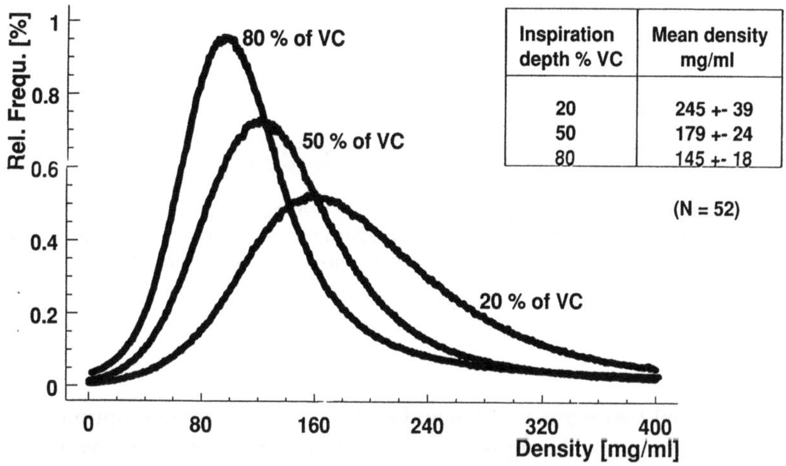

Fig. 1. Lung density as a function of inspiration. Mean lung density decreases and the histogram is flatter and shifted towards lower computed tomography values as inspiration depth increases. *VC*, vital capacity

and the right lung, determination of mean lung density and an extensive histogram analysis. Histogram analysis is here intended as a crude estimate for lung structure. We presently focus on the evaluation of arbitrary histogram percentiles; the useage of further histogram parameters and arbitrary segmental analysis is planned for but not yet implemented.

The selection of a "normal" reference population is not an easy task at all as both the definition of normal is not trivial and recruiting respective individuals is difficult. We have established a questionnaire, defining both inclusion and exclusion criteria to define and select "lung-healthy" individuals. For example, in order to be included individuals had to reach lung function test results with vital capacity >80% of age-matched normals and an FEV^1/VC ratio 0.7. Exclusion criteria were diseases of the lung, pleura and upper airways, severe trauma or surgery in the thoracic region and occupational exposure to dust. It was required for each center to scan the three representative sections (Table 1) at 50% of vital capacity (VC); the

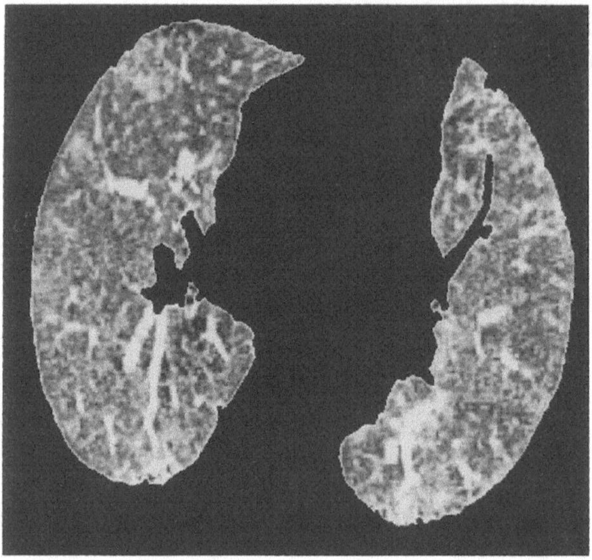
a

Fig. 2a–c. Clinical example: PULMO CT examination of a patient with lung fibrosis. **a** CT image, triggered at 50% vital capacity. **b, c** Mean density (**b**) is increased by 5.0 SD; the histogram (**c**) is flatter and shifted to the right. Density alone allows for correct classification.

additional two scans at 20% and 80% VC were declared optional as there was no consensus yet on the significance of measurements at varied inspirational levels. Up to now, 153 individuals have been included in the study (Klinikum r. d. Isar, Munich, Germany: 100; Klinikum Großhadern, Munich, Germany: 25; Academic Hospital, Maastricht, The Netherlands: 23; Inselspital Bern, Switzerland: 5), 52 of them were measured at different inspirational depths.

Results

Mean Lung Density

Lung density depends heavily on the degree of inspiration. This general assumption is confirmed and quantified by the measurements obtained from 52 individuals at 20%, 50% and 80% VC (Fig. 1). Lung density changes by more than a factor of two when going through a full breathing cycle from 0 to 100% VC. While no significant dependence on sex was observed in our population, there is an age-dependence in mean lung density which depends on inspirational depth. At 20% VC (expiration) we observed a loss of about 1 mg/ml per year. At 80% VC (deep inspiration), mean lung density remained nearly constant with age. At 50% VC, we observed a decrease in lung density with age of about 0.7 mg/ml per year (Fig. 4a).

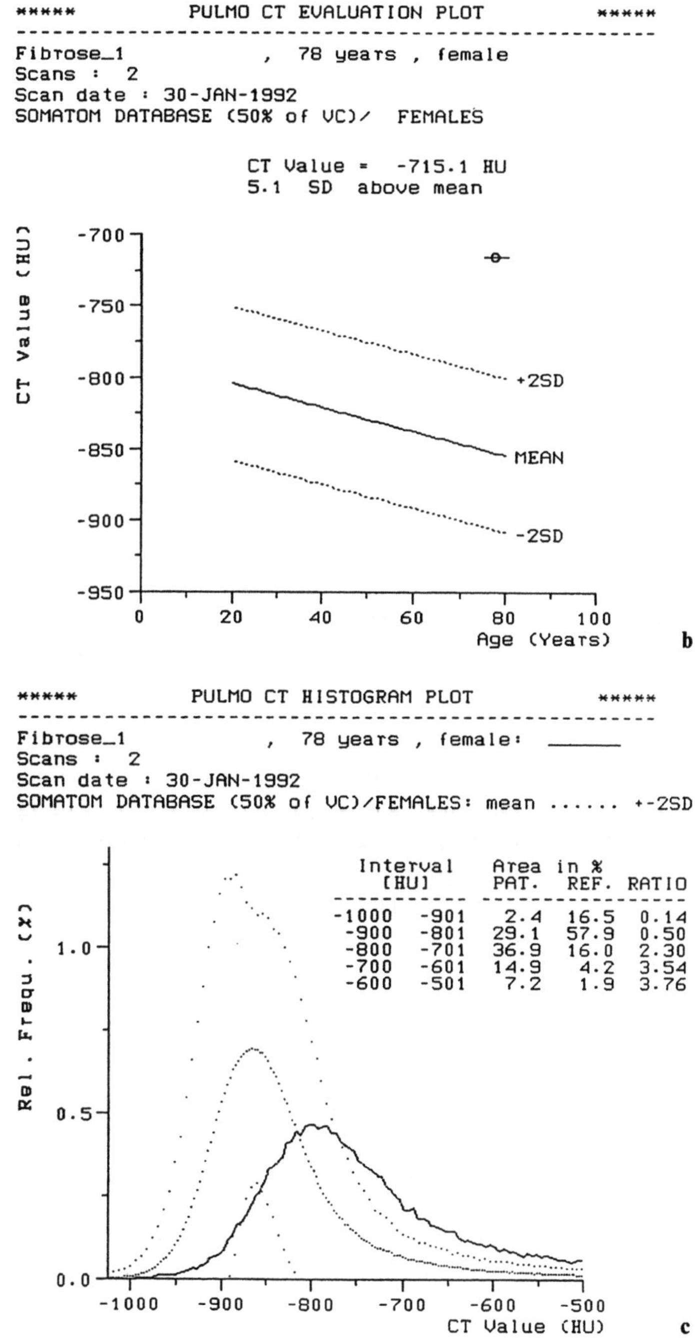
***** PULMO CT EVALUATION PLOT *****
Fibrose_1 , 78 years , female
Scans : 2
Scan date : 30-JAN-1992
SOMATOM DATABASE (50% of VC)/ FEMALES
CT Value = -715.1 HU
5.1 SD above mean
CT Value (HU)
-700
-750
-800
-850
-900
-950
+2SD
MEAN
-2SD
0
20
40
60
80
100
Age (Years)
b
***** PULMO CT HISTOGRAM PLOT *****
Fibrose_1 , 78 years , female:
Scans : 2
Scan date : 30-JAN-1992
SOMATOM DATABASE (50% of VC)/FEMALES: mean ...... +-2SD
Interval [HU]
Area in %
PAT. REF. RATIO
-1000 -901 2.4 16.5 0.14
-900 -801 29.1 57.9 0.50
-800 -701 36.9 16.0 2.30
-700 -601 14.9 4.2 3.54
-600 -501 7.2 1.9 3.76
Rel. Frequ. (%)
1.0
0.5
0.0
-1000
-900
-800
-700
-600
-500
CT Value (HU)
c

Fig. 2b, c

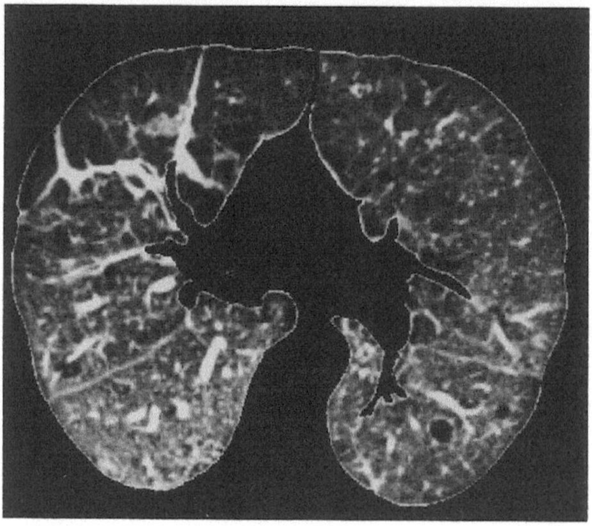

a

Fig. 3a–c. Clinical example: PULMO CT examination of a patient with lung emphysema. **a** Computed tomography image, triggered at 50% vital capacity (*VC*). **b, c** Mean density (**b**) is decreased by only 1.3 SD; the histogram (**c**) is shifted to the left. Most significant, however, the histogram interval from –1000 HU to –950 HU is overrepresented in the case of emphysema

Lung Density Histograms

Similar to the results on mean lung density, we did not find a dependence of histogram shape on sex and only insignificant dependence on age. Therefore, only one "reference histogram" is provided (Fig. 4b) which is considered representative for all sex and age categories. This decision will have to be reviewed when larger case numbers are available. The histogram is stored in digital form so that for arbitrary percentile analysis a comparison between clinical cases and the reference population can be given.

Clinical Examples

Only two examples are presented here for illustration purposes; extended clinical studies which will be using reference data are in preparation. In Fig. 2, the case of a patient with fibrotic lung disease is shown. Mean lung density is increased by more five standard deviations (SD) as compared to the reference population. In Fig. 3, a case of manifest emphysema is shown. While mean lung density is reduced only by 1.3 SD, histogram percentile analysis yielded a striking difference in the relative representation of the HU interval from –1000 to –950.

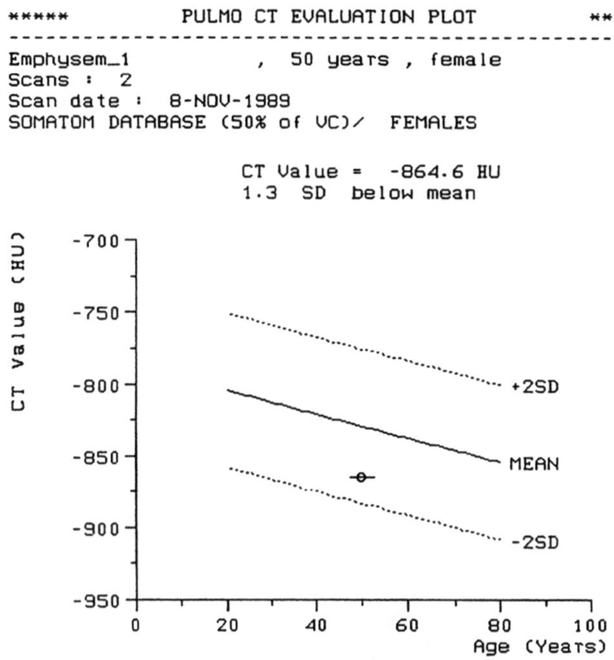
***** PULMO CT EVALUATION PLOT *****
Emphysem_1 , 50 years , female
Scans : 2
Scan date : 8-NOV-1989
SOMATOM DATABASE (50% of VC)/ FEMALES
CT Value = -864.6 HU
1.3 SD below mean
CT Value (HU)
-700
-750
-800
-850
-900
-950
+2SD
MEAN
-2SD
0
20
40
60
80
100
Age (Years)

b

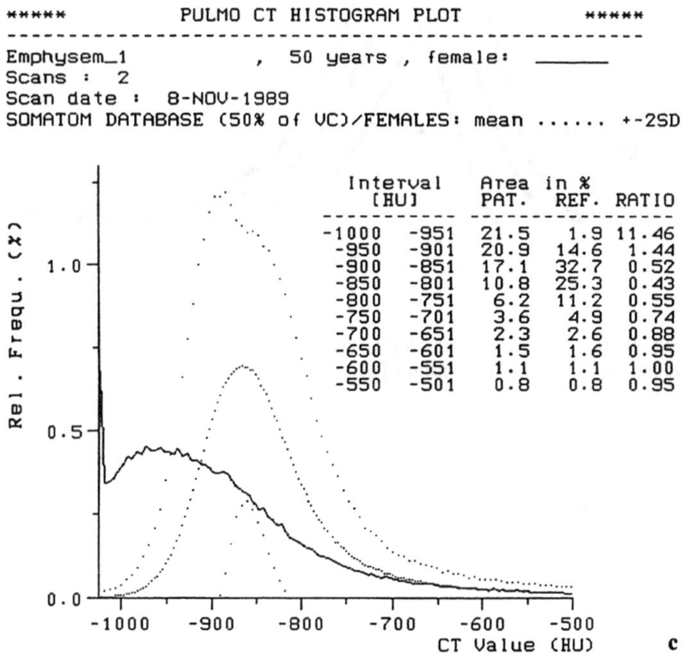
***** PULMO CT HISTOGRAM PLOT *****
Emphysem_1 , 50 years , female:
Scans : 2
Scan date : 8-NOV-1989
SOMATOM DATABASE (50% of VC)/FEMALES: mean ...... +-2SD
Interval [HU] | Area in % PAT. | REF. | RATIO
-1000 -951 | 21.5 | 1.9 | 11.46
-950 -901 | 20.9 | 14.6 | 1.44
-900 -851 | 17.1 | 32.7 | 0.52
-850 -801 | 10.8 | 25.3 | 0.43
-800 -751 | 6.2 | 11.2 | 0.55
-750 -701 | 3.6 | 4.9 | 0.74
-700 -651 | 2.3 | 2.6 | 0.88
-650 -601 | 1.5 | 1.6 | 0.95
-600 -551 | 1.1 | 1.1 | 1.00
-550 -501 | 0.8 | 0.8 | 0.95
Rel. Frequ. (%)
1.0
0.5
0.0
-1000
-900
-800
-700
-600
-500
CT Value (HU)

c

Fig. 3b, c

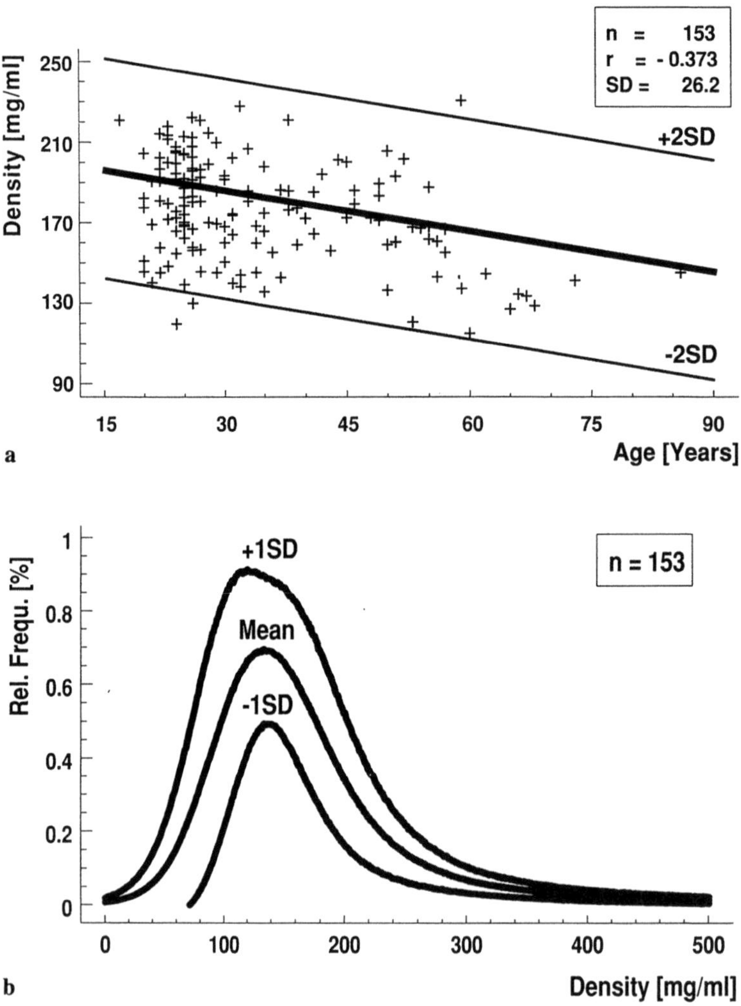

a

b

Fig. 4a, b. Reference values for mean lung density and histograms at 50 % vital capacity. **a** Lung density decreases as a function of age at a rate of about 0.7 mg/ml per year. **b** Reference histogram, averaged over all age groups

Discussion

Noninvasive in vivo measurements of lung density by quantitative CT have a high potential for clinical diagnosis and follow-up of therapy since lung function tests are often inconclusive. We have now reached a stage where such measurements are adequately supported on CT equipment to allow for reproducible and accurate measurements and for comfortable and dedicated evaluation (Kalender et al. 1990a, b). Reference values of mean lung density and reference histograms will further enhance these capabilities. It is our intention to provide a European data base. At present, the data collection is still in progress; so far, only one center has finished their self-assigned task.

The data on mean lung density as a function of inspirational depth clearly indicate that spirometric control is absolutely necessary for reproducible measurements and for a meaningful comparison of patients to a reference population (Fig. 1). Even in cooperative patients it is very hard to establish and control inspiration levels (Kalender et al 1990). Even if they might reproduce their inspiration sufficiently well, there is no objective basis for comparison to other patients or normal controls. For patients who cannot cooperate reasonably well, the need for spirometric control is even more obvious.

The distribution of density values carries more information than mean density alone. This trivial fact can be of valuable help in the diagnosis of diseases, and percentile analysis has accordingly been advocated in the literature (Rienmüller et al. 1991, 1992; Gevenois et al. 1992). It has been part of the PULMO CT evaluation software from the very start (Kalender et al. 1991).

Our preliminary results seem to confirm the predictive power of histogram parameters. In pneumoconiosis, fibrosis and other diseases of the lung which tend to increase mean lung density, a clear separation of healthy and diseased may be possible based on lung density alone. The role of histogram analysis still has to be established here. In emphysematic disease, in particular in its early stage, a selective determination of the percentage of area which lies below a certain threshold, e.g. −950 HU, appears to be a very promising approach (Gevenois et al. 1992; Goddard et al. 1982; Mueller et al. 1988).

References

Gevenois PA, De Vuyst P, Littani M, Zanen J, De Franquen P, Yernault JC (1992) CT quantification of pulmonary emphysema - correlation with pulmonary function tests: Preliminary results on 15 patients. In: Felix R, Langer M (Eds.) Advances in CT II, Springer, Berlin Heidelberg New York, pp. 3–7

Gilman MJ, Laurens RG, Somogyi JW, Honig EG (1983) CT attenuation values of lung density in sarcoidosis. J Comput Assist Tomogr 7:407–410

Goddard PR, Nicholson EM, Laszlo G, Watt I (1982) Computed tomography in pulmonary emphysema. Clin Radiol 33:379–387

Kalender WA, Rienmüller R, Seissler W, Behr J, Welke M, Fichte H (1990a) Measurement of pulmonary parenchymal attenuation: Use of spirometric gating with quantitative CT. Radiology 175:265–268

Kalender W, Rienmüller R, Behr J, Seissler W, Fichte H, Welke M (1990b) Quantitative CT of the lung with spirometrically controlled respiratory status and automated evaluation procedures. In: Fuchs W (Ed.) Advances in CT. Berlin: Springer Verlag, pp. 85–93

Kalender W, Fichte H, Bautz W, Skalej M (1991) Semiautomatic evaluation procedures for quantitative CT of the lung. J Comput Assist Tomogr 15:248–255

Kalender W, Svatos M, Niendorf E (1993) Calculation of effective dose in CT. Radiology 189(P): 347

Mueller NL, Staples CA, Miller RR (1988) An objective method to quantitate emphysema using computed tomography. Chest 94:782–787

Rienmüller RK, Behr J, Kalender WA, Schatzl M, Altmann I, Merin M, Beinert T (1991) Standardized quantitative high resolution CT in lung diseases. J Comput Assist Tomogr 15: 742–749

Rienmüller R, Altmann I, Behr J, Krombach F, Kalender WA (1990) Spirometrically standardized quantitative high resolution CT of interstitial lung diseases. In: Fuchs WA (Ed.) Advances in CT. Springer, Berlin Heidelberg New York, pp. 102–108

Rienmüller R, Behr J, Beinert T, Mehnert F, Kalender WA (1992) Evaluation of CT histograms determined by spirometrically standardized high resolution CT studies of the lung in man. In: Felix R, Langer M (Eds.) Advances in CT II, Springer, Berlin Heidelberg New York, pp. 17–24

Van Dyk J, Hill RP (1983) Postirradiation lung density changes as measured by computerised tomography. Int J Radiat Oncol Biol Phys 9 : 847–852

Lung Density Measurements of Asbestos-Exposed Persons with PULMO CT

S. Tuengerthal, P. Herb, H. Schmitteckert, G. Tropf, H. Bülzebruck, V. Schulz

Introduction

Persons occupationally exposed to fibrogenic dust may develop lung fibrosis [1]. The extent of the disease is usually classified on the plain-chest film, according to ILO-80 regulations [2]. In asbestos-related disease the ILO Classification allows a semiquantative calculation of the small irregular opacities s/t/u in four main groups or 12 subgroups [3]. The asbestos-related lung fibrosis is in most cases mild and the radiologic classification ranges in the main groups ILO 0 or 1 [4]. The classification of the low grade abnormalities and the discrimination from "normal" is difficult and especially in these cases interobserver variance remains a problem, even for trained film reades [5, 6].

With high resolution computed tomography (CT) the morphologic basis of the disease may be shown and subtle changes may be seen on 1-mm scans [7], but scoring the stage of the asbestos-related lung fibrosis based on the visual characteristics is not yet established. Therefore density measurements promise to be an objective method for quantification, because computer calculation avoids interobserver variance [8]. To prove this, we studied a group of occupationally asbest-exposed persons and compared the results of ILO classification with the results of standardized lung densitometry using the spirometric gated PULMO CT which was developed in 1991 by Rienmüller and Kalender [8, 9].

Material and Methods

Eighty-eight patients with a documented asbestos exposure at least 20 years ago underwent a chest X-ray. The ILO classification was done by two experienced ILO readers in a consensus meeting. The results of the ILO classification for small irregular opacities (when positive, s,t in the middle and lower lung fields in both lungs) is shown in Table 1 (see also Fig. 1). All patients underwent high resolution CT on a SOMATOM PLUS (SIEMENS) CAT scanner. An additional three scans (slice thickness 5 mm) were taken at the level of the aortic arch, the carina, and intermediate between carina and diaphragm. Patients underwent lung function tests before the CT examination. The expiratory vital capacity (VC) value was the basis for the PULMO scans, which were exposed at VC 50% level. At VC 50% respiratory cycle in a few cases the diaphragm was visible. When it was cut on both sides, the scan was repeated at a higher level, when visible only on one side, density measurement was calculated on the other hemithorax.

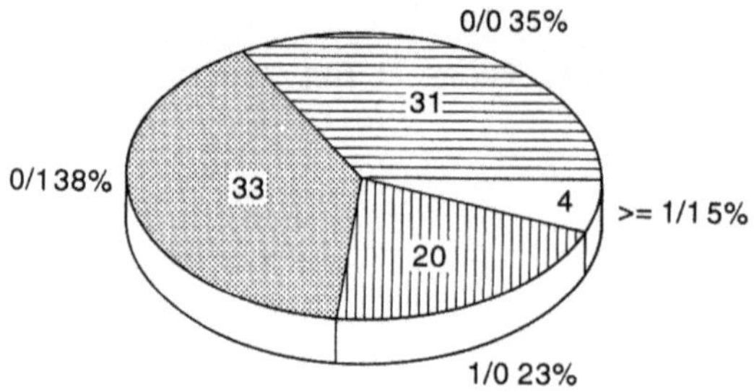

Fig. 1. Persons ($n = 88$). Distribution of ILO classification

Table 1. Mean density values at VC 50% in ILO Groups 0/0, 0/1 and ≥1

ILO 0/0	ILO 0/1	ILO ≥1/0
UF −849	−837	−815
MF −849	−836	−813
LF −831	−825	−797

Kruskal-Wallis-Test

UF			MF			LF		
	2	3		2	3		2	3
1	−	+	1	+	+	1	−	+
2	+		2	+		2	+	

VC, vital capacity.

Technical details of the PULMO CT:

SOMATOM PLUS:
Sl = 5 mm, t = 1 s, kV = 137, mA = 275, high-resolution kernel AB 7571

Densitometry:

The density calculation was performed with two methods:
1. Mean density
2. Area %

Both methods are installed on the PULMO CT Software package and run as routine procedures semiautomatically.

The *mean density* values in both lungs were calculated separately in the three lung areas. The irregular region of interest (ROI) was predefied by the voxel values from −1024/−200 HE

The *distributions of area %* were calculated in the same ROI in the three density ranges: −1024/950 HU, −949/−700 HU and −699/−200 HU.

Statistical Analysis:

Mean Density: For significance analysis two ILO groups were formed. Group 1 ("normal") consisted of ILO 0/0+ILO 0/1, group 2 ("pathologic") ILO 1/0 + ≥ 1/1).

Table 2. Mean density at 50% VC: Group 1 vs Group 2 in UF, MF, LF

ILO 0/0 and 0/1 (normal)			ILO ≥1/0 (pathological)		
UF	−843 HE	SD 21,1 HE	UF	−815 HE	SD 29,0
MF	−843 HE	SD 20,2 HE	MF	−813 HE	SD 24,0
LF	−828 HE	SD 21,4	LF	−791 HE	SD 22,1

Wilcoxon test normal vs. pathological
UF $p > 0.001$
MF $p > 0.001$
UF $p > 0.001$

VC, vital capacity

Table 3. Distribution area % in three ILO groups in OF/MF/LF

	−1024/−950 HU	−949/−700 HU	−699/−00 HU
ILO 0/0			
OF	1.42	91.91	6.16
MF	1.99	91.24	6.35
UF	2.20	88.76	8.0
ILO 0/1			
OF	1.23	91.00	7.40
MF	1.44	90.26	7.72
UF	1.70	88.84	8.46
ILO ≥ 1/0			
OF	0.77	89.00	10.07
MF	0.62	89.08	10.45
UF	1.06	85.50	12.33

Significance was calculated using the Wilcoxon rank test with two variates using the median data.

Area %: For calculation significane area % versus ILO 0/0, 0/1, and ≥ 1/0 the multivariate Kruskal-Wallis-Test was applied.

Results

The values of density measurements and the results of the statistical analysis are shown in Tables 1, 2 ad Figs. 2, 3.

The distribution of area % and the statistical analysis is shown in Tab. 1, 3 and Figs. 2–7.

Discussion

The group of 88 occupational asbestos dust-exposed persons had a male sex ratio 7:1, because only a few female textile workers were included. The mean age 62.3

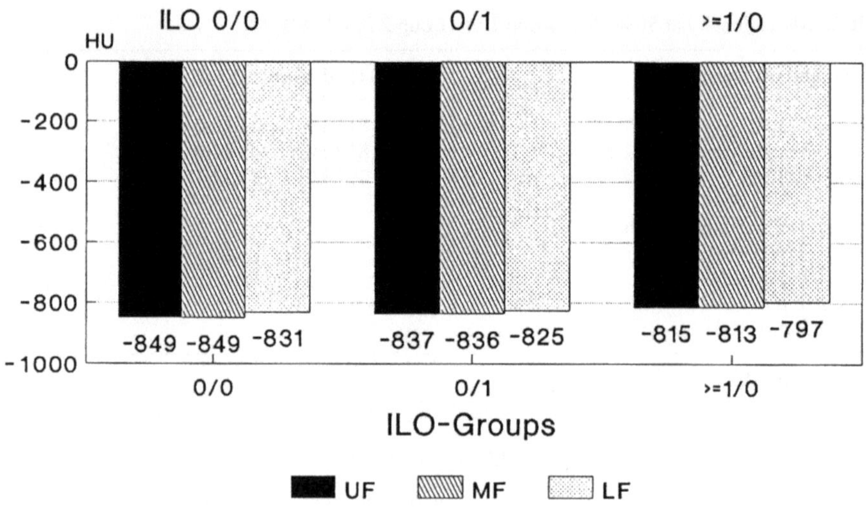

Fig. 2. Mean lung density values at vital capacity (VC) 50

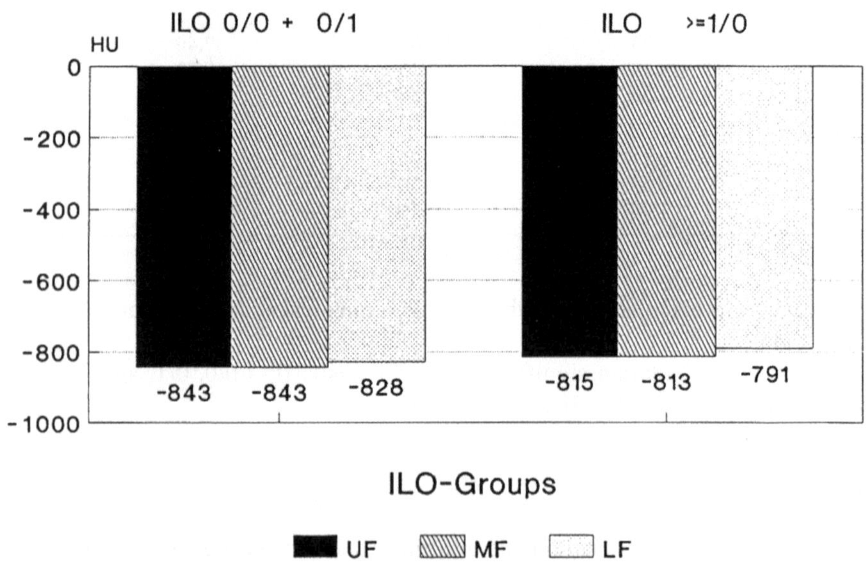

Fig. 3. Mean lung density values at vital capacity (VC) 50 ILO 0/0+0/1 ILO ≥ 1/0

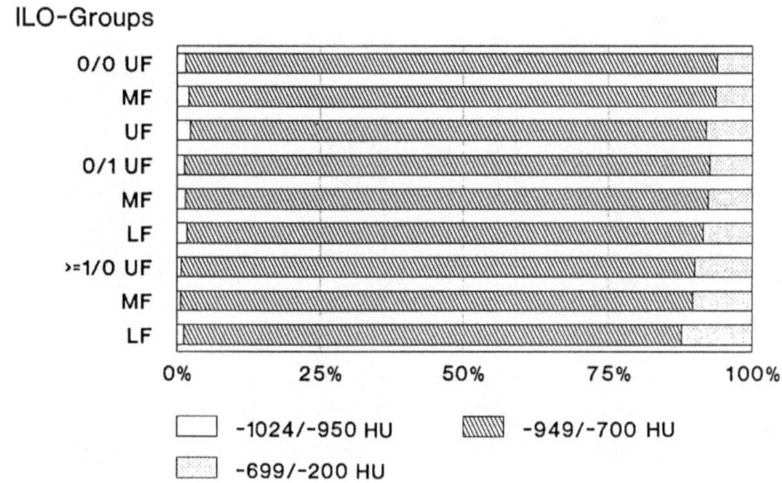

Fig. 4. Distribution of area % in UF, MF and LF in the ILO groups 0/0, 0/1 and ≥ 1/0

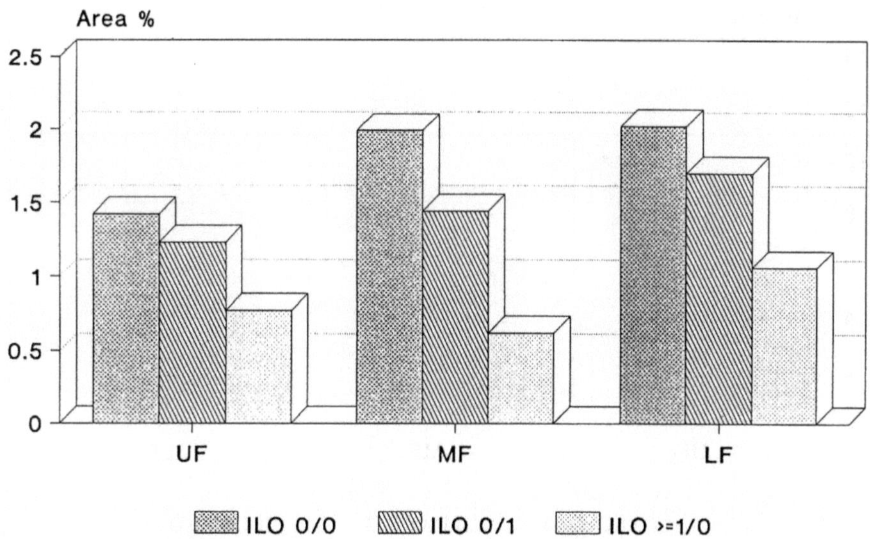

Fig. 5. Distribution of area % in ILO groups. Area of density: –1024/–950 HU

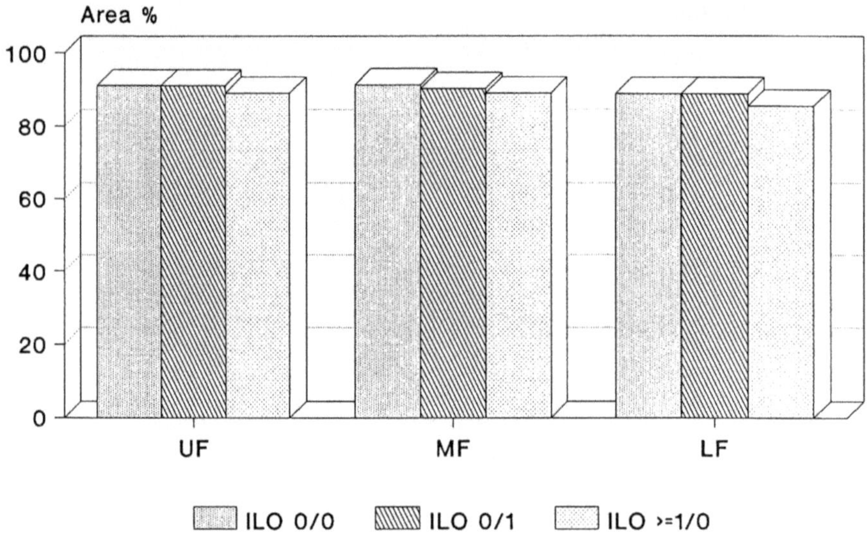

Fig. 6. Distribution of area % in ILO groups. Area of density: –949/–700 HU

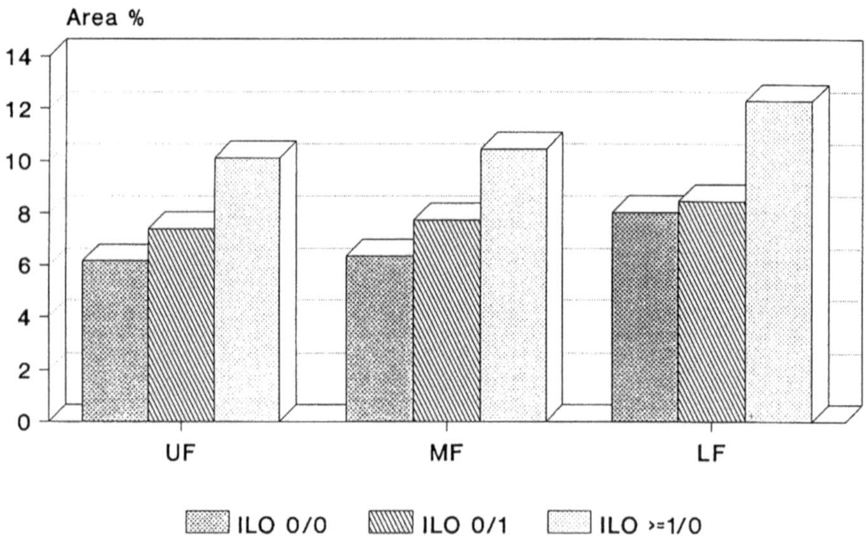

Fig. 7. Distribution of area % in ILO groups. Area of density: –699/–200 HU

years is relatively high, because the selection criteria was asbestos dust exposure beginning at least 20 years ago. Despite the long lasting exposure history the plain chest film of the elderly persons were classified in 2/3 to be normal (main group 0), (here of $n=31$ ILO 0/0, $n=33$ ILO 0/1 (slightly increased, irregular pattern, s or t). Only 24 persons are classified to have a more pronounced stage of irregular opacities of ILO main group 1. From these only $n=$ four had a distribution of ILO 1/1 or more. Similar low ILO classifications values report Staples et al. [4]. Because the number of ILO $\geq 1/1$ was too small for statistical evaluation, we put together ILO 1/0 and ILO $\geq 1/0$ to the group "pathologic". These three ILO groups were homogenous, with respect to age and sex (ILO 0/0 62.6 years, ILO 0/1 61.5 years, and ILO $\geq 1/0$ 62.2 years).

All persons had physical examination and lung function tests before the CT examination and were able to perform the respiratory maneuver during the PULMO-CT. Only a few had difficulties to exspire to the proposed respiratory level of $VC_{50\%}$ in the horizontal position, which was a condition for standardized lung density measurements. This spirometric gated scanning is necessary to get comparable results, because the pulmonary density values are changing during the respiratory cycle [11].

In the early beginning of pulmonary densitometry we made the experience, that some patients had increased density values, but normal plain chest film examination. In this cases we observed on the CT image marked hypostasis. Therefore we changed the CT procedure: Now we begin the chest examination with the PULMO-CT and start the standardized scans immediately after positioning the patient. To minimize the patient's time on the CT table helps to avoid hypostasis in the dorsal lung fields, which disturbs lung density measurements.

Technical Factors

Rienmüller proposes PULMO CT with 1- or 2-mm slice thickness [9], but we continue to perform pulmonary densitometry with Sl 5 mm. We consider that the statistical noise of a thicker slice CT image is lower and therefore the calculation of density values of the lung tissue should be more accurate. But until now this is not proved and to my knowledge studies on this subject are not yet done.

Mean Density at VC 50%

In the ILO groups 0/0 and 0/1 the mean density values in the UF and MF are nearly the same (−843) and increase in the lower lung field (+15 HU). This is not caused by lung fibrosis in the lower lung field, but due to the increased number of vessels in this area. The density values in the group ILO $\geq 1/0$ were approximately 30 HU higher in all lung fields, which is proved to be highly significant by Wilcoxon-Rank-Test ($p<0.0001$). This might be the result of an increased interstitial marking, which was visible on the chest film and therefore classified as ILO $\geq 1/0$. But it is not proven, wether this increased mean density is asbestos related or reflects other pulmonary diseases, which may look similar on the plain chest film.

The significance level between ILO classification was very high and the discrimination between the main groups ILO 0 and ILO 1 was done with a high confidence level. These results seem to be strange and do not comply with other studies. While in contrary to normal patient population in our group smokers were a minority and emphysematous lung disease was seen in the high resolution CT in two individuals only, we consider our results to be correct. The values of mean density measurements in most lung diseases are indifferent, because high values in fibrotic areas and low values in the emphysematous lung were calculated together [7, 8].

Area %

With the calculation of the area % the described disturbing effects in mean density measurements can be avoided. The calculation of area % enables to analyse the different components of the lung tissue by calculating the sum % of voxels in predefined HU levels [10]. So the increase of area % –1025/–950 represent an increase of air in the lung or emphysema [8], and area % –700/–200 represent increased lung density due to fibrosis or other reasons. Our results show that the density area %, which are calculated by the computer do not sum up to 100% exactly, as expected. We have no explanation for this fact. Nevertheless, we use the data and calculate the significance levels. The distribution of area % in the three density groups (–1024/ –950 HU; –949/–601 HU and –600/–200 HU) is different. In ILO 0/0 and 0/1 approximately 1.4–2.2% belong to the group 1 (–1024/–950 HU) and 6–8.5% to the group III (–699/–200 HU). In Persons with ILO ≥ 1/0 the percentage of lower density values is 0.6–1.06%, but the area % in density group 3 is increased to 10–12%.

With the Kruskal-Wallis multivariate test significant differences in area % were demonstrated in the groups ILO 0/0 and 0/1 vs. ≥ 1/0 in all lung scans in the three density groups with a significance level $p < 0.001$. In the area –699/–200 it was possible to discriminate 0/0 and 0/1 only in the middle field, with a significance level $p < 0.002$. In the ranges (–1024/–950 HU and –949/601 HU) significance could not be found between ILO 0/0 and 0/1 or ILO 0/1 and 1/0. The calculation of "normal" (ILO 0/0 + 0/1) vs "pathologic" (ILO ≥ 1/0) was significant at a lower significance level of $p = 0.002$ (1024/–950 HU) and $p = 0.003$ (–949/–601 HU) in the cranial scan, but highly significant ($p < 0.001$) in the range (–600/–200 HU) and all other lung areas and density ranges.

Conclusions

The PULMO CT soft- and hardware, running on a SOMATOM PLUS (Siemens) CAT scanner is a usefull tool to investigate elderly persons. The semiautomatic measurement and density calculation of the respiratory gated scans allows quantification of density changes without the problems of interobserver variance. In a cohorte of 88 asbestos dust-exposed persons the three different ILO groups "normal" (ILO 0/0), "subtle" (0/1) and "pathologic" (≥ 1/0) could be discriminted by lung densitometry with high confidence levels. With two different evaluation methods (mean density measurements and determination of area %) it was possible to separate persons which showed on a chest film increased small irregular opacities from persons who had normal or subtle increase of density on the chest X-ray. Whereas in chest radiology you need experienced experts to classify the degree of increased markings, the PULMO CT provides an exellent method to distinguish "normal" from "pathologic" in the early stage of the asbestos-related lung disease.

References

1. Bohlig H und Otto H Asbest und Mesotheliom. Fakten, Fragen. Umweltprobleme. Thieme Verlag Stuttgart 1975
2. International Labour Office (ILO) Genf: Guidelines for the use of ILO International Classification of Radiographs of Pneumoconioses. Revised Ed. 1980 Occupational Safety and Health Series No 22 (Rev 80) Genf 1980
3. Bohlig H et al. (1981) Die Weiterentwicklung der Internationalen Staublungenklassifikation und ihre Konsequenzen für die arbeitsmedizinischen Vorsorgeuntersuchungen staubgefährdeter Arbeitnehmer (ILO 1980/Bundesrepublik). Prax Klin Pneumol 25: 1075–1154
4. Staples CA et al. (1989) High resolution computed tomography and lung function in asbestos exposed workers with normal chest radiographs. Am Respir Dis 139: 1502–1508
5. Epstein DM et al. (1982) Application of ILO classification to a population without industrial exposure: findings to be differentiated from pneumoconiosis. AJR 142: 53–58
6. Browne KJ et al. Radiology of asbestos related disease. A supplement to the ILO standard set and a check on its validity et al. VI Internationale Pneumoconiosis Conference 1983 Bochum Vol 2 pp 882–887
7. Webb WR, Müller NL, Naidich DP High Resolution CT of the Lung. Raven Pres New York 1992 chapt. 5 pp 62–70
8. Müller NL Density mask An objective method to quantitate emphysema using computed tomography. Chest (1988) 94: 782–787
9. Rienmüller RK et al. (1991) Standardized quantitative high resolution CT in lung diseases. J Ass Tomography 15: 742–749
10. Kalender WA et al. Measurements of pulmonary parenchymal attenuation: Use of spirometric gating with quantiative CT. Radiology (190) 175: 265–268
11. Robinson PJ and Kreel L (1979) Pulmonary attentuatin with computed tomography: comparison of inspiration an exspiration scans. J Comp. Tomography 3: 263–143

Quantitative Assessment of Lung Density by CT in Navy Personnel exposed to Asbestos*

M. REUTER, I. HOLLING, L. EMDE, E. BETTINGHAUSEN, M. HELLER, D. SZADKOWSKI

Introduction

Occupationally induced interstitial lung fibrosis can be objectified by computed tomography (CT) for earlier stages than in conventional X-ray examinations. Usually diagnosis results from a qualitative assessment of lung parenchyma. In an attempt to detect the earliest stages of parenchymal abnormalities in asbestosis we extended standard high resolution CT for a quantitative evaluation by measurement of lung density.

Material and Methods

Subjects

The group under investigation consisted of 29 marine servicemen with differing board duties. All sailors served on ships were asbestos was used in construction. A low exposure to dust is assumed. The exposition time corresponded to the length of duty on board and was an average of 22 years. The latent period is given with an average of 35 years. The mean age is 54 years. Only five nonsmokers belong to the investigated group. The chest radiographs made within the framework of an occupational medicine preventive medical examination showed exclusively low profusion scores (0/1 and 1/0, ILO 1980) and were suggestive of asbestos-related pleural disease (1a to 3a, ILO 1980) in 15 subjects.

Pulmonary Function Studies

Vital capacity (VC) and forced expiratory volume in 1 s (FEV 1) were determined using a portable or stationary spirometer (VCT-P2A or pneumoscope, both manufactured by Jäger, Würzburg, Germany). VC less than 80% of the predicted value and FEV 1 less than 70% of VC are considered as impairment of lung function.

---

* With support of the Minister of Defence.

Computed Tomography

The CT examinations were carried out in dorsal position using a Somatom Plus-S from Siemens. The following scan parameters were employed for the measurement of pulmonary density: 1 s scan time, 275 mA tube current, 137 kVp voltage, 1-mm section thickness. The shots were reconstructed in high resolution mode. During the CT scanning the subject breathed through a hand-held pocket spirometer. By automatic blocking of the respiratory air supply during the radiographs – one at the level of the carina and one each 5 cm above and below (Kalender 1990) – an inspiratory depth of 50% of the actual vital capacity is attained (Kalender et al. 1990). A semiautomatic fast contour-tracing algorithm (Kalender et al. 1991), was used for isolation of the pulmonary parenchyma. In doing so, in addition to the thoracic wall, any pleural thickenings, the mediastinum and the central bronchovascular structures were exluded as well.

For qualitative evaluation of the pulmonary parenchyma, subsequent to the density measurements thin-layer radiographs (2-mm section thickness) were taken in maximal inspiration from the apex to the base of the lung by a table feed of 20 mm, reconstruction in high resolution mode.

Reference Data

For an objective evaluation of our quantitative findings (whole lung density) we calculated individual age-matched normative values. For this calculation provisional statistical parameters (regression curve equation) from a nonexposed reference population ($n = 153$) were available (Kalender 1994).

Statistical Analysis

The results of the various density measurements or VC determinations were tested for significance using a two-sided paired *t*-test. A correlation between differend variables was tested using Spearman's rank correlation coefficients. Differences between measurements and correlation coefficients between variables were considered significant at the 5% level ($p < 0.05$).

Results

Pulmonary Function Studies

Apart from two subjects with slight VC reductions to 71% of the predicted value and normal FEV 1 (% VC), no impairment of lung function was observed (Table 1). There was no correlation between the pulmonary function parameters and exposition or latent periods.

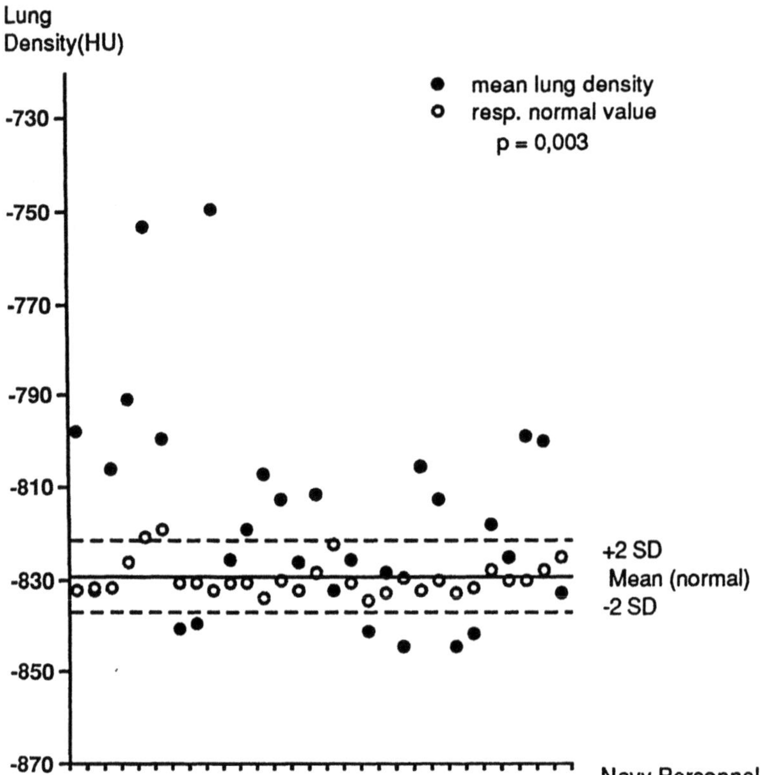

Fig. 1

Table 1. Results of lung function masurements

	VC	VC (% pred)	FEV1	FEV1/VC (%)
Mean	4.5	95.7	3.6	81.7
Range	3.2–6.6	70.8–126.9	2.5–5.1	72–98
SD	0.8	15.7	0.6	6.5

VC, vital capacity; FEV, forced expiratory volume; pred, predicted

Pulmonary Density Measurements

The servicemen exposed to asbestos exhibited a significantly higher global density value ($p < 0.01$; Fig. 1) with a mean HU value of −816.0 compared to the calculated age-matched mean normal value of −829.8 HU. Individually the measurements in 19 servicemen revealed differing degrees of a predominately marked elevation in the pulmonary density, while in ten cases the density values were within the normal range or slightly lower. Two servicemen with HU values of −753.1 and −749.5 have

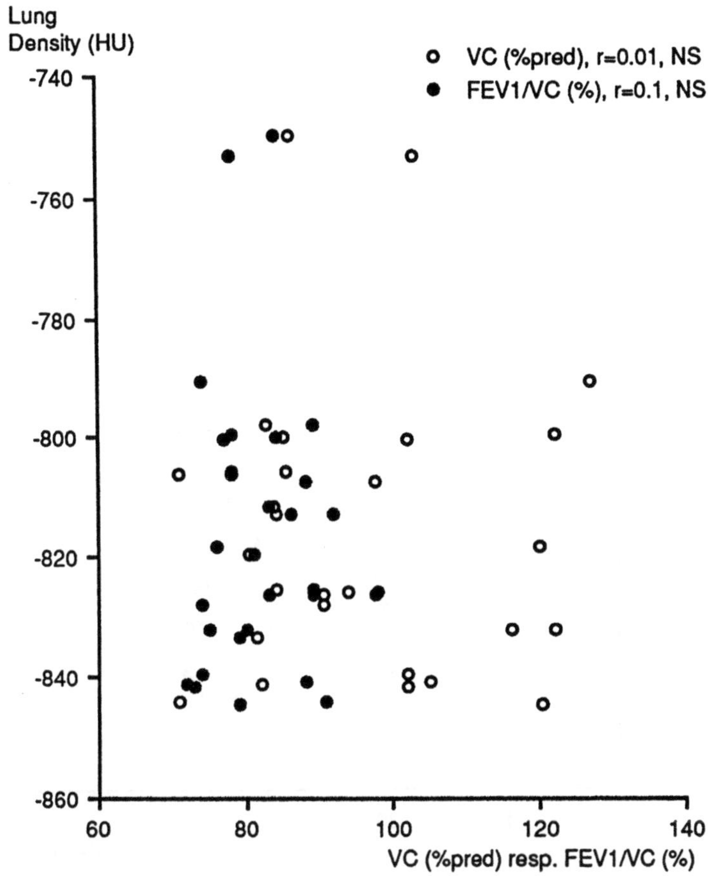

Fig. 2

conspicuously high density values. The HRCT radiographs reveal discrete persisting fibrotic densifications in the prone position in only one case.

There were no correlations between the pulmonary density measurements and the pulmonary function parameters (Fig. 2) as well as the exposition and latent periods (Fig. 3).

High Resolution CT

Discrete signs of a localized interstitial fibrosis were only found in six servicemen (Fig. 4), in one case a small bullous emphysema was observed. Asbestos-typical pleural alterations were documented in nine persons (Fig. 5).

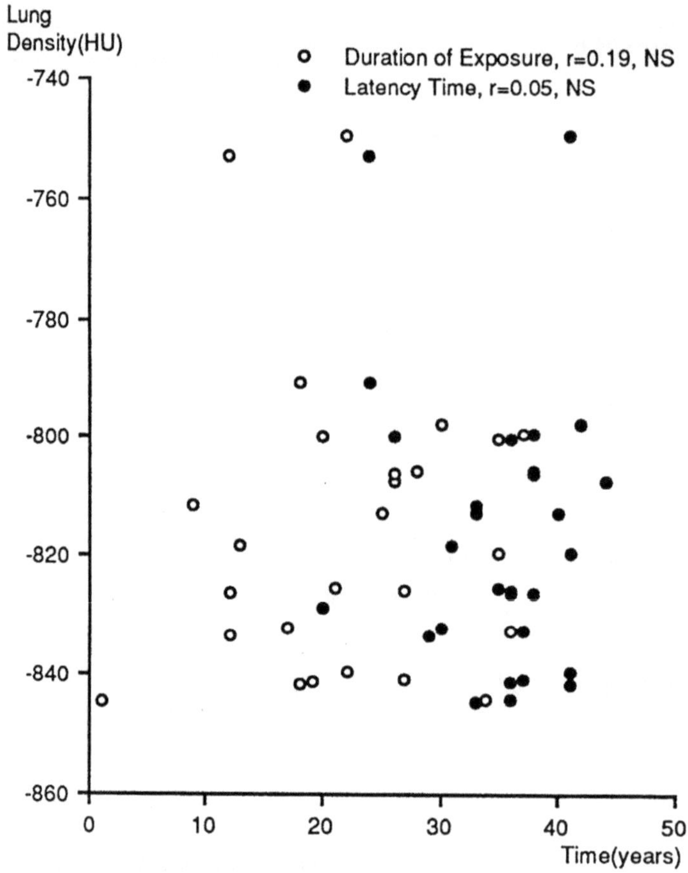
Lung
Density(HU)
Duration of Exposure, r=0.19, NS
Latency Time, r=0.05, NS
-740
-760
-780
-800
-820
-840
-860
0
10
20
30
40
50
Time(years)

Fig. 3

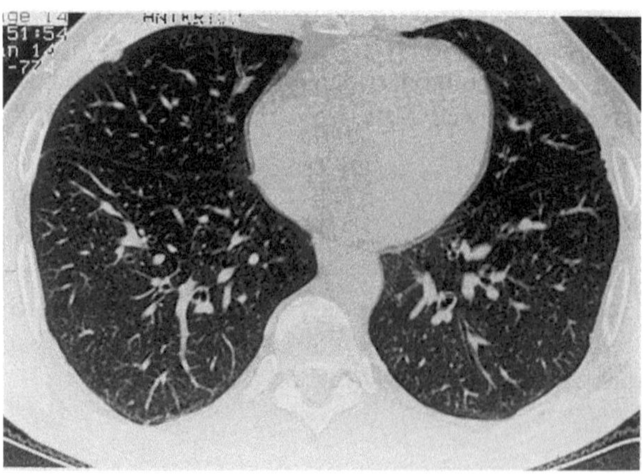

Fig. 4

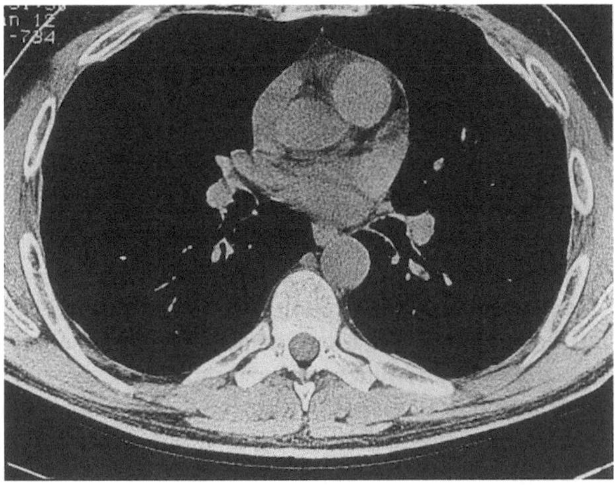

Fig. 5

Discussion

In comparison to other collectives with similar or even longer exposition or latent periods (Aberle et al. 1988; Friedman et al. 1988; Akira et al. 1991; Gamsu et al. 1991; Odsa et al. 1994), in the present investigation on asbestos-exposed marine servicemen the largely inconspicious pulmonary architecture observed with high resolution CT (HRCT) is triking. This circumstance can be traced back to the comparatively low exposure to dust. The decisive radiological indicator of a previous exposure to asbestos was therefore the computer tomographic pleural findings seen in nine of the servicemen. The investigated collective is apparently suitable for the testing of another – likewise CT – procedure for assessing the early phase of asbestos dust-induced interstitial pulmonary alterations, in this case even preceding the appearance of characteristic morphologic alterations in the HRCT. For this we supplemented the HRCT by recording quantitative measurements from which the lung density is calculated. Since lung density is decidedly influenced by the respiratory status (Wegener et al. 1978; Rosenblum et al. 1980; Vock et al. 1987; Robinson and Kreel 1979; Goddard et al. 1982), older studies on lung density measurements are characterized by inadequate reproducibility. This problem is countered in the present study by the use of spirometer-directed respiratory gating (Kalender et al. 1990).

Our measurements on 29 asbestos-exposed sailors revealed a statistically significant elevation of the global pulmonary density in contrast to the calculated normal values in the corresponding age. It is conspicious that discrete signs of fibrosis were detectable with HRCT in only four of these 19 persons. Wollmer et al. (1987) also detected a significant increase in density in investigation on 33 workers from an asbestos cement factory, however in contrast to our study a slight impairment of pulmonary function was correlated with the elevation in density. Considering the almost inconspicuous pulmonary architecture in HRCT and the unimpaired pulmonary function we interpret our results as an expression of a very early parenchymal reaction to the previous asbestos exposition. In comparison, in their quantitative investigation Wollmer et al. (1987) documented an advanced parenchymal alteration with the commencement of impaired pulmonary function.

Conclusions

1. With quantitative computed tomography early parenchymal alterations preceding the appearance of morphological alterations in HRCT are sensitively detected.
2. The measured elevations in denstiy are subclinical alterations in the face of inconspicuous pulmonary function.
3. The respiratory gated CT forms in the basis for reporducible investigations of the course by asbestosis tending to progression. (Akira et al. 1991; Ehrlich et al. 1992).
4. The normal values for pulmonary density must be set on a broader basis.

References

Aberle DR, Gamsu G, Ray CS (1988) High-resolution CT of benign asbestos-related diseases: clinical and radiographic correlation. Amer. J. Roentgenol. 151: 883–891

Akira M, Yokoyama K, Yamamoto S et al. (1991) Early asbestosis. Evaluation with high-resolution CT. Radiology 178 : 409–416

Ehrlich R, Lilis R, Chan E et al. (1992) Long term radiologial effects of short term exposure to amoisite asbestos among factory workers. Br. J. Ind. Med. 49 : 268–275

Friedman AC, Fiel SB, Fisher MS et al. (1988) Asbestos-related pleural disease and asbestosis: a comparison of CT and chest radiography. Amer. J. Roentgenol. 150 : 269–275

Gamsu G, Salmon CJ, Warnock ML (1991) High-resolution CT: pathologic correlations in asbestosis. Radiology 181 : 117

Goddard PR, Nicholson EM, Laszlo G et al. (1982) Computed tomography in pulmonary emphysema. Clin. Radiol. 33 : 379–387

Kalender WA, Rienmüller R, Seissler W et al. (1990) Measurement of pulmonary parenchymal attenuation: use of spirometric gating with quantitative CT. Radiology 175 : 265–268

Kalender WA (Editor) (1990) Determination of normal values for lung density and structure by quantitative computed tomography (QCT)-a european multicenter study. Siemens Medical Systems, Erlangen

Kalender WA, Fichte H, Bautz W et al. (1991) Semiautomatic evaluation procedures for quantitative CT of the lung. J. Comput. Assist. Tomogr. 15 : 248–255

Kalender WA (1994) Personal communication

Oksa P, Suoranta H, Koskinen H et al (1994) High-resolution computed tomography in the early detection of asbestosis. Int. Arch. Occup. Environ. Health 65 : 299–304

Robinson PJ, Kreel L (1979) Pulmonary tissue attenuation with computed tomography: comparison of inspiration and expiration scans. J. Comput. Assist. Tomogr. 3:740–748

Rosenblum LJ, Mauceri RA, Wellenstein DE et al. (1980) Density patterns in the normal lung as determined by computed tomography. Radiology 137 : 409–416

Vock P, Malanowski D, Tschaeppeler H et al. (1987) Computed tomographic lung density in children. Invest. Radiol. 22 : 627–631

Wegener OH, Koeppe P, Oeser H (1978) Measurement of lung density by computed tomography J. Comput. Assist. Tomogr. 2 : 263–273

Wollmer P, Jakobsson K, Albin M et al. (1987) Measurement of lung density by X-ray computed tomography. Relation to lung mechanics in workers exposed to asbestos cement. Chest 91 : 865–869

Spiral CT of the Thorax with Significant Reduction of Contrast Material: A Comparison of a 60-ml, 45-ml and 30-ml Bolus

L. P. Emde, J. Link, S. Müller, M. Heller

Introduction

Dynamic incremental computed tomographic (CT) examinations of the chest are usually performed with 120 – 150 ml of intravenously administered contrast material to discriminate between normal mediastinal structures, hilar vessels and pathologic processes. The amount of contrast media used allowed for a sufficiently long scanning interval with adequate vascular enhancement (Sagel and Glazer 1989).

CT systems with cycle times of 1 s or less led to the acquisition of volumetric data sets, when a patient is continously moved through a continously rotating X-ray beam. Images can be reconstructed at any arbitrarily chosen table positions and with a number of different algorithms (Villafan et al. 1991).

Currently tube heating specifications for the Somatom Plus S (Siemens AG, Erlangen, Germany) allow continous scanning at 210-mA tube current and 120 kVp for 32 s. Based on a slice thickness of 1 cm a volume of 32 cm (table speed 1 cm/s, pitch 1) or 64 cm (table speed 2 cm/s, pitch 2) in length can be scanned. Examination of the entire thorax (including the adrenal glands) is achievable with this technique (Kalender et al. 1990; Vock et al. 1990).

Reduction in examination time has several advantages. First, the patient is examined during suspended respiration. Motion artefacts are practically eliminated and detection of pulmonary nodules is greatly improved. Reconstruction at smaller intervals additionally increased the yield (Costello et al. 1991; Remy-Jardin et al. 1993). Second, a reduction of contrast material while still achieving a high degree of vascular opacification. Lund and mediastinal image quality was deemed equal or better as compared to conventional CT (Costello et al. 1992). The need for reliable and standardized contrast media boli arises. The purpose of this study was to develop, compare and assess three contrast media boli for routine spiral CT examinations of the thorax during a single-breath-hold maneuver. An attempt was made to minimize the amount necessary to achieve opacification of great hilar vessels without sacrificing diagnostic information.

Materials and Methods

A total of 100 consecutive patients (age 9 – 88, mean 54) referred for chest CT were examined with 45 ml of contrast material, 50 patients (age 16 – 82, mean 59) with

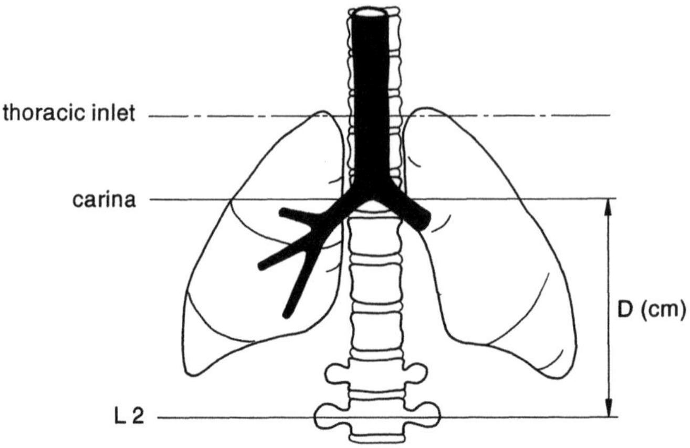

Fig. 1. An a.p.-topogram used to calculate the distance to be scanned from below

60 ml and 35 patients (age 21 – 80, mean 55) with 30 ml. Referrals were made from all in- and outpatient departments. Only patients requiring contrast material for chest CT were included. Patients were excluded for insufficient venous access, inability to hold their breaths for 32 s (or 16 s, respectively) or lack of contrast delivery. Intensive care patients were included, since artificially induced breath hold could be applied in most cases.

The chest was examined from the thoracic inlet to the level of the adrenal glands in a cranio-caudal fashion, except when 30 ml were given the direction was reversed.

Scan parameters: 120 kVp, 210 mA, slice collimation 10 mm, table speed 10 mm/s (60 ml) and 20 mm/s (30 and 45 ml). Reconstruction interval was 8 mm. Iopentol (Imagopaque, 300 mg/ml iodine, Nycomed, Norway) was administered through a 18-gauge catheter via an antecubital vein.

A programable power injector (Ulrich Pumpe, Ulrich, Ulm, Germany) was used to inject the three boli. Scan delay was 16 s for the 45- and 60-ml bolus. Timing for the 30-ml bolus was individually calculated by the actual time needed to scan the volume between lung base and carina from an a.p-topogram (Fig. 1). Adjustments were made for a different intravenous access.

Vascular opacification was measured with a region of interest (ROI) in the subclavian artery at the level of the thoracic inlet, aortic arch, ascending and descending aorta at the level of the carina, main pulmonary artery and thoracic artery at the level of the diaphragms.

Results

Scan duration varied between 32 s (60 ml) and 17 – 19 s (30 and 45 ml), respectively. All patients were able to hold their breath during scanning. No adverse effects were observed. Vascular enhancement was on average more than 100 HU (Table 1). The increase is far above the level of unenhanced vessels (Fig. 2a – c).

Table 1. Results of mean vascular enhancement (HU)

	Contrast bolus (ml)		
	60	45	30
Subclavian artery	164	170	143
Aortic arch	180	181	136
Ascending aorta	192	198	142
Descending aorta	192	190	134
Main pulmonary artery	184	194	148
Lower thoracic aorta	142	177	86

Where there are only minor differences between the 60- and 45-ml boli, the enhancement at 30 ml is significantly less, but still far above non-contrast studies. Since the examination with 30 ml started at the lung base enhancement of the lower thoracic aorta was failry low.

Mediastinal and lung-image quality were considered adequate for diagnosis in all cases (Fig. 1a–c, Fig. 3a–b).

Discussion

The introduction of spiral CT technology allows scanning of complete body regions during suspended respiration (Kalender et al. 1990).

While X-ray tube output is currently not optimal for abdominal examinations, examination of the thorax with 210 mA and 120 kVp produces an image quality which is comparable to conventional CT (Costello et al. 1992; Hacking and Dixon 1992). Doubling table speed compared to slice thickness (pitch 2) shortens examination time further, but increases the effective slice thickness and pixel noise values (Kalender et al. 1991; Polacin et al. 1992; Brink et al. 1992), leading to some image degradation. However, tube output can be more than doubled due to shortened data aquisition time (e.g. 250 mA for 20 s). In our study we found that even with a pitch of 2 image quality was adequate for diagnosis at 210 mA. Radiation exposure is reduced by half for a pitch of 2.

Previous studies have shown effectiveness of spiral CT of the thorax with reduced volume of contrast material (Costello et al. 1992). Due to 8-mm slice collimation and a pitch of 1 only 17.6 cm of the chest were scanned in one breath-hold. Examination with 1-cm slice thickness and a pitch of 2 required different boli and timing. Flow rates needed were determined in prelimary experiments.

Results indicate that a high degree of vascular enhancement is achievable with considerably lower amounts of contrast material than has been used in the past with conventional chest CT. Opacification of hilar vessels was regarded as crucial. Due to the short and early scanning interval enhancement of venous structures, other than the ones opacified by inflowing contrast media could not be expected.

Increased table feed has led to sucessful reduction of contrast material to 45 ml. In an attempt to further reduce contrast volume caudo-cranial scanning was intro-

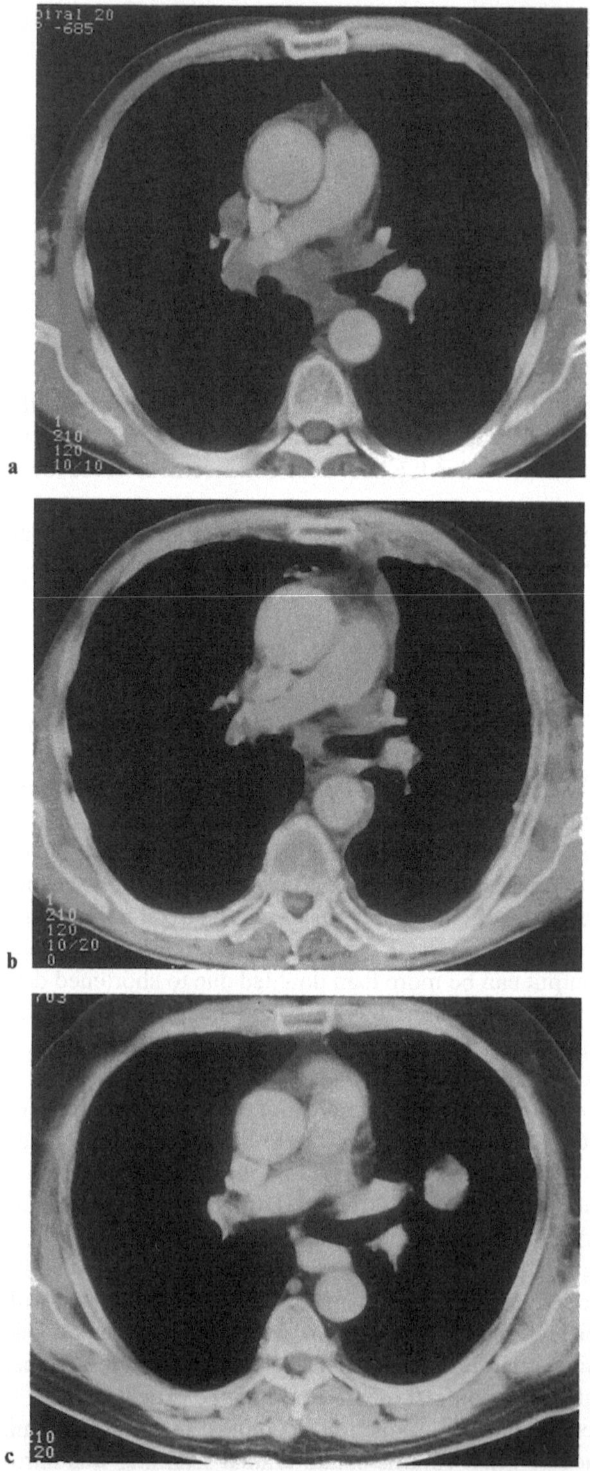
a
b
c

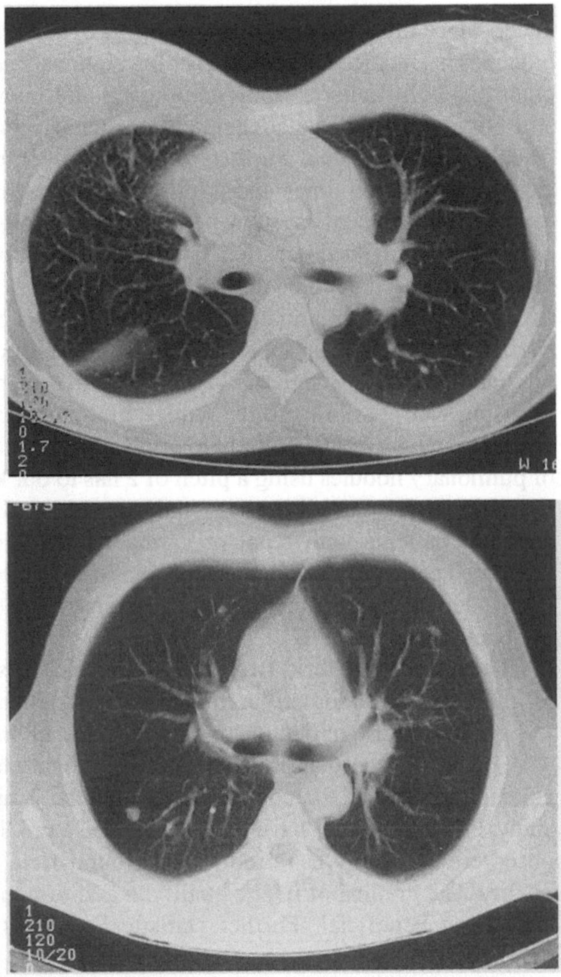

a

b

Fig. 3 a, b. Lung-image quality in high-resolution algorithm. **a** A 15-year-old girl referred for computed tomography of the chest for a large anterior mediastinal mass. Scanned with a ptich of 1 and 60 ml. **b** A 60-year-old patient with pulmonary metastasis from a malignant seminoma. Examined with a pitch of 2 and 45-ml bolus

Fig. 2 a – c. Enhancement of hilar vessels. **a** A 61-year-old patient with carcinoma of the lung and right hilar and mediastinal lymphadenopathy. Staging examination with 60 ml of contrast media, pitch of 1. **b** Same patient 5 months later for restaging post-therapy. Examined with 45 ml bolus, pitch of 2. **c** A 59-year-old patient presenting with left hilar mass for computed tomography of chest. Examined with 30 ml of contrast material. In all three cases discrimination of lymph nodes and vascular structures is possible duced, since the main pulmonary artery is opacified shortly before the aorta and its branches is enhanced. The 30-ml bolus obviously shows less enhancement than the other two boli. Using a tailored approach and improved tracking of the bolus it is still possible to achieve adequate hilar opacification without predetermination of actual circulation time. Further reduction in contrast dose is questionable, since varying circulation times and dilution of contrast material with blood in the heart cavities, even during first-pass, poses physical limits. At this point a 30-ml bolus can only be recommended in patients with optimal intravenous access and in whom only hilar structures need to be opacified.

The increase in nominal slice thickness with doubling of table speed posed no significant problem, since overlapping reconstruction with different algorithms provided excellent image quality without gap or motion artefacts. Caudo-cranial scanning can possibly further reduce motion artefacts, which are most likely to occur at the lung bases. A study to grade lung-image quality and assess detectibility of pulmonary nodules using a pitch of 2 has to our knowledge not been undertaken.

Rapid, high-quality CT examinations with small doses of contrast are advantageous in patients with renal or cardiac impairment, intensive care patients and ventilated patients, in whom suspension of respiration is possible. The risk of contrast-induced nephropathy and other adverse reaction declines (Gomes et al. 1989; Bush and Swanson 1991).

The option to perform two contrast-enhanced examinations of different regions (e.g. thorax and abdomen) in immediate succession has improved efficiency.

Less overall use of contrast material can result in substantial cost savings.

A control group that underwent conventional chest CT to derive values of vascular enhancement for comparison would be a useful addition to the foregoing study. Previous studies have only introduced a grading system, used by independent observers. No study has used actual Houndsfield values as a criterion for image quality. The grading of image quality in addition to the current investigation would have been beneficial. Further statistical analysis will be performed as patient numbers rise.

Thoracic CT has been revolutionized with the advent of spiral CT. Image quality and vascular enhancement of hilar structures is comparable, if not better, to conventional CT. Motion artefacts are practically eliminated. Use of contrast material can be reduced for up to 80% of previously necessary doses. Increase in pitch leads to only insignificant image degradation. The refined technique requires sensible patient selection and occasionally a different approach, if venous opacification is desired. All patients benefit from smaller contrast doses and short examination times. Cost is reduced and efficiency improved. We now routinely use a bolus of 45 ml in all thoracic imaging requiring administration of contrast material.

References

Brink JA, Heicken JP, Balfe DM, Sagel SS, DiCroce J, Vannier MV (1992) Spiral CT: Decreased Spatial Resolution in Vivo Due to Broadening of Section Sensitivity Profile. Radiology 185 : 469–474

Bush WH, Swanson DP (1991) Acute reactions to intravascular contrast media: types, risks factors, recognition, and specific treatment. AJR 157 : 1153–1161

Costello P, Anderson W, Blume D (1991) Pulmonary nodule: Evaluation with Spiral Volumetric CT. Radiology 179 : 875–876

Costello P, Dupuy DE, Ecker CP, Tello R (1992) Spiral CT of the Thorax with reduced Volume of Contras Material: A Comparative Study. Radiology 183 : 663–666

Gomes AS, Lois JF, Baker JD, McGlade CT, Bunnell DH, Hartzman S (1989) Acute Renal Dysfunction in High-Risk Patients after Angiography: Comparison of Ionic and Nonionic Contrast Media. Radiology 170 : 65–68

Hacking JC, Dixon AK (1992) Spiral versus conventional CT in soft tissue diagnosis. Europ J of Radiol 15 : 224–229

Kalender WA, Polacin A (1991) Physical performance characteristics of spiral CT scanning. Med. Physics 18(5): 910–915

Kalender WA, Seissler W, Klotz E, Vock P (1990) Spiral Volumetric CT with Single-Breath-Hold Technique, Continous Transport, and Continous Scanner Rotation. Radiology 176 : 181–183

Polacin A, Kalender WA, Marchal G (1992) Evaluation of Section Sensitivity Profiles and Image Noise in Spiral CT. Radiology 185 : 29–35

Remy-Jardin M, Remy J, Giraud F, Marquette CH (1993) Pulmonary Nodules: Detection with Thick-Section Spiral CT versus Conventional CT. Radiology 187 : 513–520

Sagel SS, Glazer MS (1989) Thorax: technique and normal anatomy. In: Lee KJT, Sagel SS, Stanley RJ (Eds.) Computed body tomography. Raven, New York, pp. 169–243

Villafan T (1991) Technological advances in computed tomography. Curr. Opin. Radiol. 3 : 275–283

Vock P, Soucek M, Daepp M, Kalender WA (1990) Lung: Spiral Volumetric CT with Single-Breath-Hold Technique. Radiology 176 : 864–867

Spiral CT of the Chest of Premature Children and Newborns

R. KURSAWE, C. DEWEY

Introduction

Conventional radiography of the chest is the most frequently used imaging method to diagnose and follow up complicated obstructive pulmonary disorders. However, in many cases only a few roughly findings lead to the real morphological structures and so to final diagnosis. Thus, there are multiple diagnostic questions, which can not be answered by conventional chest radiography.

Clinical use of standard thoracic computed tomography (CT) is restricted by multiple artefacts based on body movement as well as respiration. Introducing spiral

a

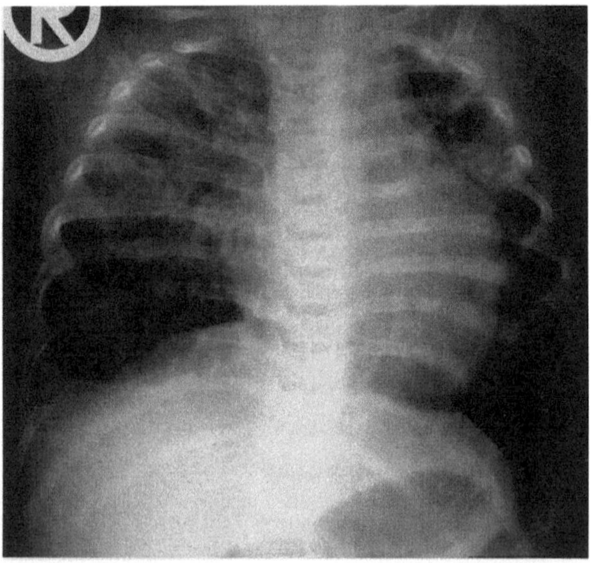

Fig. 1a, b. Female newborn, premature birth (28th week of pregnancy, 940 g), long-time artificial respiration, chronical obstructive bronchitis. **a** Chest X-ray (postnatal): asphyxia and pneumonia, suspicion of bronchi-pulmonary dysplasia. **b** Spiral computed tomography: to prove the extension of pathological findings: uniform dispersion of fibrosis and over-inflated parts of both sides of the lung. Large fibrosis of the right lung (*segments 2, 3, 8 and 9)* and left lung (*segments 5, 6, 8–10*). Multiple pneumatoceles (maximum 3.2 cm), right lung (*segments 7 and 10*), left lung (*segments 8–10*). No evidence of florid pulmonary infiltration

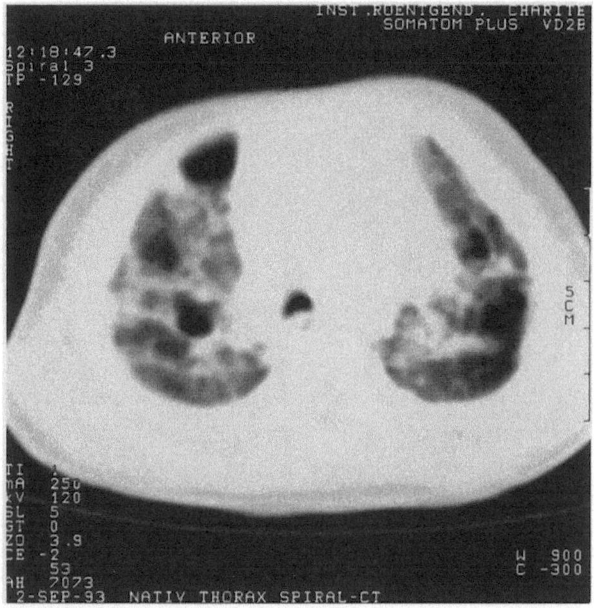
INST.ROENTGEND. CHARITE
SOMATOM PLUS VD2B
ANTERIOR
12:18:47.3
Spiral 3
TP -129
RIGHT
5 CM
mA 250
kV 120
SL 5
GT 0
ZO 3.9
CE -2
53
AH 7073
2-SEP-93 NATIV THORAX SPIRAL-CT
W 900
C -300

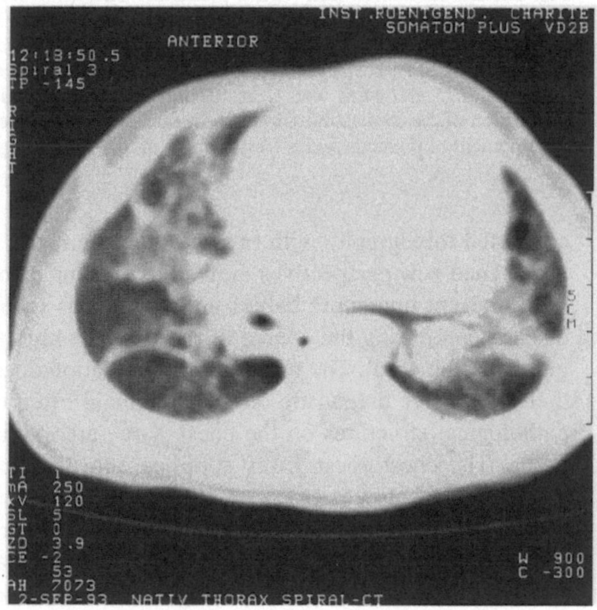
INST.ROENTGEND. CHARITE
SOMATOM PLUS VD2B
ANTERIOR
12:18:50.5
Spiral 3
TP -145
RIGHT
5 CM
TI 1
mA 250
kV 120
SL 5
GT 0
ZO 3.9
CE -2
53
AH 7073
2-SEP-93 NATIV THORAX SPIRAL-CT
W 900
C -300

Fig. 1b

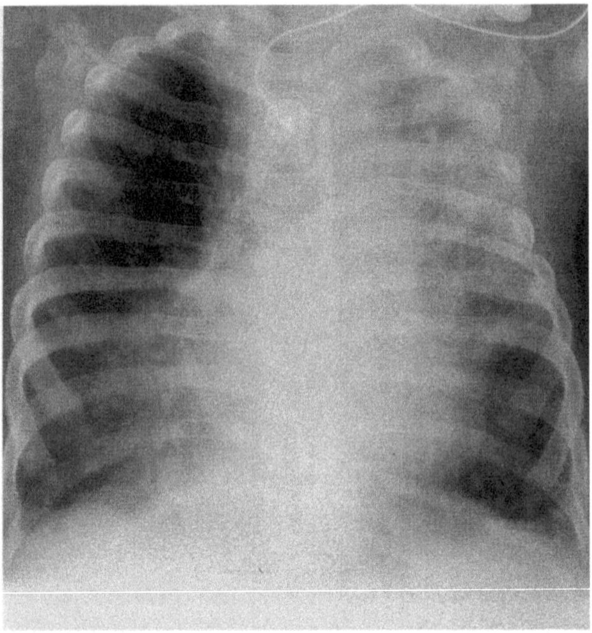

a

Fig. 2 a, b. Female newborn (twin), premature birth (26th week of pregnancy), acute respiratory distress syndrome, long time artificial respiration. **a** Chest X-ray (postnatal): acute respiratory distress syndrome (IV°). follow up: bronchi-pulmonary dysplasia. **b** Spiral computed tomography (8th month of life): Extensive bronchi-pulmonary dysplasia with large fibrosis in the right lung (*segments 4, 5 and 8*) as well as in the left lung with shrinking of the upper lobe. Irreversible dislocation of the mediastinum to the left, further on extensive over-inflated parts of the lung with development of pneumatoceles (*segments 2–6, 8, 9* on the *right, 8–10* on the *left*)

computed tomography with breath hold volumetric scanning in clinical radiology has opened new perspectives in diagnosing lung disorders.

At present premature babies and new-borns with complicated obstructive lung diseases get during the course of the illness a high number of conventional radiographs of the chest. The resultant high radiation does is not inconsiderable. Nevertheless decisive diagnostic questions remain often unanswered. It is possible that pathological structures on the chest X-ray are overlapped by patent neighbouring tissue. The chest chest X-ray supplies only less specific findings for the actual morphological structures.

The purpose of this clinical study was to compare the diagnostic value and the accuracy of the spiral CT in contrary to conventional chest X-ray and to find correlation's between diagnostic findings and clinical symptoms in order to improve the therapeutic management of these children.

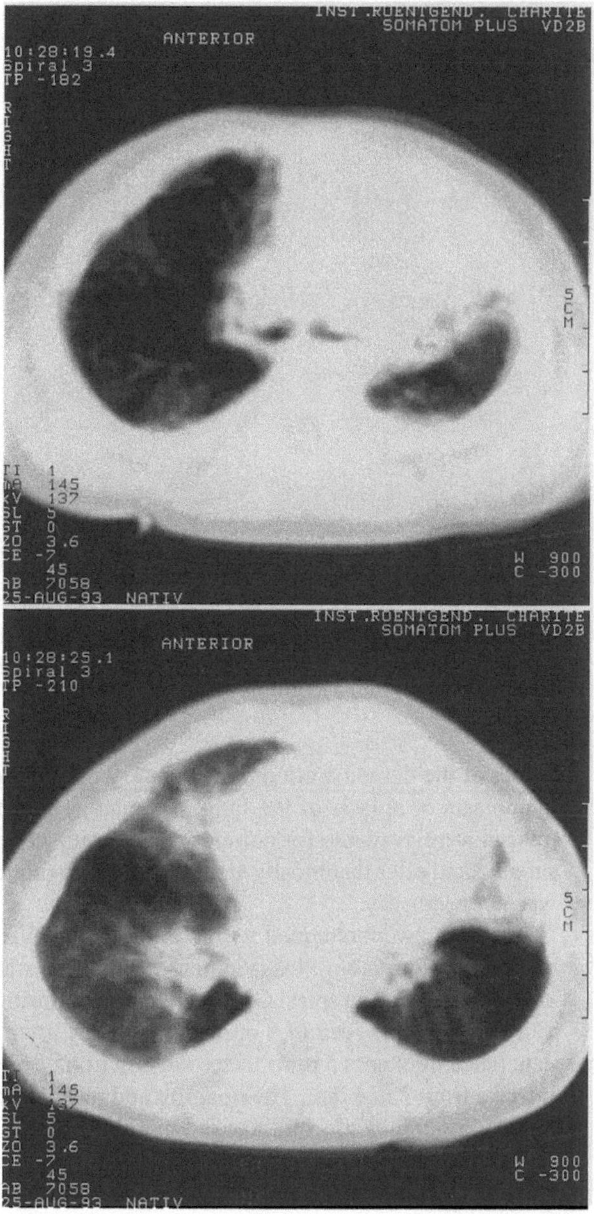

Fig. 2b

Material and Methods

In 14 newborn children (5 premature birth) 18 examinations were performed with spiral CT. The youngest child was 8-h old and the oldest one 12 months. Clinical indications to perform spiral CT were to grade a bronchipulmonary dysplasia as a common complication in the course of respiratory distress syndrome of premature

a
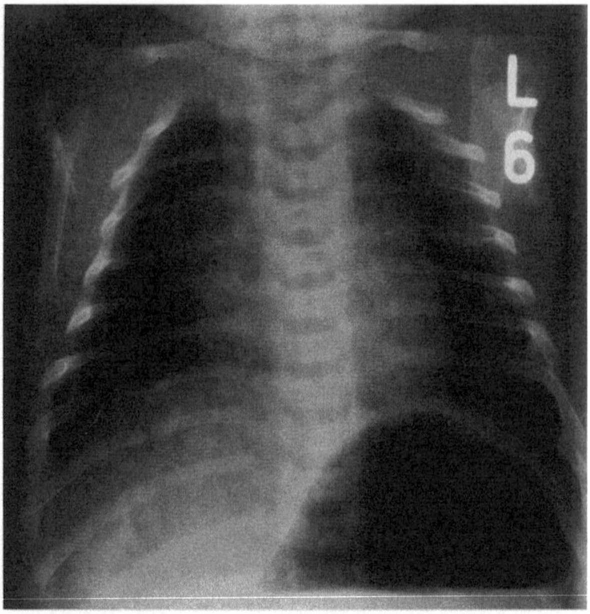

Fig. 3 a, b. Male newborn (hypertrophy, 4680 g), prenatal sonographical suspicion on lung cyst. **a** Postnatal: no evidence of lung cysts by conventional chest radiography. **b** Spiral computed tomography (first day of life): extended cystic malformation of the right lower lobe of the lung

babies or the demonstration of pulmonary malformations (e.g. cystic degeneration, hypoplasia or aplasia of the lung, oesophago-trachea fistula). Magnetic resonance images were available for comparison in some cases. A sedation procedure for the satiated and after that mostly sleeping children (not underwent artificial respiration) was not necessary.

The scans were obtained with commercially available, continuously rotating CT equipment (Somatom Plus, Siemens Medical Systems). In patients who underwent artificial respiration spiral CT was performed during an apneic phase of the child in 12 s using a table feed of 5 mm. Immediately after finishing the acquisition of CT data (slice thickness 5 mm) the reconstruction of images was proceeded with a slice interval from 2 to 4 mm. The imaging and reconstruction parameters for spiral computed tomography are summarised in Table 1.

Two radiologists red out all the chest X-ray films and hard copy documents of the spiral CT examinations and evaluated the accuracy of the imaging data obtained.

Results

Ten patients were newborns or premature children, some of them with complex malformations (e.g. vitium cordis) under critical clinical conditions with respiratory distress syndrome. The complications of the respiratory distress syndrome could be completely detected by spiral CT. On the base of a long time artificial respiration

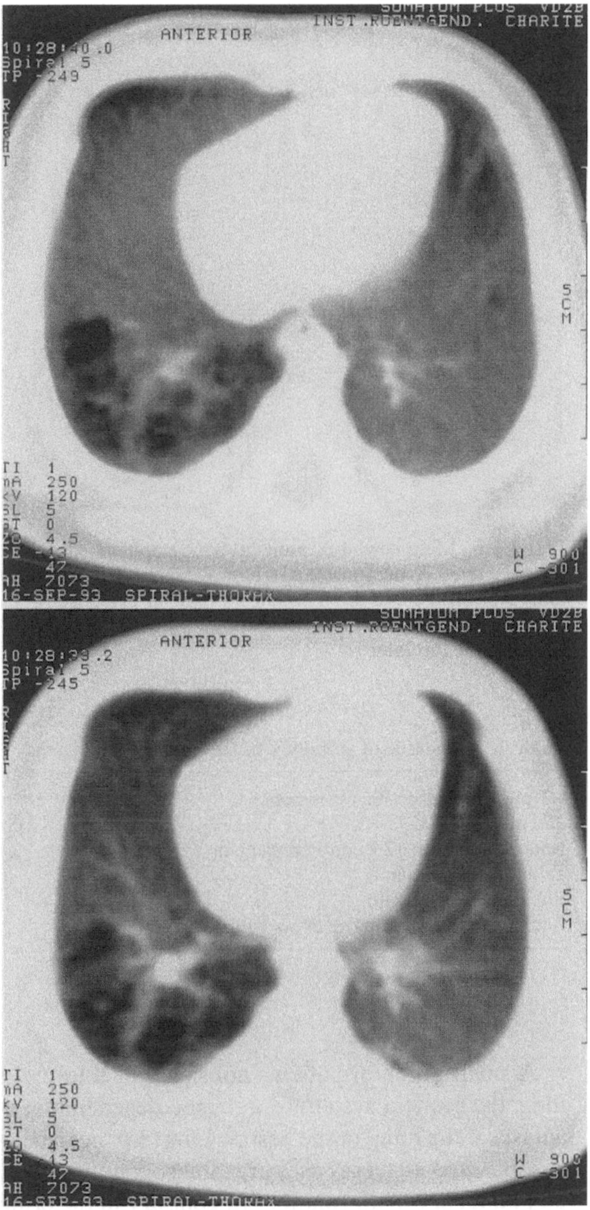

Fig. 3b

some patients with respiratory distress syndrome developed a bronchi-pulmonary dysplasia in the course of the illness. In four cases the children with bronchi-pulmonary dysplasia underwent follow-up examination using the spiral CT. The extension of the bronchi-pulmonary dysplasia, for instance with lung fibrosis, pneumatocele, obstruction or dislocation of the bronchi system and florid pulmonary infiltration could be described (Fig. 1, 2).

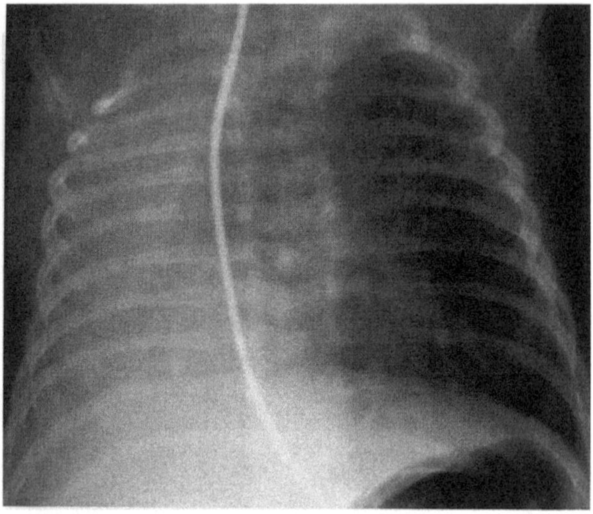

a

Fig. 4 a, b. Male newborn, prenatal sonographical suspicion on lung agenesia on the right side. **a** On the chest X-ray (postnatal): homogeneous decrease of the transparency on the right side, left lung over-inflated, at the moment no clinical evidence of an acute infection. **b** Spiral computed tomography (sixth day of life): no lung tissue on the right, no sequestration, good ventilated lung tissue on the left lung

Table 1. Technique of spiral CT of the chest of new-borns

CT unit: Somatom Plus (Siemens)
250 mA, 120 kV
Data acquisition: 12 s contiguous (1 or 2 times)
Table feed: 5 mm/s
Slice thickness: 5 mm
Reconstruction of images: 2- to 4-mm slice interval

CT, computed tomography

A small group of patients consisted of four children with malformations of the lung, the bronchi system (e.g. cystic degeneration of the lung lobes, hypoplasia or aplasia of the lung) or the oesophagus (e.g. oesophago-tracheal fistula, atresia of the oesophagus). In these cases prenatal sonography was performed and led to suspicion on pulmonary malformation. In contrary to the critical clinical state of the children the conventional chest X-ray postnatal could not confirm the prenatal obtained sonographical results. Only the spiral volumetric computed tomography led to final diagnosis (Fig. 3–5). The information obtained resulted directly in decisions of paediatric surgeons.

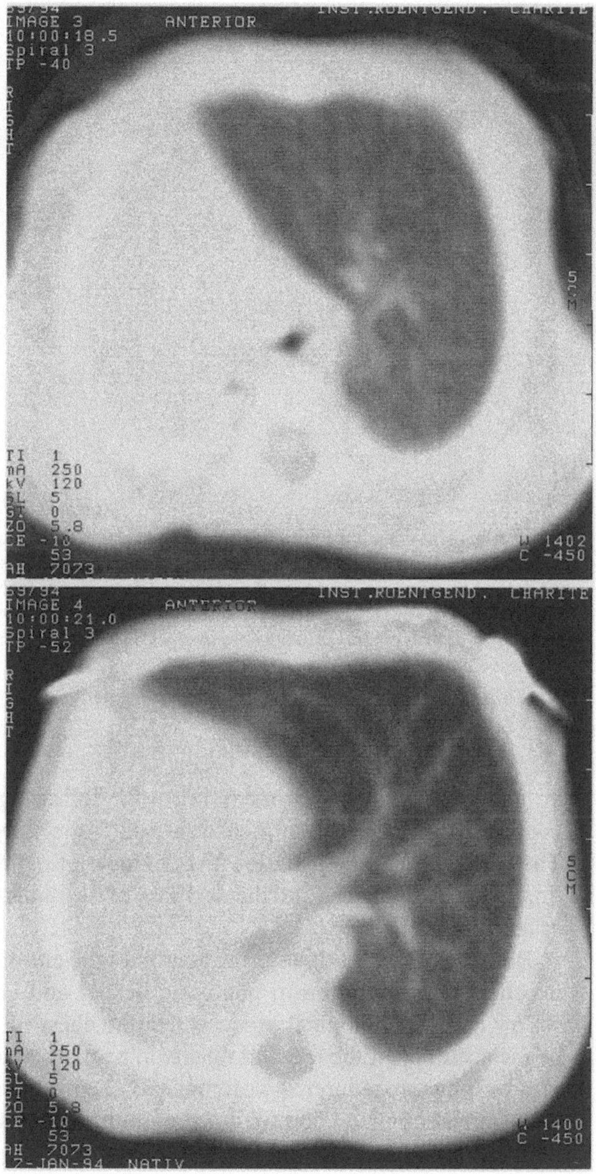

Fig. 4b

Discussion and Conclusion

The results of spiral CT of every patient provided a perfect differentiation of morphological structures in the chest due to non overlapping anatomical slices. The pulmonary changes at bronchi-pulmonary dysplasia and the thoracic malformations of the lung and the bronchi system could be well proved by using the spiral CT. The extension of irreversible pathological findings was exactly fixed. The spiral CT was

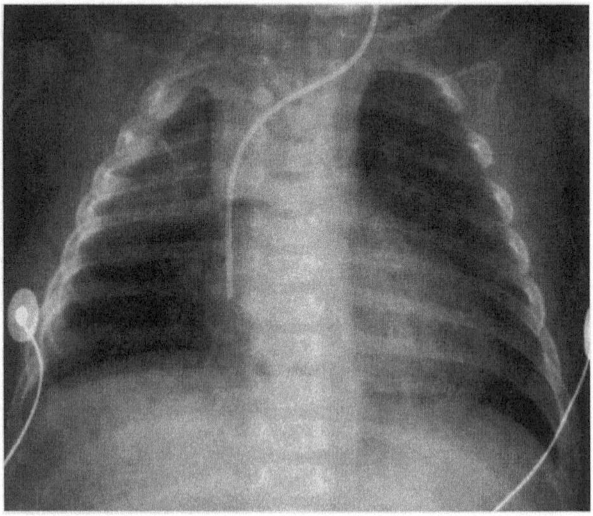

a

Fig. 5a, b. Male newborn with oesophagus-atresia (II); in the second month of life surgery of the oesophagus following by an insufficiency of the anastomosis and formation of a fistula. Clinical weakened respiratory sound on the right. **a** Chest X-ray (second month of life): decrease of the transparency of the right upper lobe of the lung. **b** Spiral computed tomography: atelectasis of (*segments 1 to 3*, thin pleural effusion latero-dorsal realised by drainage

an important diagnostic precondition for following therapeutical procedures, for instance planning of the surgical treatment, especially in the cases of malformations. The method could be used for this clientele of patients, because of the short duration of the examination and the decrease of the radiation dose compared to the single scan CT.

Because of the contiguous evaluation of the entire chest the spiral CT provides an excellent demonstration of anatomic details and is valuable for imaging and the follow up of pathological processes in the chest of small children. The high diagnostic accuracy of the method results in a remarkable reduction of the conventional radiographic procedures too often used. The promising results of our study suggest that spiral computed tomography of pulmonary diseases may become a useful diagnostic imaging method for new-borns.

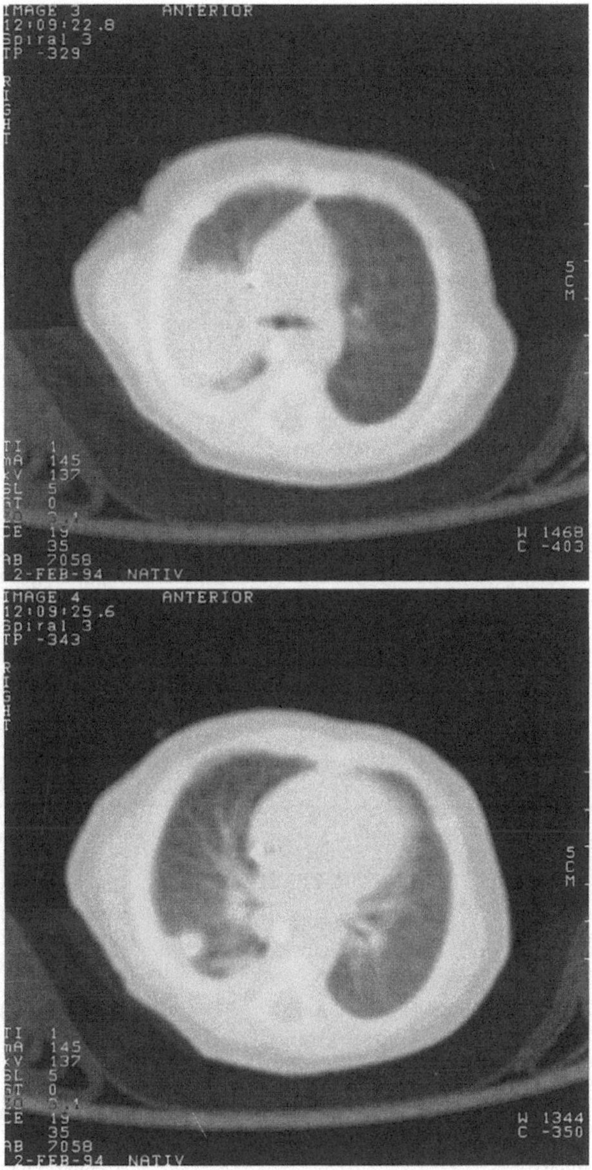
ANTERIOR
12:09:22.8
TP -329
145
137
W 1468
C -403
7058
NATIV
IMAGE 4
ANTERIOR
12:09:25.6
TP -343
145
137
W 1344
C -350
7058
NATIV
5 CM

Fig. 5b

Subject Index

MIX
Papier aus verantwortungsvollen Quellen
Paper from responsible sources
FSC® C105338

If you have any concerns about our products,
you can contact us on
ProductSafety@springernature.com

In case Publisher is established outside the EU,
the EU authorized representative is:
Springer Nature Customer Service Center GmbH
Europaplatz 3, 69115 Heidelberg, Germany

Printed by Libri Plureos GmbH
in Hamburg, Germany